MW01283257

Bone, Ivory, and Horn
Identifying Natural Materials

Michael Locke

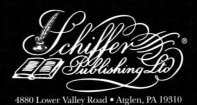

Schiffer Publishing Ltd

4880 Lower Valley Road • Atglen, PA 19310

Dedication

I dedicate this book to my wife Janet for keeping me happy during its genesis, to my oncologist, Dr. Leonard Minuk, for keeping me alive long enough to finish it, and to places like Stones'N Bones Museum, Sarnia, Ontario, Canada, which stimulated my interest.

Other Schiffer Books on Related Subjects:
Asian Ivory. Jeffrey B. Snyder. ISBN: 978-0-7643-2728-5. $79.95

Cover design: Bruce Waters
Type set in Bernhard Modern BT/Arrus BT

ISBN: 978-0-7643-4307-0
Printed in China

Published by Schiffer Publishing, Ltd.
4880 Lower Valley Road
Atglen, PA 19310
Phone: (610) 593-1777; Fax: (610) 593-2002
E-mail: Info@schifferbooks.com

For the largest selection of fine reference books on this and related subjects, please visit our website at **www.schifferbooks.com**. You may also write for a free catalog.

This book may be purchased from the publisher. Please try your bookstore first.

We are always looking for people to write books on new and related subjects. If you have an idea for a book, please contact us at proposals@schifferbooks.com

Schiffer Books are available at special discounts for bulk purchases for sales promotions or premiums. Special editions, including personalized covers, corporate imprints, and excerpts can be created in large quantities for special needs. For more information contact the publisher.

Michael Locke

I have enjoyed the work of others but the errors are mine.

"Not pikt from the leaves of any author, but bred amongst the leaves and tares of mine own brain."

Sir Thomas Browne, (1605–1682)
Religio Medici Pt. 1.35

Contents

Preface..4

1. Introduction...5

2. The Biology of Natural Structural Materials.............................9

3. The Cylindrical Form...18

4. Bone, the Internal Skeleton of Vertebrates 24

5. Antler, External Bone 38

6. Ivory, Teeth Large Enough to Trade 55

    1. Introduction 55

    2. Physeter and Orca 60

    3. Narwhal 69

    4. Pearly Concentrations—Ivory Pearls 75

    5. Walrus 75

    6. Pigs, Suidae 79

    7. Hippopotamus 88

    8. Elephants, Mammoths, and Mastodons 99

    9. Discussion—Laminar Architectures 122

    Conclusions 123

7. Keratin, the External Skeleton of Vertebrates.......................124

    1. Introduction, Keratin Eaters 124

    2. Keratin Derivatives 126

    3. Skin, Vellum, and Leather...128

    4. Scales and Tortoiseshell...134

    5. Hooves, Claws, and Beaks 138

    6. Horns 142

    7. Hair, Wool, and Quills...158

    8. Whale Baleen 164

    9. Rhinoceros Horn..170

    10. Feathers 175

8. Other Materials..178

9. Artifacts and Antiques 182

10. Curating, Restoring, and Repairing 249

11. Glossary...255

12. References...265

13. Acknowledgments..274

14. Conclusion...275

15. Index..276

Preface

Prose is traditionally divided into fiction and non-fiction, but this does not tell the whole story. Fiction is not about anything that happened. The reader's interpretation is as valid as that of the writer who is thereby encouraged to be vague, impressionistic. Approval by the reader is often narcissistic, the excellence being in his own interpretation of what the author might have meant. Non-fiction is characterized by clarity of expression, the object is to inform, but it is of two very different kinds. Both use the scientific method of interpreting data in the most probable way, but differ in their subject matter. Most non-fiction is about things or events that we have created—biographies, histories, art critiques. It is non-fiction about human creations, things that vary from being pure fiction such as art works, to things that have some reality such as biographies. A minority of non-fiction is about the non-human part of the universe, the natural environment—astronomy, chemistry, biology for example. It is pure non-fiction. This book contains elements of both, descriptions and hypotheses about man-made artifacts and the pure science descriptions of natural materials.

For the scientist, every observation is a question waiting to be answered. For those interested in structure, this defines the difference between anatomy and morphology. Anatomists describe the structure, giving names to distinctive components. Morphologists explain the causes that have given rise to that structure—genetic, evolutionary, developmental, adaptive, mechanical. The anatomists job is completed by the naming. Unfortunately many anatomists in the nineteenth century usurped the position of morphologists, filling morphology journals with anatomy, writing as though naming rather than explanation was the scientific end. Their fog of names has continued into the twenty-first century. Textbooks with impenetrable nomenclature giving no clue to causes for the structure. The result is a waste of student's time devoted to rote learning a language that has little relation to histology or morphology or to their professional futures. Wherever possible I have avoided using the old terminology of anatomists in favor of the descriptive words of the morphologist that illuminate function.

Chapter 1

Introduction

"Some books are to be tasted, others to be swallowed, and some few to be chewed and digested."

Francis Bacon, 1625, (quoted in (81)*

This book is about the natural materials used to make functional objects in the days before synthetic plastics. It is not about beautiful works created by artists for the rich now displayed in museums. Bone, antler, ivory, horn, and tortoiseshell used to be essential commodities with guilds of skilled craftsmen working long hours to create the goods that everyone needed in their daily lives. Before mass production, craftsmen made enduring objects for people with fewer, but more appreciated, possessions. Things that are now made from plastic, brushes and combs, knives and forks, things that we take for granted, were valued objects in everyday life. Such artifacts have their own beauty, an elegance derived from the simplicity of design needed for efficient function. We still get pleasure from that beauty, but we also get satisfaction from the stories they tell about life in the times of their creators and users.

Artifacts also tell stories about the biology of the animals that supplied the materials. How did they live and grow, what are the properties of the materials that they provided and how did those properties evolve that make them so useful to us? A scientist tells stories, but has a much harder job than the writer of fiction. That scientist may not make up the elements of the story, which must come from observations of the natural world that takes him on a journey of exploration. His role is to put his observations together in the most probable way to complete the travelogue. Just so in this book, which describes a trip inside

bones and tusks and horns to understand their structure

Artifacts have stories to tell. How did the artist-craftsmen who worked the materials acquire their skills, where did they work, what tools did they use? How did owners use their objects, and what do they tell us about the way they lived their lives? Things made then that we no longer use have a special value in that they tell us of forgotten fashions and ways of life. Yesterday is another country, the borders of which are now closed, but the inhabitants have left us their artifacts, which may tell us how they lived.

This book is also about collecting. The collector is a researcher discovering new information from the juxtaposition of his finds. Selecting an object for a collection has less to do with its individual merit than with its potential relationship to other objects already acquired. This is what makes the collection of greater interest than the sum of individual pieces. Just as the onlooker derives pleasure from juxtapositions in the best museum displays, so too does the collector. His perception of relationships brings him joy, elevating collecting to a creative act with the goal of discovering a story. The collector is also a puzzle seeker and solver. Nothing gives him more delight than to find an artifact with an unknown function. It becomes a conversation piece leading to many hours of speculation and discussion. When finally it reveals its secret—bone rings as pattern markers in knitting, for example—there is an

---

* All references are numbered as shown here. (81) refers to the eighty-first reference, displayed in Chapter 12 References, see page 266.

instant of joy, the data suddenly fit together, just as they do when making a scientific discovery.

This is a practical book. Discovery is not the only joy that drives students of natural materials. There is also satisfaction in working and conserving in the ways of traditional craftsmen. Present day craftsmen can emulate the skill and industry of their predecessors using techniques that are even better than those available earlier. It is also now much easier to care for artifacts to ensure that they may last for several hundred years more, not just because they were made to last, unlike their present day plastic counterparts.

Identification is an essential part of studies of natural materials. Antiques for sale are often incorrectly identified; I have seen bone labeled as ivory, even in major museums. This book shows how to identify natural materials, how to tell bone from ivory, horn from tortoiseshell, old from new.

In 1784, Samuel Johnson wrote *"... all truth is valuable and all knowledge pleasing in its first effects, and may subsequently be useful"* (58). Structure is the datum, the base on which all these studies rest, but it is not an end in itself. As Charles Darwin pointed out many years ago in a letter to Henry Fawcett, September 18th, 1861, (27) *"... all observation must be for or against some view if it is to be of any service."* A morphologist sees every elucidation of structure as a collection of answers to questions that may not yet have been asked. He makes his anatomy into the science of morphology by making it answer questions. Sadly, this has not always been the objective. In the eighteenth century, followers of Carl Linnaeus gave Latin names to everything that lived and left it at that. In the nineteenth century, the objective was to give one's name to some new structure or cell type—Henle's layer, Huxley's layer, etc.—with little regard for function or development. By the twentieth century, the textbooks were so full of nomenclature for its own sake that science was lost and needed a new start. The objective of this book has been to simplify descriptions to show how questions and answers, from molecular biology to ultrastructure, histology, and basic biology, help us to understand natural materials. To meet this objective I have tried to use pictures rather than text. As the American photographer Minor White (1908–76) said *"One should photograph objects, not only for what they are, but for what else they are."* Pictures contain their own commentary.

I have tried not to use the Internet as a source, because it is readily available to everyone. There are many excellent articles, but they change rapidly and are not consistently reliable, since most have never been reviewed. Wikipedia is generally very good, but "Googling" is not research. I have used my own research to create unambiguous pictures and diagrammatic interpretations of material that has been largely overlooked.

On the Interpretation of Images

See how Nature is a living book,
    Misunderstood but not beyond understanding.

                                            Goethe 1774

"Do not decide that something is the case until you know it is the case." Mma Ramotswe in Tea Time for the Traditionally Built, Alexander McCall-Smith, 2009, quoting Clovis Andersen The Principles of Private Detection.

When we examine a three-dimensional object we guess at the internal structure by extrapolating from what we see on the surface. The guess may often be wrong. The inside of a bone may not resemble what we see on the outside, so we cut new surfaces to look at. This procedure of cutting sections has been outstandingly successful in microscopy. Sections thin enough to be translucent enable us to look at the structure in profiles, having any orientation we choose. However, this technique brings its own problems. Profiles in a single plane can be misleading. To understand the three-dimensional structure we need to have profiles in all three dimensions. Researchers sometimes leap to conclusions about three-dimensional structure from observations in a single plane, assuming that the appearances in other planes are like the one they have been studying.

When examining a surface, either in a section or the flat face of a block, the most important thing to keep in mind is the probability of finding the two-dimensional profile of the three-dimensional structure postulated to exist. Illustrations are the data used by morphologists. They do not lie. It is only our interpretation that may be in error. Figure 1.1 shows some mistakes that seem elementary, but they can all be found in the scientific literature. For example, parallel lines are more likely to be profiles of paired sheets than longitudinal sections of a cylinder (Figure 1.1E).

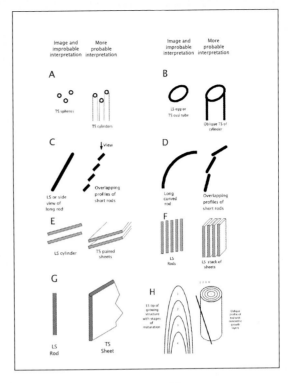

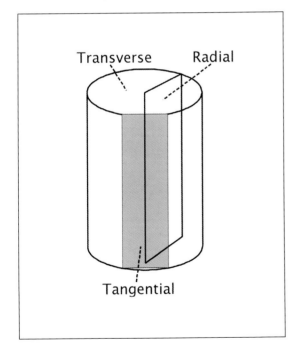

Figure 1.2. The three profiles of cylindrical structures used in this book for the reconstruction of three-dimensional images: transverse, radial, and tangential. The page orientation has been standardized for all illustrations. **Transverse profiles** have the periosteal edge to the top. **Tangential profiles** orient the length of the object with the length of the page. **Radial profiles** are transverse to the page.

Figure 1.1. The interpretation of images: patterns seen on surfaces or in sections only show one profile of the object. These diagrams illustrate some of the pitfalls in attempts to guess the structure from profiles in a single plane, all of which can be found in the literature. The real structure, the most probable interpretation of such images, can only be determined by reconstruction in three dimensions. **A.** Circular or round objects are most probably transverse profiles of rods or tubes. **B.** Oval objects are most probably oblique profiles of tubes (oblique profiles of dentinal tubules have been mistakenly interpreted as cross sections of oval tubes). **C.** Rods are most unlikely to be sectioned longitudinally. Images that appear to be long rods are more likely to be overlapping images of many rods oriented parallel to one another as in transverse profiles of teeth with radial diagonal dentinal tubules. **D.** If rods as in C are angled to one another in successive layers then the overlapping images may appear to be curved as in dentinal tubules in radial profiles of elephant tusks. **E.** Paired lines are unlikely to be longitudinal profiles of cylindrical structures such as osteons in bone. They are much more likely to be transverse profiles of paired sheets like those in laminar bone. **F.** Aligned rods are unlikely to be longitudinal profiles of a multiple fiber and more likely to be stacks of sheets as in the radial laminae of dentine (complicated by the laminae being composed of laterally aligned dentinal tubules) or nesting keratin sheets as in horn. **G.** Single rod-like images are unlikely to be rods but may be transverse profiles of layers as in tangential profiles of the keratin sheets of horn. **H.** Longitudinal profiles of the tips of structures maturing by the successive accretion of layers (such as secondary osteons that may grow at their tips) are unlikely, but would resemble incomplete oblique profiles of cylindrical structures with concentric growth layers such as tusks or the formation of secondary osteons in laminar bone.

Another common source of error lies in the number of observations made. Morphologists find it very easy to assume the nature of a structure and then search for an illustration to back up their assumption. It has been said that osteons in antlers are smaller than those of bone, but it depends how and where the sample is taken. Sample size and selection are as important in morphology as in statistics.

In studying micro-architecture it is important to know exactly the relation between the different planes being observed. Research described in this book uses transverse, radial, and tangential profiles to reconstruct three-dimensional structure as in Figure 1.2. The page orientation has been standardized for all illustrations. Transverse profiles have the external edge, such as the periosteal surface in a bone, to the top. Tangential and radial profiles orient the length of the object with the length of the page. Conclusions on structure are presented as diagrams wherever possible, for diagrams are a visual précis of complex three-dimensional ideas.

On Observation

When a subject spans a range of sizes from the molecular to objects held in the hand, it may often be difficult to visualize the scale of things. The table at the end of the glossary may help to put things in perspective. See page 262.

Chapter 2
The Biology of Natural Structural Materials

Introduction

Human beings were lucky that materials with properties ideally matched for tool-making were readily available during their early evolution. Natural materials that have contributed most to human evolution, both social and genetic—through brain changes, have come mainly from other vertebrates in the form of bone and ivory (calcified collagen), hair, horn, tortoiseshell (keratin), and sinews and skins (uncalcified collagen). Together with wood, stone, and mollusc shells, they share mechanical properties unsurpassed until the modern introduction of metals, carbon fibers, glass, ceramics, and reinforced plastics. Apart from stone, the properties that made them ideal have evolved over many million years as an evolutionary response to the need for tough, rigid, protective materials unrelated to the human requirement. Wood and shell have been important, but vertebrates have contributed the most materials. Calcified collagen and keratin are defining features of vertebrates. Bone has had half a billion years to bind collagen proteins and calcium salts together into an ideal material with respect to toughness and ability to bear loads. Ivory, the dentine constituent of vertebrate teeth, has similar constituents and a history almost as long, evolving to meet the need for strength and hardness in a material resistant to cracking. Keratin, the stable protein making up horn and other epidermal skin derivatives, is another vertebrate success story. It is waterproof and unsurpassed for its toughness and crack resistance when dry. Uncalcified collagen, a constituent of connective tissue in dermal skin and tendons, is superbly resistant to tension while remaining pliable. As leather we have made it waterproof. These are the raw materials that allowed humanity to start on the road to tool-making. Their use continued with little competition until the advent of synthetic plastics. It could be argued that human evolution might have taken a very different course if vertebrates had not evolved keratin and collagen, the raw materials used in technologies developed by our ancestors (ignoring the fact that we ourselves are dependent on these materials for our own construction). How might we have evolved if those technologies had been restricted to wood, shell, stone, and plant fiber?

Overview of collagen and keratin

The initial chemical steps in evolution involved two special structural proteins, collagen and keratin, in response to two very different needs—recycling and inertness. Collagen was a building block that remained for the most part within the body's metabolic pool. It could be used in growth and then broken down to be reused elsewhere. Keratin, tough and chemically inert, had a different role. Once deployed for protection from the environment it was dead, outside the body's metabolic pool.

Bone forms by the secretion of calcium binding molecules (polysaccharides on collagen proteins, (112, 141)) into a compartment inside the body space of vertebrates. The periosteal layer defines this compartment to create an environment separate from that of the rest of the body that can be suitable for collagen accumulation and calcification. The shape of these compartments controls the form and properties of the skeleton. Since they are inside the body, bones remain alive, with their own blood vessels and nerves (except for antlers, which grow outside and die after maturity). They are alive in the sense that they are in a dynamic state, continuing to be resorbed and redeposited throughout life. The properties of the bones of ancestral vertebrates were determined when they left the water, creating the need to resist compression and shear in order to support weight that had previously been buoyed up by water. Mammal bones in particular needed strength and rigidity to resist bending and support weight held above the ground. Bird bones required lightness and are a marvel of design for achieving a high strength to weight ratio. The bones of many vertebrates have been used as construction materials by humans.

Ivory is dentine, the main inner constituent of teeth, which began after the evolution of jaws in the earliest vertebrates some 400 million years ago. Skin denticles in the margins of these earliest jaws became teeth by enlarging and developing differently from those over the rest of the body. Dentine lies between protective enamel on the outside and the cells depositing it that line a pulp cavity containing nerves and blood vessels on the inside. Dentine, like bone, is calcified collagen, but except for the resorption of milk teeth, it is outside the metabolic pool. A tooth grows only from its base with little structural change once formed. Although there may be some mineral exchange, dentine is dead in most senses. Ivory has evolved to be tough, resisting physical and chemical attack for a lifetime. All teeth contain ivory, but only those from about ten of our largest mammals are big enough to have been commercially useful.

Keratin is the main protein of horn, hair, feathers, tortoiseshell, scales, and outer layers of the skin. Both (keratin filaments and ® keratin sheets form inside epidermal cells, the layers of cells at the outer surface of the skin. Eventually whole cells fill with keratin and die. The evolution of intracellular structures to protect large surfaces presents a problem —how to prevent the individual keratin containing cells from separating. The solution has been to unite such cells with junctions called desmosomes. If there were a way to destroy desmosomes, then a keratin structure could be made to fall apart in a heap of pieces like an unassembled three-dimensional jigsaw puzzle. There is a rare human genetic deficiency that affects desmosomes in this way. The slightest touch causes tears in the skin of those who suffer from it. The chemical properties of keratin and the orientation of its component fibrils and sheets give epidermal derivatives their unique properties of toughness, rigidity, chemical inertness, and water repellency. Mature keratin structures are dead, even more than ivory, but the death is accomplished by masses of cells dying as the structure matures (some horn does have small blood vessels). In contrast to bone and ivory, the loss of keratin by the organism is considerable; for example the average person loses about 9 lbs [4 kg] of dead keratin containing skin cells per year.

Developmental Origins

The distribution of collagen and keratin is reflected in vertebrate development (Figure 2.1). Cells in the early embryo are totipotent, they can become any part of the adult. Most cells then become one of the three germ layers—endoderm (forming the gut), mesoderm (forming internal organs), and ectoderm forming chiefly the epidermis, the outer protective layer. Their synthetic capabilities reflect this differentiation. Some mesoderm encloses the bone compartment in a capsule having a surface of finger-like projections of blood vessels, bone, and connective tissue (72). Within the bone compartment, other mesoderm cells secrete collagen that calcifies to make bone. Dentine is also secreted by a mesodermal epithelium but into a compartment bounded on the outer face by an ectodermal epithelium that

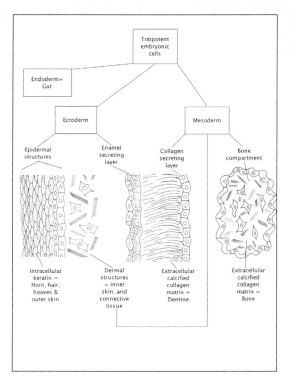

Figure 2.1. The fundamental difference between collagen and keratin forming structures begins with their development. Keratin is deposited within cells of ectodermal origin, which form dead structures outside the body's metabolic pool (outer skin layers, "tortoiseshell," hair, horn, scales, and feathers). Collagen is secreted by cells of mesodermal origin, either in isolated compartments where metastable solutions of calcium and phosphate permit hydroxyapatite crystal growth in the formation of dentine or bone, or throughout the body without calcification as in dermis and connective tissue.

secretes enamel. Both bone and dentine occupy spaces or compartments that allow separate control of their environments. Connective tissue such as tendons and the dermis contain collagen that is not sequestered in compartments separate from the body cavity and does not calcify. Keratin structures are made in a very different way. Keratin is not secreted but synthesized inside cells where it accumulates until they die.

Collagen and keratin come to us after a long evolution as parts of all vertebrates. They are not unique to vertebrates—collagen occurs widely in other phyla—but no other groups have exploited them to the extent that has made them defining vertebrate characteristics. They are proteins, polymers of amino acids linked together in long polypeptide chains. They are examples of molecules with properties that have emerged after multiple replication, like the unforeseen properties that emerged when single rocks used to break windows were piled into heaps and used to build houses. Keratin and collagen fibers both arise by the aggregation of their component molecules (Figures 2.2 and 2.5). Collagen especially has the property of precipitating calcium salts. To understand how evolution has shaped collagen and keratin, it is helpful to know something about their properties—chemical, physical, and architectural—as well as their developmental origins. Their chemical and physical properties are outlined below. Architecture is the subject of chapter 3, "The cylindrical form."

The molecules concerned:

Collagen

Tropocollagen is the starting molecule for bone, ivory, and connective tissue. Cells assemble amino acid chains into tropocollagen particles that pass externally into extracellular compartments where they become collagen. The discovery of the aggregation of tropocollagen into collagen fibers was one of the first successful studies of kinetic subunits, that is, particles with all of the properties needed to assemble spontaneously into complex structures outside cells. In the 1950s, Jerome Gross described collagen formation and illustrated beautifully some of the principles by which gross structures can arise spontaneously as a result of the properties of their subunits (13, 48).

The starting point is an ⟨ chain, a unit length of a helical polypeptide of about 1050 amino acids that remains after a terminal globular sequence has been cleaved off (Figure 2. 2 A, B). Glycine makes up about one in three amino acids in these a chains, allowing the formation of a regular repeating structure that stabilizes both in the length of the ⟨ helix and laterally with other ⟨ helices. Three similar but not identical ⟨ helical chains wind around one another into the much larger triple helix of tropocollagen (Figure 2.2. C). Each tissue has its own kind of collagen in addition to species differences: eighteen different classes of collagen have been described at the last count. The differences come about in two ways: differences in sequence allow different kinds of 〈 helix, and assembly of different groupings of 〈 helices into triple helices characterize each tissue. Skin, tendon, bone, and dentine share one of the major types of collagen in which two of one kind of 〈 helix wind around one of another kind. The 1050 amino acid sequences of the three 〈 helices repeat themselves along the length every 280nm to form the basic tropocollagen molecule Figure 2.2.D).

The sequence is polarized, giving each tropocollagen molecule a head and a tail. The sequence has another characteristic important in fiber assembly—it is subdivided into four similar 70nm regions. The head and tail allow it to string together in long filaments while the similarities along its length give it the interesting property of aligning side-by-side in the quartile staggered fashion that gives the characteristic 70nm repeat banding pattern of collagen fibers (Figure 2.2.E, F).

Tropocollagen molecules are kinetic subunits, that is, units that can build larger structures spontaneously, depending only on the information contained within them and the environment in which they find themselves. Since they exist in an almost infinite variety, depending on their amino acid sequences and the grouping of chains in the triple helix, they have a similar potential to create many different structural forms. Cells secrete tropocollagen into a local environment (e.g., the dentine or bone compartments, Figure 2.1) where conditions allow realization of that potential to emerge in the patterns and orientations of their aggregation.

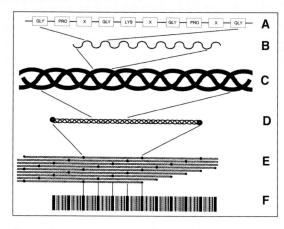

Figure 2.2. The structure of collagen. A. Collagen is characterized by abundant glycine (about 25%), proline (about 15%), and lysine (about 4%). It is almost unique in having hydroxyproline (about 14%) and hydroxylysine (about 1%). Glycine in every third position and hydroxylation of the proline encourage the formation of a regular helix as in B, much of it being composed of repeating sequences of (Gly – Pro – X)n, X being some other amino acid. C. Tropocollagen is composed of 3 a helices like those in B wrapped around one another in a much larger right handed triple helix. Specificity comes from minor differences in the sequences, making particular kinds of a helix and from the proportions of each kind of a helix in the triple helix. Skin, tendon, bone, and dentine have a common type of collagen in which two of one kind of a helix wind around one of another kind. D. The basic tropocollagen molecule consists of three 280nm left-handed a helices of about 1050 amino acids each wound together into a right handed coil. E. Collagen fibers arise from end-to-end and side-to-side alignment of tropocollagen subunits. Because the amino acid sequence is similar every 70nm, tropocollagen has a quartile lateral alignment giving rise to the characteristic 70nm repeat banding pattern of collagen fibers seen in F.

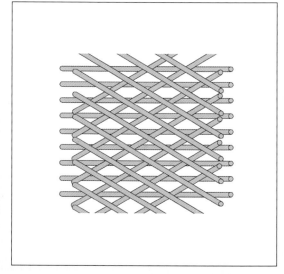

Figure 2.3. Collagen fibers often align parallel to one another in sheets with the orientation changing from sheet to sheet like plywood.

Collagen Arrangement

Collagen filaments may form a meshwork, a matrix in which other ordered filament arrangements are embedded. More often, especially at surfaces, the filaments align side-by-side into sheets, the orientation of which changes from layer to layer like plywood (Figure 2.3). In laminar bone these plywood-like layers or lamellae are flat sheets parallel to the laminae. In osteonic bone, they wrap around the vascular spaces in concentric cylinders. In ivory, collagen filaments form tubules resembling osteons in being cylindrical but ten to a hundred times smaller. The properties of cylindrical structures that results in them being used at many different levels in biological architecture is explored in the next chapter.

Calcification of Collagen

The general mechanism for calcification involves the creation of an environment where calcium salts are supersaturated, precipitating them from solution at particular locations on collagen fibers, defined by calcium binding polysaccharides (112, 141). The salts can reach critical levels because they are secreted into compartments (Figure 2.1) independent from the general body. Regions of bone or dentine differ in their calcification within these compartments, showing that the calcium salt level is only permissive: the precise location of calcification being determined by the location of the collagen regions that host the calcium-binding polysaccharides. Within the dentine compartment of hippo canines, for example, calcification varies in different positions within a band. The explanation may lie in the unique high hydroxylated lysine and proline that characterize collagen (Figure 2.2). They could serve as calcification sites in specific positions by being platforms for the N-linked oligosaccharides that carry -NH rich amino acids.

Keratin

Amino acid chains inside cells may form proteins by balling up into globules (e.g., microtubules) or align side-by-side and lengthways to form fibers (e.g., microfilaments).

Structures made by most of these proteins are in equilibrium with more soluble precursors: microtubules form a changeable scaffolding, while microfilaments, constructed of a protein similar to the actin in muscles, are involved in shape change. In contrast, synthesis of another class of intracellular fibrous proteins, the Intermediate Filaments, is a one-way trip. Once made, they are semi-permanent inhabitants of the cell. The keratins are a subclass of these intermediate filaments, with which they share about a quarter of their sequences. They are not fibrous proteins in the sense that collagen is a fibrous tensile material. Keratins are rigid polymers embedded in an amorphous cross-linked matrix, the main component of vertebrate epithelia, hair, wool, feathers, horns, hooves, and nails (132). They are characterized by having a high content of the amino acid cysteine, typically 10–15% in hair. Cysteine is an unusual amino acid in that it contains an –SH group that sticks out to the side when it becomes part of a polypeptide chain, allowing linkage to –SH groups of cysteines in adjacent chains through the formation of multiple disulfide bridges (Figure 2.4). Keratins are of two kinds, varying in their sulfur content. ® keratins have most cross linking –SH groups,

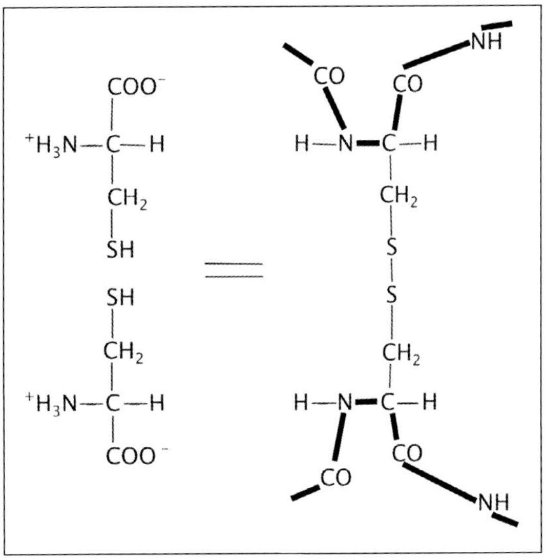

Figure 2.4. Cysteine is the most abundant amino acid extracted from hydrolysed keratin. Two cysteine amino acids in adjacent polypeptide chains (shown in bold type) can form disulfide bridges to make cystine. Such disulfide bridges are responsible for much of keratin's stability.

creating the inflexible keratins of horns, claws, hooves, and nails and the hard keratins of beaks and claws. 〈 keratins have fewer disulfide cross-links, which gives them the elasticity to stretch and return after relaxation of tension. Both kinds of keratin may be made harder by the incorporation of calcium salts.

Keratin filaments share a basic structure of four conserved regions with a combined length of about 40nm (Figure 2.5D). R groups stabilize their chains in the axial direction by hydrogen bonding to form 〈 helices (Figure 2.5A, B). Conserved regions differ from tissue to tissue and are genetically distinct while retaining a basic similarity in their amino acid sequences. Homologies between 〈 keratin and intermediate filaments and between different keratins are restricted to these 〈 helical regions. In contrast, the non-helical regions separating them are variable. The sequence of four helical regions separated by variable regions repeats indefinitely in long strands, linking together through one of the non-helical regions. The structure of the helical regions allows three strands to twist together with crystalline precision into ropes of left-handed super helices of indefinite length (Figure 2.5C,D). The filaments shown in keratin structures by microscopy are bundles of these triple helices (Figures 2.5E, 2.8).

Ⓡ keratins form sheets (Figure 2.6). In Ⓡ keratins the polypeptide chains shown in Figure 2.5A are extended in a flat zig-zag rather than coiled in a helix. Chains unite with neighbors oriented in the opposite, antiparallel, direction by hydrogen bonds (N – H ···· O = C) in the plane of the sheet to create a pleated sheet (Figure 2.6A). Stacks of these sheets are united through disulfide bridges (- S – S-) between cysteines like those uniting 〈 helices in 〈 keratin (Figure 2.6B). Ⓡ keratin is densely packed with crystalline precision, giving it the useful properties of hardness, insolubility, chemical inertness, and hydrophobicity (most of the reactive side chain groups are involved in cross linking the chains and sheets).

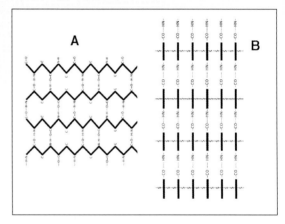

Figure 2.6. The sheet structure of b keratin. Simplified view of the pleated sheets of A. b keratin forms pleated sheets, where each extended polypeptide is linked by hydrogen bonds side-by-side with its neighbors having an antiparallel orientation. The R groups of cysteine carrying the SH groups project at right angles to the plane of the page. B. Simplified view at 900 to A, showing end on views of the peptide chains as thick bars united through hydrogen bonds in the plane of the pleated sheet and disulfide bridges between the sheets.

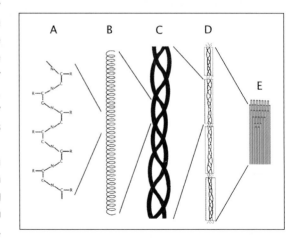

Figure 2.5. The filamentous structure of a Keratin. A. A polypeptide chain showing how the R groups of amino acids pointing away from the chain can form stable links with similarly aligned neighboring chains as in the 2 cysteines 1 cystine reaction in Figure 2.3. Other R groups stabilize the chains in the axial direction by hydrogen bonding in an a helix. B. The polypeptide chain in a keratin is mainly an a helix giving it structural rigidity. Four conserved helical regions are separated by short variable non-helical segments. C. Three a helices combine in a left-handed super helix giving even more rigidity. D. The four a helical regions separated by non-helical segments are aligned in the superhelix. E. Bundles of the three stranded super helical ropes of indefinite length form keratin filaments of the kind revealed by microscopy inside epithelial cells.

A full understanding of the chemistry of collagen and keratin encompasses many of the principles of cell biology such as secretory pathways and protein assembly and also genetics. Proteins may be secreted outside the cell or accumulate within it. Collagen is a secreted protein synthesized into the lumen of the endoplasmic reticulum from bound ribosomes before being modified as it passes through the Golgi complex to secretory vesicles carrying it outside the cell. Keratin is synthesized on free ribosomes and accumulates in the cytoplasm as an intracellular protein. Folding lengths of ⟨ helices and ® sheets into three-dimensional structures is an activity of most proteins. Both collagen and keratin are species specific, that is their genes differ in small ways from one kind of animal to the next, and also tissue specific, there are different genes coding for the collagens and keratins in each tissue. In humans, for example, there are fifty-four different keratin genes. These complications lie far beyond the scope of this book.

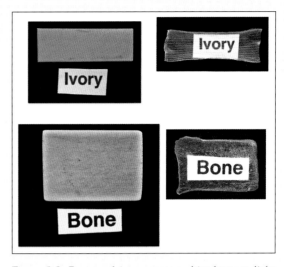

Figure 2.8. Bone and ivory appear white because light passing through them is scattered by regions of different refractive index—calcium salts, organics such as collagen, and water. After dilute acids have removed calcium salts and drying has removed water, the residual collagen is completely translucent. The titles Bone and Ivory can easily be read when placed underneath the calcium extracted 2mm thick sheets of bone and ivory.

Physical Properties

The colors of natural materials

The color of most natural materials tends to white—bone, ivory, unpigmented skin, and horn. The reason is that they are composites of materials with several different refractive indexes. Bone and ivory can contain calcite, RI 1.65 and 1.48, and hydroxyapatite, RI 1.65 and 1.64 interspersed with materials having lower refractive indices—organic materials 1.5, water 1.3, and air 1.0. Light passing through such mixtures is scattered much as sunlight passing through clouds appears white after bouncing repeatedly from air to water droplets. When bone or ivory is treated with dilute acids to dissolve the calcium salts, it loses its stiffness and becomes rubbery. It also becomes more translucent

Collagen

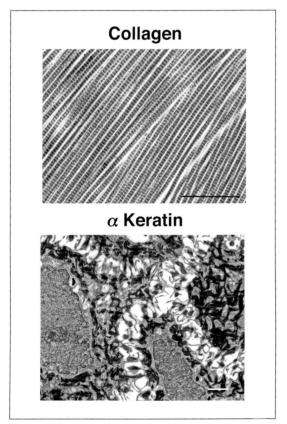

α Keratin

Figure 2.7. Collagen is an external secretion that assembles into these banded fibers. Keratin is an internal cell component showing up here as densely stained fibers. See Figures 2.2 and 2.5. Scale bars = 1mm. By kind permission of Dr. James McMahon, Cleveland Hospital.

as scattering between water/collagen and the high refractive index inorganic salts is reduced. But it is still opaque. It becomes completely translucent after drying out and collapse of the water spaces removes the cause of light scattering (Figure 2. 8).

The colors of horn and hair are due to melanin granules deposited inside the cells together with the keratin. Melanin is a condensation product of polyphenols with the aid of phenol oxidase enzymes, notably tyrosinase. The color ranges from yellow through orange to brown and black, depending on the nature of the precursors and the enzymes concerned in the condensation. The granules themselves are not produced by the cell in which they finally reside. Melanocyte pigment cells pass granules on to keratin forming cells by a kind of natural tattooing process. Skin color is only partly due to continual pigment production in melanocytes and transfer to epidermal cells. Melanin is conserved in melanocytes in the basal layers between the dermis and epidermis where the tattooist aims to inject his pigments. If it were not for this, the tattooists efforts would be transitory, due to the shedding of skin. Human skin color is due to the melanosome content of the melanocytes, not their frequency.

Material	Density μ SD
Ivory	
1. Mammoth	1. 70 μ 0.05
2. Elephant	1. 78 μ 0.07
3. Narwhal	1. 88 μ 0.03
4. Walrus	1. 92 μ 0.05
5. Hippopotamus	1. 93 μ 0.06
6. Warthog and other pigs	1. 93 μ 0.03
7. Sperm whale	1. 99 μ 0.05
8. Killer whale	2. 05 μ 0.02
Cementum	
Mammoth	1. 89 μ 0.06
Elephant	1. 89
Enamel	
Hippopotamus	2. 36
Bone	
Peripheral laminar cow longbone	2. 04 μ 0.05
Antler	
White tailed deer, peripheral region	1. 79 μ 0.06
Jet	
Whitby jet	1.3

Densities of Natural Materials

Table 2.1. Densities of natural materials

Density

Bone and ivory, with densities of 1.7 – 2.05 when dry (Table 2. 1), are much denser than typical organic materials that range from about 1.1 to 1.6 (Table 2. 2). The difference is due to varying degrees of calcification. The low density of mammoth ivory (1.70) compared to that of elephants (1.78) is due to the reverse of calcification. Depending on the preservation, variable amounts of both organic and inorganic constituents dissolve into the bog water and melted permafrost. Dried less well preserved specimens are porous and readily take up water. Density and preservation is not directly related to color which may range from off white to deep brown caused by water-bourn tannins. Mammoth and elephant ivory cementum have similar densities as would be expected for cementum being enamel low in calcium. Of the eight ivories measured, three —those of the walrus, hippopotamus, and warthog (and other pigs)—were not statistically different from one another (1.92–1.93). All the others were significantly or highly significantly different from one another and from these three. The differences are probably due to the degree of calcification, but structure may also play a part. Sperm whales and killer whales have the most dense ivory (1.99 and 2.05) that is characterized by having solid dentinal "tubules." Differences in density could confirm the kind of ivory used to make an artifact, although the structure should usually be all that is needed for identification.

Thermal Conductivity

Dry ivory or bone with its finely dispersed air chambers is a poor conductor of heat, making it desirable as an insulator for handles on pots and kettles.

Material	Density
Celluloid, Cellulose acetate	1.27 – 1.60
Cellulose nitrate	1.35 – 1.60
Epoxies	~ 1.1
Melamine-formaldehyde, Melamine resin	1.51
Methacrylates, Lucite, Plexiglass, Perspex	~ 1.16
Phenol-formaldehydes, Bakelite, Formica	1.31 +
Rubber, vulcanized,	1.1 – 1.2 +

Densities of Synthetic Plastics

Table 2.2. Densities of synthetic plastics. Densities are often increased by additions of inorganic compounds to increase weight or hardness or to change color, but they are usually below bone and ivory. Data from (119).

Chapter 3
The Cylindrical Form

Introduction

Many natural structures involved in mechanical support are cylindrical. Long bones are not solid, they have a center of soft marrow where fat is stored, or in birds, air sacs. Antlers have a shell of hard, strongly calcified bone supported by an elastic core of spongy trabeculae with little calcification. Horns may be solid at their tips, but through most of their length they are thin keratin cylinders laid over spongy bone. The strength to weight ratio in the cylindrical rachis of feathers is unsurpassed, a requirement for the evolution of flight. Insects, in fact the whole phylum Arthropoda, have evolved with all their limbs and bodies constrained within tubular exoskeletons. At the microscopic level the scaffolding of cells is made from microtubules. In dentine, the supports for calcification of teeth are dentinal tubules of collagen about 5mm in diameter. They have a role like that of the steel rods in reinforced concrete. Hollow forms have a special place in both living and man-made structures. Weight for weight, a cylinder is the most economical way to create strength in an elongated structure. The reason for this is easy to visualize. Imagine what happens inside a rod when it is bent (Figure 3.1). The surface layers are compressed on one side and stretched on the other, balancing out in the middle, which is neither stretched nor compressed. Since the center of the rod carries no load, it can be a cylinder with little loss of strength but great economy in material. In a similar argument, torsion at the surface of a cylinder results in progressively less stress from the periphery to the center where it disappears, allowing a cylinder to be almost as strong as a rod in resistance to twisting. Millions of years of evolution have refined many massive supporting structures into delicate hollow shells. It is a remarkable fact that organisms exploit the properties of cylinders at so many different levels, three in the materials discussed in this book. At the gross macroscopic level, long bones, horns and tusks are cylinders around a space used for other purposes; at the microscopic level, bones may be constructed from longitudinal stacks of cylindrical osteons. At an even finer level, the dentine of ivory consists of radial arrays of dentinal tubules (Figure 3.2).

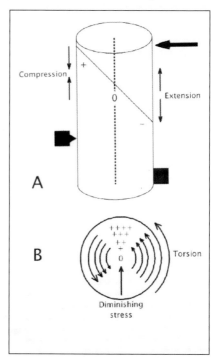

Figure 3.1. Many natural structures can be cylinders with little loss of strength compared to rods (bones, exoskeletons, horns, teeth, microtubules, dentinal tubules, feathers, plant stems, bamboo, hair). A. The center of a restrained rod subjected to a lateral force is unstressed. Since the center of the rod carries no load it can be a cylinder with little loss of strength while economizing on material. B. Torsion at the surface of a cylinder results in progressively less stress from the periphery to the center where it disappears, allowing a cylinder to be almost as strong as a rod in resistance to twisting.

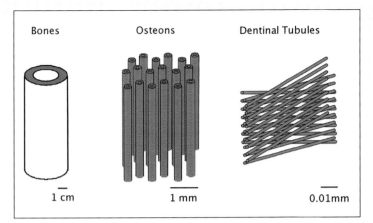

Figure 3.2. Organisms exploit the cylindrical form at many different levels. On a large scale such as the shafts of long bones, the strength of a cylinder allows the core to be used to store lipids and make blood cells. On a microscopic scale bundles of osteons strengthen the walls of such bones while using their cores to transport blood. On an even finer scale dentinal tubules strengthen the dentine of tusks.

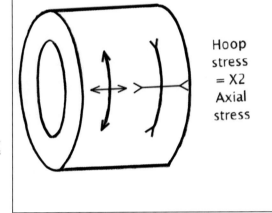

Hoop stress = X2 Axial stress

Figure 3.3. In a cylinder under uniform internal pressure, the hoop stress is twice the axial stress. Cracks or tears from such stresses are therefore longitudinal.

Stress in cylindrical structures

Table 2.1. Densities of natural materials

Table 2.2. Densities of synthetic plastics. Densities are often increased by additions of inorganic compounds to increase weight or hardness or to change color, but they are usually below bone and ivory. Data from (119).

Almost any very old bone, tusk, or antler is likely to be cracked. The polished surface of a rib from a 32,000 year old mammoth (Figure 3. 4A) shows the typical pattern. Antlers also crack in longitudinal radial patterns after shrinking due to drying out (Figure 3. 4B). We see such longitudinal surface cracks so frequently that we take them for granted without thinking about how they have come about, and yet they result from the operation

of an engineering principle that has important consequences for the design of tubular structures in biology. In a cylinder under uniform internal hydrostatic pressure the hoop stress is twice the axial stress (Figure 3.3) (46, 132). This is why exploding boilers split along their length rather than blowing off their ends and may be the reason why the stretch marks of pregnant women who are not too corpulent (ie cylindrical rather then spherical in form) tend to be up and down. When the material composing a cylinder shrinks the negative pressure and the stress it produces in the circumference is also twice that in the axis. Cracks to relieve the stress therefore also appear in the radial-longitudinal direction at right angles to the greatest stress. To the extent that tusks and bones are homogeneous material this simple mechanical principle explains why they crack with a longitudinal axial pattern.

This is not to say that the orientation of components does not influence the direction of cracking. It clearly does, as in the crack patterns of elephant ivory described in Chapter 6. The mammoth rib bone (Figure 3. 4A) is slightly unusual in that it is composed of axially oriented osteons with a spongy core (Figure 3. 4C). It might be argued that the axial cracking is solely a response to the axial orientations of these components. However, when a thin slice of such bone is cut transversely and freed from the restraints of being part of a cylinder before being allowed to dry out and crack, the crack pattern becomes random in the axis (Figure 3. 4D). In these instances, the cracks are influenced both by the hoop stress and by the arrangement of components. Cracking is radial/axial around the longitudinally arranged osteons until the hoop stress component is removed when it is both radial and circumferential in the axis. When the structure and properties are similar in the axis and circumference as in laminar bone, the hoop stress dominates and cuts through the laminae (Figure 3. 4E). When such bones are cut in thin transverse slices to remove the hoop stress, shrinkage causes circumferential/axial cracks between adjacent layers of laminae (Figure 3.4F). Surface layers with similar structure in the axis and circumference therefore provide some protection against hoop stress cracking. We see this in some deer antlers that have a wide shell of laminar-like bone around a core of osteons and spongy bone. Shrinkage results in axial/longitudinal cracking in the osteonic layer but is prevented by the laminar layers from reaching the surface. This is an advantage for antlers with surfaces exposed to a dry environment that may not be needed by rib bones protected inside the body.

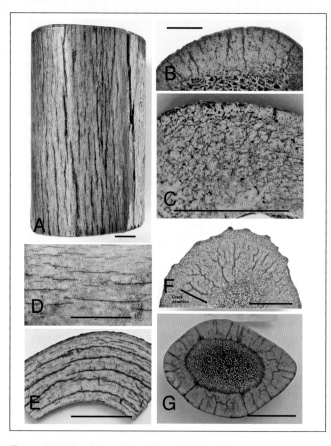

Figure 3.4. Cracks resulting from shrinkage in tubular organic structures tend to be axial because the hoop stress is twice the axial stress. A. The crack pattern in a 32,000 year old mammoth rib bone has numerous longitudinal cracks. B. A transverse profile of A shows the radial longitudinal arrangement of cracks although the osteons forming the bone are symmetrical in the plane of the surface. C. After removing the hoop stress by cutting a thin transverse section of osteonic bone similar to B, shrinkage cracking is random/axial rather than radial. D. Laminar bone cracks longitudinally/radially although the structure is similar in the plane of the surface. Cow femoral bone. E. After removing the hoop stress by cutting a thin transverse section of osteonic bone similar to D, shrinkage cracking is circumferential/axial rather than radial. F. Surface layers of laminar bone are less susceptible to shrinkage cracking than the osteonic bone below them. Transverse profile of Moose antler. G. Antlers with less laminar bone crack like the mammoth rib bone in A that also lacks laminar bone. Transverse profile of white tailed deer antler tine.

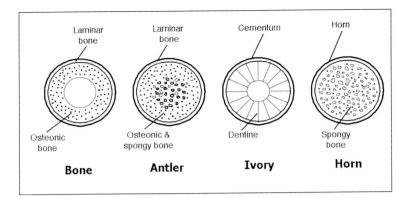

Figure 3.5. Surface shells with uniform properties in the plane of the surface may have evolved at least partly to limit cracking of components below, as in laminar bone in long bones and antlers, cementum in ivory tusks, and keratin around the bone core in horns

The requirement for many tubular structures to resist particular stresses, for example compression and bending, may not be the most appropriate to resist cracking. For example, the longitudinal orientation of osteons in bones may resist bending but encourage longitudinal cracking. It is probably for this reason that surface shells have evolved, laminar bone in long bones and antlers, cementum in ivory tusks and keratin around the bone core in horns (Figure 3.5). The shells are made from components with uniform properties in the plane of the surface providing protection from the hoop stress tending to initiate longitudinal cracking in core components below them oriented to resist bending. In this book, **Shell** will be used as a general term to describe surface layers of tubular structures structurally and functionally distinct from the cortices below them.

When studying stresses experimentally, it is important to start with a stress free surface; cracks can easily be initiated from tears produced at right angles to the blade of a blunt saw. Saw marks must be ground out and the surface polished before treatments that allow cracks to indicate stress and structure. The nature of cracks in an artifact can be a clue to its authenticity.

We can conclude that these two engineering principles—that rods can be hollow with little loss of strength and that the hoop stress in a cylinder is twice the axial stress—have far-reaching consequences in the evolution of the design of skeletal structures.

Growth in cylindrical structures

Cylinders may be efficient in terms of strength for the material used, but they present problems for the living systems that make them. Organisms make things by secretion at the surfaces of layers of cells (epithelia). If this takes place on the outside of the cylinder, the surface of living cells dies when deposition is completed because it is exposed to the environment (as in antler formation). If it is on the inside, the diameter cannot increase, and the epithelia ultimately get squeezed to a narrow rod (the tips of horns and teeth). The other problem is that coverings tend to be rigid for protection. Laying down material inside the original surface restricts change in size and shape (this is why insects and other arthropods can only grow by casting off their old skins and blowing up their new ones before they harden). Protective surfaces are therefore either pliable (skin) or restricted to scales allowing growth around the edges as in the flat epidermal coverings of turtles ("tortoiseshell"). The development of tortoiseshell is a good place to begin, because it leads on easily to the growth of horns. Turtles protect their insides with a carapace of interlocking polygonal bones supported on their ribs. Above these bones, in a different pattern, lie a polygonal patchwork of tortoiseshell scales. The animal grows by increments around the edges of the bones and around the edges of the keratin scales (Figure 3.6 A, B). Horns are cylindrical derivatives of this kind of structure. In bovids (cattle, sheep, goats) bone outgrowths from the head form a template on which the epidermis forms the cylindrical horn. How can the horn cylinder grow in diameter when it is secreted from the outside? It does so by growth from the base, allowing increase in breadth and length (Figure 3.7).

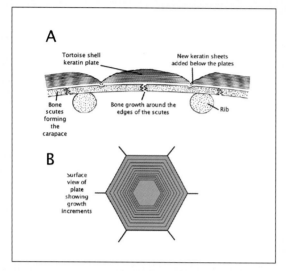

Figure 3.6. A, B. Tortoiseshell scales form a polygonal patchwork supported on a carapace of interlocking polygonal bones. Growth is by increments around the edges of the keratin scales. Horns are cylindrical derivatives of this kind of structure.

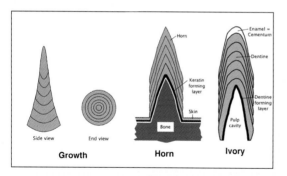

Figure 3.7. Growth in external tubular structures. Horns are deposited outside a bone core. They increase in length and diameter by growth from the base. Dentine forming ivory in a tooth is protected on the outside by enamel or cementum and can only grow on the inside. It solves the problem of growth like horn, growing from the inside, but unlike horn the dentine forming layer lies above a core of pulp rather than bone.

The problem of growth in cylindrical long bones is solved in a different manner by recycling material removed from the inside and redepositing it on the outside (see figure 4.8 in Chapter 4). Long bones are mainly cylinders of up to several hundred laminae deposited one upon the other from the outside. If this were all, it would result in a solid rod with a tiny core, but vertebrates have better uses for this space as marrow to store fats and as a place to manufacture some kinds of blood cells. During growth, the inner surface of bones is irregular, as though bone of all kinds is being eroded. This is smoothed over in mature bones where the surface often cuts diagonally across circumferentially oriented layers of laminae, showing that erosion follows a different pattern from deposition. The final shape of a bone depends upon the specific patterns and extent of erosion as much as growth on the outer surface. Most bone deposited early in development is replaced during growth. For example, transverse profiles from the middle of the femur and humerus of pigs about two months old can fit completely inside the bones at six months. In summary, the problem of forming a cylinder while depositing bone on the outside during growth is solved by the old small diameter inner face being constantly eroded while laminae of the new large diameter outer face are deposited. Antlers grow like other bones. They differ only in that their outer formative surface dies at maturity and the core is filled with a special elastic matrix designed for maximum resistance to shock.

Ivory is the dentine from tusks, cylindrical elongated teeth adapted to resist lateral deformation. The problem of tusk growth is similar to that in horn except that it is formed in layers secreted by two different epithelia. The outer covering of cementum (= modified enamel) is secreted from the outside, allowing growth by increase in diameter or length. Dentine is secreted on the inside from a conical growth zone. Layers of conical dentine shells are deposited like the layers in an elongated onion (Figure 3.7).

Increasing the diameter from the tip is by the addition of layers at the periphery of this conical growth zone. Growth in length occurs from the base, where many layers may be secreted at the same time in a conical growth zone. Further down a tusk, the extended cones become almost cylindrical, appearing in cross section like the growth rings of a tree. A cross section of an elephant tusk where the diameter has reached its maximum, has the oldest rings at the periphery. Unlike tree rings, the most recently formed layers are on the inside next to the pulp cavity. Also unlike tree rings, the conical or cylindrical layers corresponding to these rings viewed longitudinally are formed in sequence from the tip to the base. The absolute age of a layer will vary with its position along the length.

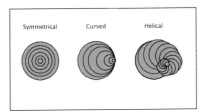

Figure 3.8. In both horns and teeth, straight cylindrical structures arise when growth is evenly distributed around the basal growth zone. Curved structures arise when growth is greater on one side. Progressive movement of such greater growth zones around the perimeter results in curved helical structures as in this left-handed helix.

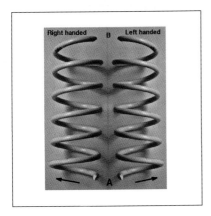

Figure 3.9. The handedness of helices: the direction of the turn in a helix is independent of the direction of viewing. In a right-handed helix viewed from A, the turn is clockwise away from the viewer towards B. A left-handed helix is a mirror image of this, following a curve away from the viewer in an anticlockwise (counterclockwise) direction and towards the viewer in a clockwise direction.

On Curves

Cylindrical structures are only straight if their growth rate is evenly distributed around the basal growth zone. Faster growth on one side leads to curved structures (Figure 3.8). Consistent, even growth to one side leads to symmetrical curves like those in the horns of an Oryx or the upper canine teeth of pigs. When the position of the increased growth rate moves progressively to one side, the result is a curved helical structure like that of a rams horn.

On Helices

Cylindrical structures lend themselves to the formation of helices. Several keratin structures (horns), ivory tusks (narwhal, elephants, mammoths, and pigs), and dentinal tubules arrangements (elephants and hippos) are helical. Reconstructing these arrangements in three dimensions in the mind is not easy, but it is important for understanding their structure. Anyone who can picture helical structures intuitively has a very superior intellect. For the rest of us, the following description may help.

A right-handed helix follows a curve away from the viewer in a clockwise direction. Conversely, it follows an anticlockwise (counterclockwise) curve as it proceeds towards the viewer. A left-handed helix is a mirror image of this, following a curve away from the viewer in an anticlockwise direction and towards the viewer in a clockwise direction. The direction of the turn is independent of the direction of viewing. In a right-handed helix viewed from **A**, the turn is clockwise away from the viewer towards **B** (Figure 3.9). Viewed from **B**, the turn is also clockwise away from the viewer towards **A**. However, this same clockwise movement viewed from **A** becomes anticlockwise because the direction has been reversed by the observer's position.

Chapter 4
Bone,
The Internal Skeleton of Vertebrates

Introduction

Unlike ivory and horn, which have been under researched, there is much literature on the structure of bone, both contemporary and classical. Structures carrying the names of their discoverers are illustrated in most histology and general biology textbooks by beautiful pictures derived for the most part from nineteenth century studies of ground or decalcified sections. Studies are mainly on mature human bones and those from common experimental mammals rather than the various bones of commerce that are the emphasis here. Except for the work of Enlow (31–33), who surveyed bone structure in a wide array of animals, and workers who emphasize mechanical properties (132), most publications overemphasize the role of osteonic bone and ignore laminar bone. Some textbook diagrams also confuse lamellae with laminae. Lamellae are components of laminar and osteonic bone. Such errors have been passed on to Internet descriptions. The following overview shows that laminar and some osteonic bone is primary, but most osteonic bone is secondary, and that laminar bone profiles have often been mistakenly portrayed as lamellae or longitudinal profiles of osteons (74). The simplified description here should help the reader to assess the textbook drawings more critically.

Observation Technique

Because bones are hard and opaque, their study has usually involved the tedious process of grinding sections thinly enough to allow the transmission of light. This is no longer necessary for transmission electron microscopy where diamond knives are used for sectioning or for the observation of surfaces by scanning electron microscopy. It is also not necessary for light microscopy, where direct observation of polished surfaces can yield much information with little effort in preparation. The observation of polished surfaces also makes three-dimensional reconstruction easier by linking together what is seen on all faces of a block, whether by microscopy or observations with a hand lens.

Bone samples can be prepared as cubes, as in Figure 1.2, to preserve faces with known orientations (72, 74). In only a few seconds the bone compartment and vascular spaces can be displayed by painting the polished surface with a black marker pen and removing surplus ink by an alcohol wipe. The simplicity of this technique makes it useful for anyone studying bone and bone artifacts.

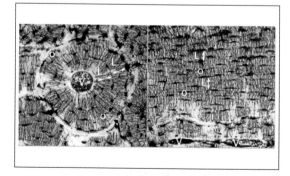

Figure 4.1. The basic structure of bone consists of layers or lamellae (L) of calcified collagen with lacunae (spaces) containing osteocytes (O) linked by fine cell processes called canaliculi. A. In osteonic bone the lamellae form cylinders around tubular external compartments (V, vascular spaces) containing capillaries and nerves. B. In laminar bone the lamellae form flat sheets outlining the external compartment containing capillary network sheets (V). Bar scale = 100mm.

Basic structure

The major component of all kinds of bone consists of long variably calcified collagen fibers 50–100nm thick laid down in 10–50mm wide lamellae that are either in cylinders around tubular vascular spaces in osteonic bone, in laminae separating reticular capillary network sheets (Figure 4.1 A, B) or in thin shells or twigs in spongy bone. The basic structure is that of a compartment limited on the outside by the periosteum made from osteoblast cells and connective tissue, and on the inside by their endosteal equivalent. Osteocytes occupy lacunae (spaces) in the bone lamellae within the compartment and link together through canaliculi (fine channels). Osteoblasts secrete precursors to the bone lamellae into the compartment where osteocytes maintain them. There are two variables: shape of the compartment and orientation of the collagen fibers within it.

The form of the bone is determined by the shape of the compartment, how the sheets or cylinders twist or turn or lay flat and straight. Surface folding from the periosteal and endosteal faces allows blood vessels and nerves closer proximity to the contents of the bone compartment. In laminar bone, the surface folds are in reticular sheets connected to one another and to the surface. In osteonic bone they are tubes (Figure 4.2). The infolds in spongy bone are a coarse reticulum of thin walled chambers surrounded by thin walled bone shells.

Fiber orientations change from lamella to lamella like the layers in plywood, giving orientations characteristic for each kind of bone. The collagen sheets are flat in laminar bone and curve into cylinders in osteonic bone.

In development and throughout life there is a dynamic interplay of destruction and replacement of different kinds of bone giving rise to many intermediates between osteons, laminae, and spongy structures (24, 136, 137).

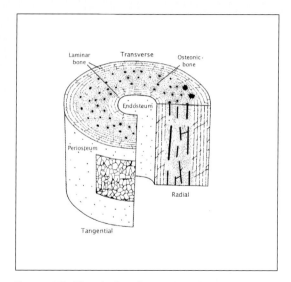

Figure 4.2. The shafts of most long bones are made primarily from circumferential sheets of lamellar bone. Network sheets containing capillaries separate each layer. Blood vessels penetrate connective tissue of the periosteum on the outside and on the inside where the endosteum marks the boundary with the bone marrow. Secondary osteonic bone, consisting of cylinders of lamellae around a central blood vessel, may replace laminar bone to varying degrees. Osteons can also form primary bone. Radial blood vessels connect each capillary sheet and the vessels in osteons. Osteocytes lie in over dispersed lacunae in the lamellae of both kinds of bone as in Figure 4.1.

On Osteons and Haversian Systems

Clopton Havers (1657–1702) was a physician, a Doctor of Medicine from both Oxford and Utrecht and a Fellow of the Royal College of Physicians (29). He was elected to the Royal Society at the age of twenty-nine while Samuel Pepys was President. Robert Hook (1635–1703), regarded as the founder of Cell Biology from his clear picture of the cells of cork published in *Micrographia* in 1664, was a contemporary, elected to the Royal Society at a similar age of twenty-eight years. Havers must have been influenced by Hook and the wealth of new knowledge that microscopes were revealing. He probably read van Leeuwenhoek's note in the *Philosophical Transactions of the Royal Society*, September 21st, 1654, which said, "I have several times endeavored to observe the parts of a Bone, and at first I imagined I saw on the surface of the shinbone of a Cow several small veins …" (perhaps something like that in Figure 4.5). In 1689, Havers lectured to the Royal Society on bone structure and is remembered as a pioneer in osteogeny. In 1691, he put his lectures into a book, "Osteologia nova, or some New observations of the Bones and the Parts belonging to them, with the manner of their Accretion and Nutrition." He described something like Figure 4.1 A, but his figure lacked the crispness of Hook's illustrations. Later workers coined the term Haversian system for what he described. While the term has merit in honoring the name of the most distinguished pioneer in the field, its indiscriminate application to all long bone structure has resulted in lack of attention to the more common laminar structure. The term has become imprecise. In more recent terminology, a Haversian system might be a group of primary or secondary osteons. The basic structure of bone is either that of lamellae in the bone compartment around a straight central blood vessel creating an osteon, or sheets of lamellae separating branching blood vessels in flat reticular spaces. "Haversian system" does not fit easily into a description of what we now actually see in a bone and should be discarded as a useful term.

Structure and Development of Long Bones

There are two origins in the embryological development of mammalian bones. The clavicle or collar bone and non-appendage bones (skull, jaw) are "membrane bones," developing directly from mesoderm in the dermis. Appendage bones (humerus, femur, etc.) begin as cartilage precursors made to approximately the right shape before they become bone by "endochondral ossification" (66). They increase their length by the progressive conversion of their cartilaginous ends into shafts made mainly of compact bone while increasing their diameter by the growth of laminar bone in the way described in Figure 4.8.

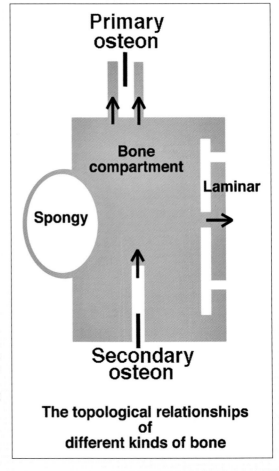

Figure 4.3. The complexity of bone structure can be derived from the arrangement of collagen in cylindrical projections out of the bone compartment (Primary osteons), around finger-like projections into the bone compartment (Secondary osteons), or in sheets parallel to flat outgrowths forming Laminar bone.

Laminar Bone

Although in primary bone formation we may think of the vascular spaces connected to the surface as functional **infolds** into the bone compartment, they arise in development as spaces between **outgrowths** of the surface. In secondary bone, on the other hand, bone **is** deposited around infolds. This leads to a simple fundamental distinction between primary and secondary bone. Primary bone is deposited around outgrowths from the bone compartment and secondary bone is deposited around ingrowths into the bone compartment. Laminar bone is primary, osteonic bone may be primary or secondary (Figure 4.3). The description below is mainly of the shafts of long bones, the bone material used for most artifacts. Long bones are made from compact bone (laminar, osteonic, or mixed), designed to bear loads, with spongy ends and core devoted to lipid storage, blood, or blood cell creation.

Structure

Laminar bone is primary bone, the first formed bone either in development or in repair. Other kinds of bone do not transform into it as, for example, secondary osteons form from laminar bone. Laminar bone consists of stacks of capillary network sheets separated by bone laminae, with each lamina being a plywood-like composite of several lamellae. It is the most common, basic, compact bone structure. Its distinguishing feature is that the calcified collagen fibers forming its lamellae lie in sheets parallel to the surface within compartments defined by the periosteum (Figures 4.1 B, 4.4). Stacks of these bone lamellae are incompletely separated from one another by reticular ingrowths from the surface that are topologically external, containing networks of blood vessels, nerves, and connective tissue (72). The shafts of long bones are usually made initially from this kind of compact bone.

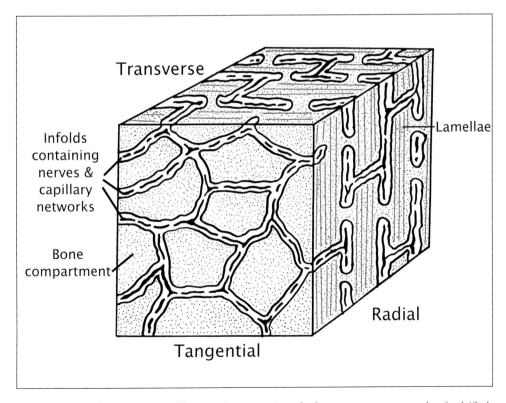

Figure 4.4. The basic structure of laminar bone consists of a bone compartment made of calcified collagen lamellae parallel to the surface alternating with reticular sheets containing networks of blood vessels, nerves, and connective tissue as in Figure 4.1 B.

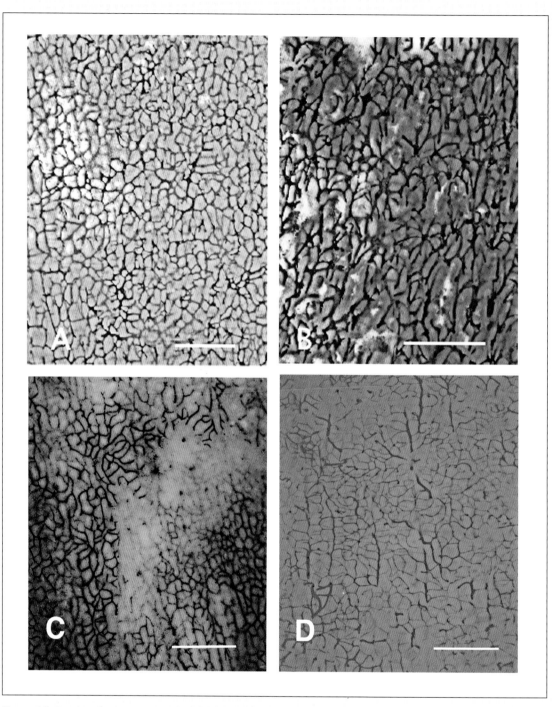

Figure 4.5. Laminar bone structure. A, B. The reticular spaces containing capillary network sheets in one layer of laminar bone from the humerus of a two-year-old cow seen in surface tangential view. C. Slightly oblique profile of the surface of a giraffe radius showing three layers of reticular spaces. D. The blood-filled capillaries in an unstained preparation similar to A. A–C. Ink-filled dry bones. D. Fresh bone. Bar scales = 1mm.

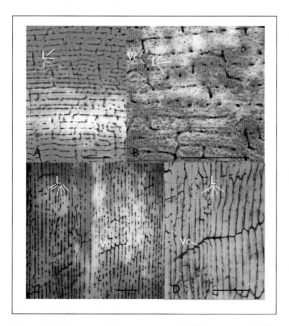

Figure 4.6. Laminar bone structure. A. Transverse profile of laminar bone from the humerus of a cow. Radial connections between laminae (Volkmann's canals) are rarely visible in transverse profiles because they are oblique to the axis. B. Transverse profile of laminar bone from the humerus of a lamb. Reticular system profiles range from circles to cylinders depending on the angle. C. Longitudinal radial profile of buffalo humerus. The profiles of the reticular system tend to be elongated axially as would be expected if the reticulum tends to be straighter axially as in Figure 4.5 B and C. The white areas are more heavily calcified and reflect light rather than being stained brown by the silver staining. D. Longitudinal radial profile of a cow humerus. The reticular system in each lamina may connect by occasional short spaces or by oblique radial extensions (Volkmann's canals). A, B, C surface views after silver staining, D, Coomassie blue stain. Bar scales = 1 mm.

Tangential views of the surface of fresh bones of many kinds show networks of bright red blood vessels filling the reticular spaces (Figure 4.5 D). These reticular spaces can be visualized experimentally in clean dry bones by staining or filling them with ink (Figures 4.5 A, B, C). The same effect occurs naturally in old bones by infiltration with dirt. These reticular patterns are very varied and can be used to characterize particular bones, species, regions, and developmental stage. Transverse profiles of preparations like those in Figure 4.5 show circumferentially arranged laminae-like tree rings (Figures 4.6 A, B). Each stained space containing blood capillaries is about 10–50mm across and is separated from the next by a bone lamina about 200mm wide. Longitudinal radial profiles show that each reticular system space is connected to the next one by radial side branches (Volkmann's canals), allowing blood flow throughout the bone. Capillaries connect from one lamina to the next as well as within each lamina (Figure 4.6 C, D). Most blood vessels are capillaries within the reticular system spaces, but some wider axial vessels and those in Volkmann's canals are more purposefully oriented. Although most laminar bone is in regular cylindrical layers, laminae sometimes divide and fold. This has given rise to the term "woven bone," a misnomer, since it encourages the impression that the constituent lamellae and collagen fibers interweave like the fibers in a cotton fabric. Woven bone is only woven in the sense that the lamellae around reticular vascular spaces have changed from a flat to a three-dimensional reticulum. Felt-like would be a more appropriate descriptive term.

Growth—Formation of New Bone

New peripheral bone compartments remain connected to the older ones, suggesting that growth is from outgrowths enlarging around new reticular vascular spaces until only the radial connections mentioned above join it to the surface (Figures 4.7 A–D, 4.8). During endochondral ossification (see below) large blood vessels from the outside penetrate the bone marrow. The reticular spaces formed between bone compartment outgrowths at first contain only an amorphous matrix (Figure 4.7 A). Only later do blood vessels branch from the inside as each new layer of the reticular system forms. The depth from the surface thus reflects the stage of development, nearest to the surface being the most recently formed. Profiles of developing laminar bone can be very confusing and difficult to interpret. Depending on the stage, there are two interdependent reticular patterns. The bone compartment is a broad reticular sheet during the middle stages of development (Figure 4.7 A, D). Vascular spaces are narrow reticular sheets in mature laminar bone (Figures 4.4 and 4.5). Tubes through the mature bone compartment connect adjacent reticular vascular spaces (Figures 4.8.1, 2, 4 and 4.7 B, C). The reticular vascular spaces are very thin, so that mature bone compartments touch and connect to each other between the vascular reticulum (Figures 4.1, 4.4, 4.8.1, 4). Early in development, new bone laminae appear as papillae on the surface of the old lamina (Figures 4.7 B, 4.8.2, 3). The appearance also depends upon the level of the profile. In mature laminae tangential profiles through the vascular space show it to be reticular. (Figure 4.8.1, 4). In the same preparations profiles closer to the surface show the bone compartment to be a coarse reticulum around the tubes connecting the vascular spaces (Figure 4.8.1, 4).

Growth at the endosteal surface

An irregular endosteal surface may relate to one of three conditions—erosion during aging or malnutrition, size, and shape change in normal development, or it may be the normal lining of spongy bone apposing bone marrow especially at the ends of long bones (see spongy bone, Figure 4.16). During aging, the endosteal surface of long bones may erode due to osteoporosis, the well-known cause of brittle bones in human seniors (Figure 4.9 A–D). At the same time, laminar and osteonic bone may lose mass by the enlargement of their vascular spaces, looking like stages in the conversion of laminar to osteonic bone. Similar changes take place during the normal life cycles of many mammals, for example in bears during hibernation and deer during calcium withdrawal for antler development.

(Opposite page)
Figure 4.7. Laminar bone formation—observations. A. The vascular space near the surface is wide and continuous while the bone compartment has many finger-like projections. During maturation towards the inside, the bone compartment becomes wider and less fragmented and the vascular space becomes narrower and more reticular. Transverse profile of developing pig humerus. See Figure 4.8. B. Surface of a forming lamina showing tubular connections between adjacent vascular spaces and bone columns traversing the vascular space to connect with the bone lamina above. Cow femur. See Figure 4.8.2. C. Ink-stained lamina surface showing a reticular vascular space and the tubular connections emerging from it through the lamina to the vascular space above. Cow femur. See Figure 4.8.1 & 4. D. Growth of the new bone compartment has begun to reduce the vascular spaces traversing laminae to tubes. Tangential view below the surface of a growing lamb femur. See Figure 4.8.3. E. Developing vascular spaces seen as circles have almost reached their final form. Tangential profile of a calf femur. B, bone compartment; V, vascular space or vascular columns uniting adjacent vascular spaces as in B; bc, bone columns uniting adjacent laminae. A, D, and E, silver stained. B and C whole mounts of dissected surfaces. Bar scales = 200mm.

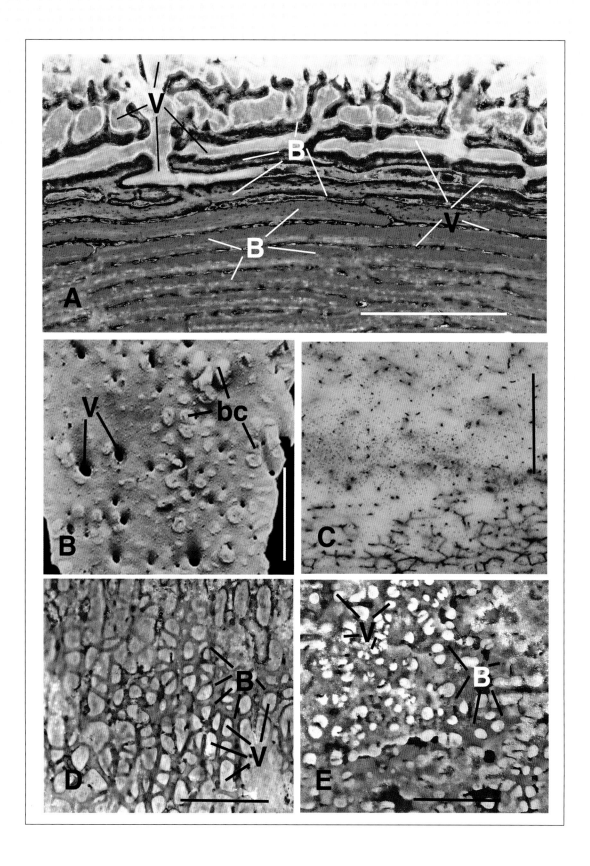

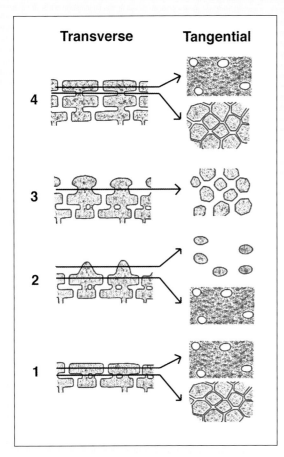

| **Transverse** | **Tangential** |

4

3

2

1

Figure 4.8. Laminar bone formation—interpretation. Transverse and tangential profiles explain the images in Figure 4.7. The surface of the bone compartment (1) bulges out (2, 3) to enclose a new vascular layer that becomes increasingly reticular by enlargement of the bone compartment (4).

If bone growth only involved the addition of new bone at the surface as described above, then old bones would be almost solid rods. In fact, young bones can easily fit within the hollow core of the old ones that they become. At the same time as growth in a bone cylinder occurs by deposition on the outside, osteons and laminae are eroded on the inside. Growth requires continuous destruction as well as deposition (72, 85, 86) (Figure 4.10). Erosion at the endosteal surface until the new diameter is reached is a prerequisite for growth (Figure 4.10 E). This erosion is not just an orderly reversal of deposition. It may follow a different path, often at an angle to the previous plane of deposition, allowing the juvenile form of a bone to be reshaped into

that of an adult (Figure 4.10 G). The complex shapes of adult bones are thus the result of equally complicated interplays of deposition and destruction, allowing for a change in shape from that mandated by the original periosteal deposition.

Whatever the erosion and secondary bone development, the end result is that the mature endosteal surface is covered by a smooth layer of laminar bone (Figure 4.10 F) or an irregular development of spongy bone (see spongy bone Figure 4.16).

Osteonic bone

Primary osteonic bone, like laminar bone, is the first formed bone either in development or in repair. Mature buffalo and cows have leg bones made from a mixture of laminae and osteons, a structure appropriate for the axial compression received from their massive body weights. Other grazers, such as deer and even young fawns, are fast moving and lighter bodied, requiring their limb bones to have extra resistance to bending and shear. From the beginning of development, their leg bones are bundles of primary osteons with a very precise arrangement (Figures 4.11, 13).

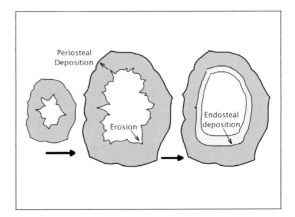

Figure 4.9. Long bones increase in diameter by deposition on the outside. Erosion on the inside maintains the economical cylindrical form.

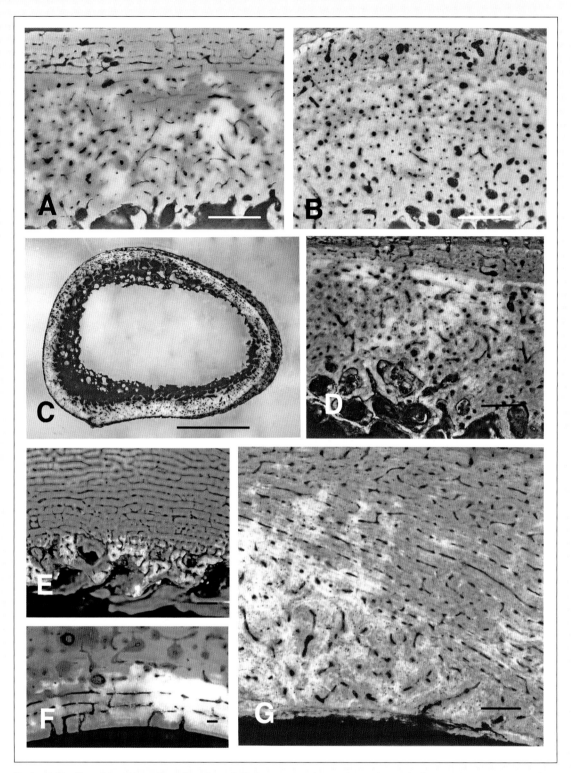

Figure 4.10. Growth at the endosteal surface. A–E, formation of irregular surfaces. A, C. Irregular endosteal surfaces with thinning of the shaft due to erosion and osteoporosis. Laminar bone is first replaced by osteons. B. Osteons are replaced by cavities in osteoporosis. D. Erosion at the inner face together with the beginnings of osteon decay. Transverse profiles of the right femur of an elderly woman. E. The endosteal surface of long bones may also be irregular due to the erosion needed to change shape in normal development. Transverse profile of a young cow bone. F, G. Completed mature surfaces may be smooth with several layers of laminar bone or irregular due to the development of spongy bone (see Figure 4.16). F. The eroded endosteal surface of a mature bone may be re-covered with laminar bone as in this transverse profile of a three-year-old buffalo femur. G. Shape change may require the plane of deposition to change as in this transverse profile of a lamb bone where new laminae are at an angle to those deposited earlier. Silver stained. C. Scale bar = 1cm, F. = 100 mm, others = 1mm.

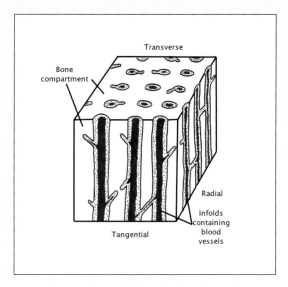

Figure 4.11. Osteonic bone consists of cylinders of calcified collagen lamellae around columns of blood vessels, nerves, and connective tissue as in Figure 4.1 A.

Primary osteonic bone, like laminar bone, arises from outgrowths of the bone compartment at the surface. In the formation of primary osteons the outgrowths of the bone compartment enclose axial folds that form osteons in the furrows between them (Figures 4.12, 13).

Much osteonic bone is secondary, formed as a replacement of both laminar and primary osteons. Bone loss is of two kinds, erosion at the endosteal surface discussed above, and resorption below the surface around laminar and osteonic blood vessels, with or without redeposition. Erosion of the reticular spaces in laminar bone allows for replacement by secondary osteons. Laminar bone may be a suitable compromise between the competing needs for growth and structural stability in a rapidly growing animal, but be unsatisfactory for the mechanical and circulatory properties required by mature bones. Osteons contain blood vessels of greater diameter than the capillaries of the reticular system that they replace. The evolution and development of secondary osteons may have two consequences. 1. The introduction of a mechanism for the local turnover of bone components without compromising the loss of strength that would occur from more generalized erosion of laminar bone, and 2. A change in mechanical properties, resistance to compression shifting to toughness in relation to torsion and bending.

Primary laminar bone rarely remains as the only component of long bones, often being replaced by secondary osteons that act as longitudinal reinforcing columns. Profiles of a human femur show an inner layer of osteonic bone surrounded by more recently deposited laminar bone (Figure 4.10 A), but even these laminae have been changed to osteons in many places (Figure 4.10 B). Lamellar sheets are replaced by stacks of cylinders that retain the lamellar spacing.

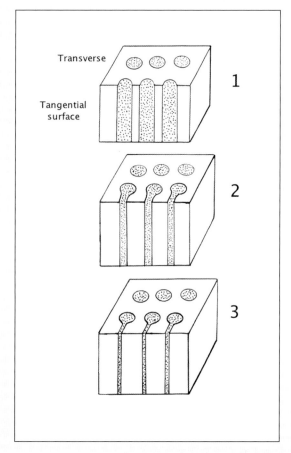

Figure 4.12. Primary osteons form as cylinders between longitudinal folds growing out from the surface. These tend to be in regular arrays and lack the boundary membranes present in secondary osteons.

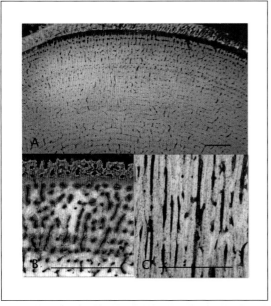

Figure 4.13. Primary Osteon formation. Longitudinal folds form at the surface of the bone compartment below the periosteum. The bundles of osteons created in this way have a regular arrangement, unlike secondary osteons that may also be overdispersed but have an irregular distribution. A. Transverse profile of a deer cannon bone formed mainly from primary osteons. B. The surface in A showing the longitudinal folds in transverse profile. C. The longitudinal arrangement of primary osteons in a tangential profile of the bone in A and B. Scale bar = 1mm.

Secondary osteons form in laminar bone by erosion of the lamellar sheets of reticular vascular spaces to make straighter longitudinal channels around which new cylindrical lamellae are deposited (Figure 4.14). The end result is that flat sheets of lamellae composing the laminar bone are replaced by cylindrical lamellae around the newly enlarged cylindrical space. New osteons at first line up with the capillaries in the reticular network that they replace, but as they mature they lose their exact parallel orientation with the original laminae in a competition for space between osteons. Development of new osteons is asynchronous. In addition to eroding laminar capillaries, late forming osteons may erode those formed earlier, creating several generations of osteons. The method of formation of secondary osteons leaves them with a distinctive difference from primary osteons. They are enclosed in a "cement layer," marking the boundary with the original laminar bone within which primary bone has been eroded and new bone deposited (Figure 4.14 K)(84).

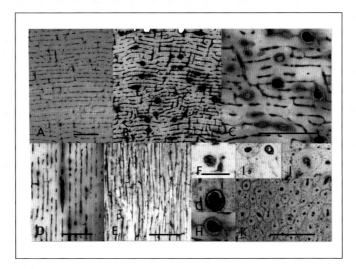

Figure 4.14. Secondary osteons form in laminar bone by erosion of the lamellar sheets of vascular spaces to make straighter longitudinal channels followed by deposition of new cylindrical lamellae. A. The laminar structure of a mature cow femur before replacement by secondary osteons. Silver stained transverse profile. B, Secondary osteons begin to replace laminar bone in a three-year-old buffalo femur. C, D. New osteons line up with capillaries from the reticular network that they replace. C. Transverse profile. D. Radial profile. Silver stained. E. Mature secondary osteons lose their exact parallel orientation with the original laminae. Radial profile of ink infiltrated giraffe fibula. F–J. The sequence from capillaries in a network sheet to secondary osteons. F. The capillary space stains intensely as the surrounding bone begins to erodes. G. The space enlarges. H. The flat sheets of lamellae composing the laminar bone are replaced by cylindrical lamellae around the newly enlarged cylindrical space. I. Development of new osteons is asynchronous. Even new osteons next to one another may be at different stages of development. J. Fully formed secondary osteon. K. Secondary osteons differ from primary osteons in being enclosed in a "cement layer" marking the boundary with the original laminar bone. Transverse profile of a giraffe fibula. Ink infiltrated. Scale bars 100mm, F–J 200mm.

Spongy Bone

Structure

Spongy bone is a structural compromise between the need for strength and economy of material. Thin walls outline spaces that can function like bone marrow (Figure 4.15). The wall thicknesses and shapes of the spaces alter in response to stresses present during development. The results vary from a roughly symmetrical foam-like appearance to sheaves of spicules.

Formation and growth in bone length

The ends (epiphyses) of bones are at first made from cartilage separated by a circular transverse bone plate (the epiphyseal plate) from the laminar bone of the shaft. Growth of these plates pushes them further apart as the bone lengthens. The plates form spongy bone (endochondral ossification) that is replaced by compact bone on the outside and marrow on the inside. In the final stages, spongy bone fills the ends of the shaft (Figure 4.15). During endochondral ossification, the cartilage at first lacks blood vessels. These penetrate from the surface into the future bone marrow.

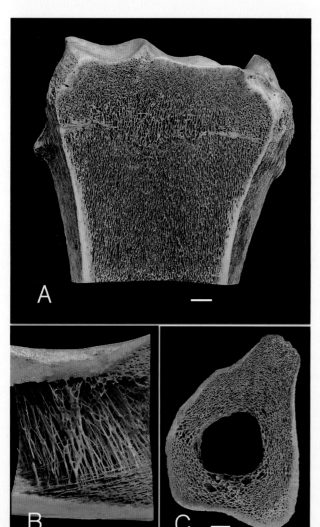

Figure 4.15. A. The ends of long bones may be made entirely of spongy bone. Longitudinal profile of giraffe radius. B. Longitudinal and transverse profiles near the ends of a cow radius. Scale bars = 1cm.

Summary of Bone Structure

In summary, three kinds of bone can be distinguished by their fiber orientation and differing vascularization, but there are many intermediates (Figure 4.16). Bone vascular systems lead either to capillary network sheets or to the relatively long straight vessels in osteons. Figure 4.2 represents the generalized structure of the shaft of most adult mammalian femora. The structure of bone is a compromise between limitations imposed by the dynamic need for deposition and resorption on the one hand, and particular mechanical properties on the other, creating an exercise in different ways that calcified collagen filaments can be assembled while remaining part of the body metabolic pool.

A purpose of this chapter has been to ensure that corrections are made in teaching the histology of bone structure. The technique of polishing a bone and showing the shape of its vascular compartments is simple enough for anyone to determine that its structure is not that described in most textbooks and many research publications. Anyone trying this for themselves will learn that primary observations are more reliable than textbook dogma.

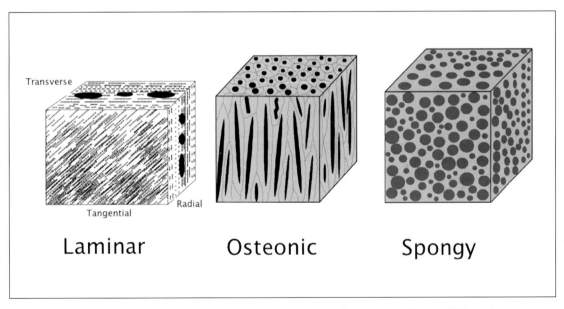

Figure 4.16. The three main categories of bone structure are Laminar, Osteonic, and Spongy. All have the same fine structure of lamellae of calcified collagen fibers. In Laminar bone the lamellar layers change in orientation to create a plywood-like structure. In Osteonic bone, this plywood structure is cylindrical. The cylinders are not exactly parallel to the long axis, reducing planes of weakness along which cracks might propagate. Lamellae in Spongy bone enclose spaces of varying shape and size increasing the ratio of strength to weight.

Chapter 5
Antler

External Bone

The preyful princess pierc'd and prick'd a pretty pleasing pricket.

William Shakespeare
Loves Labours Lost IV II 58

Some say a sore: but not a sore, till now made sore with shooting.

Ibid. 59
Pricket = two-year-old buck,
sore = four-year-old buck.

Introduction

Several features of antlers make them a commodity important both in the past and present. Antler is not harder than bone, for it is bone, but the arrangement of lamellae make parts of it tougher, and therefore much sought after for all the more robust applications for which bone might have been used. Bone was good enough for the city, country living required antler. Dinner knives had bone handles, but those for the farrier, for hunting, butchering, and carving were made of antler. In the late twentieth and twenty-first centuries, there has been a revival of craftsmanship by artisans creating knife handles and sticks for country walking, both old crafts having a contemporary resurgence. Craftsmen are helped in their preferred choice of material because the deer that make antlers discard them every year. They can be picked up in the wild or cropped annually in domesticated herds without damage to their owners. The value of venison and of velvet (growing) antlers in Oriental folklore medicine has led to many species being domesticated. There is also an industry devoted to maintaining deer for hunting with antlers as prized trophies. Antlers are now a cash crop. All these features make antlers of interest and value.

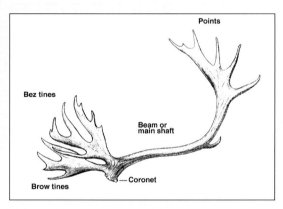

Figure 5.1. The main features of an antler illustrated by the left antler of a male Woodland Caribou (*Rangifer arcticus*). They only occur in males (except in *Rangifer* where females have smaller versions). The lower tines, called the brow, bez, and sometimes a third one called the trez or royal, project forward to protect the head. The beam points up and back, terminating in a crown of surroyals with as many as sixty-two points in some extinct deer. Points branching above the trez are "points on top." In Red Deer more than twelve points constitutes a "Royal," and more than fourteen, a "Wilson" (117). Park reared deer may have many more points. The head is bent down to point the crown forwards in use, mainly for sexual competition between stags and to control hinds. They are not for offense in general but may be used against dogs.

Species	Distribution	Record Antler Size[1]		
		Length on outside curve in cms	Distance from tip to tip in cms	Number of points [2]
Caribou, (*Rangifer arcticus*)	Northern Canada	158	102	21 + 17
Chital, (*Axis axis*)	India	98	50	3 + 3
Elk or Wapiti (*Cervus canadensis*)[3].	Northern America	178	105	6 + 6
Fallow Deer, (*Dama dama*),	Europe and Asia Minor	81	46	12 + 10
Hog Deer (*Hyelaphus porcinus*)	India	59	33	3 + 3
Irish Elk, (Cervus giganteus)	Formerly Europe, now extinct		381	7 + 7
Moose, (*Alces americana*)[4]	North America, Northern Europe and Russia	124	114	40
Mule Deer, (*Odocoileus hemionus*)	Mexico to British Columbia	81	66	21 + 19
Muntjac, (*Cervulus muntjac*)	India to Indonesia	24	13	2 + 2
Pere David's Deer, (*Elaphurus davidianus*)	Originally from China, now only in parks	84	35	8 + 8
Red Deer, (*Cervus elephas*)	Europe	104	57	7 + 7
Reindeer, (*Rangifer tarandus*)[5].	Northern Europe and Northern Asia	151	97	15 + 16
Roe deer, (*Capreolus capreolus*)	Northern Europe and Northern Asia,	33	25	3 + 3
Sambar (*Rusa unicolor*)	India and South East Asia	127	61	3 + 3
Sika, (*Cervus nippon*)	China, Japan	65	44	4 + 4
Swamp deer, (*Rucervus duvauceli*)	India	104	90	8 + 5
White tailed Deer, (*Odocoileus virginianus*),	North America	70	37	6 + 6

[1] Deer reared in Parks may have larger antlers than those from the wild.

[2] Some deer have more points than those of record size.

[3] The American Elk or Wapiti is the North American equivalent of the Red Deer to which it is closely related.

[4] The European Elk, *Alces alces*, should not be confused with the American Elk or Wapiti, *Cervus canadensis*.

[5] Reindeer are domesticated Caribou, probably not a separate species.

Table 5.1. Record sizes of antlers from the most common deer in the wild and their distribution in the world. (Resources 20, 135). Antlers from game parks frequently exceed these records.

There are about thirty-four different species and many subspecies of deer occurring on all continents, except Australia and Africa south of the Sahara. They are mammals belonging to the Order Artiodactyla (pigs, camels, antelopes, giraffes, cattle); Sub-order Ruminantia (they have chambered stomachs allowing them to chew the cud, giving their teeth a second chance at cutting up their dinner); Family Cervidae or Deer. Antlers are the characteristic feature of male deer known as bucks or harts (Figure 5.1). Female deer are hinds or does.

Unlike bone, the structure of antlers is not limited by the need for resorption, only by the problems of growth "outside" the body. They grow from the frontal bone of the skull only in males (except in Reindeer where females also have antlers) and are shed each year at the end of the rutting season. In an uncharacteristic lack of economy, Nature has allowed the raw materials used in their construction to be wasted by this annual shedding. In Red Deer, for example, 4–5 months of growth may make 7–10 KG [8–22 lbs] of antler that only has 4–5 weeks of use defending the harem before being shed. The disadvantage of carrying these unwieldy instruments throughout life outweighs the loss of material from annual shedding.

The pattern of branching in antlers varies within species and even from side-to-side. For trophy records, their size is measured along the outside curve together with the number of tines or points where the branches end. They are absent in Musk Deer (*Moschus moschiferus*). In Tufted Deer (*Elaphodus cephalophus*) they are small spikes and in Muntjacs (*Muntiacus sp.*) they are limited to two-tines. In most deer they are much larger with up to sixty tines. Their distribution,

record sizes, and shapes of their antlers are summarized in Table 5.1 and Figure 5.2. Antlers of Red Deer, Elk, Caribou, White tailed deer, Reindeer, and Moose are those most commonly used in antiquity and in more recent industry and crafts. Except in Reindeer, castration prevents antler renewal. Reindeer and Caribou also differ from all other deer in that their hinds bear antlers, although much smaller ones. Buck reindeer shed their antlers before the does, mostly before Christmas, raising the probability that Rudolph, Donner, Blitzen, and his buddies were probably Delphina, Donna, Belinda, and *their* friends.

Antler is tougher than bone. The annual joustings between stags has placed a premium on the evolution of large sturdy antlers that can be battered without cracking. The shape of multiple forked prongs allows a stag to tangle with his rival in a demonstration of strength. The object in these duels is to "lock horns" and cause the assailant to back away or fall. Three features characterize antlers: annual growth on pedicles, design of the forks, and the structure that determines the properties of the material.

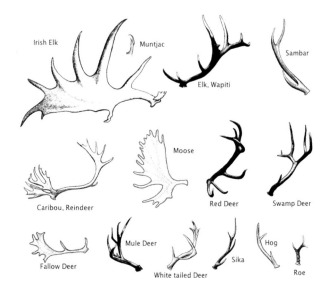

Figure 5.2. Antler shapes in some well known deer species, see Table 5.1. In Reindeer, Caribou, Irish Elk, and especially in Moose, the beam is flattened, palmate, like a hand with tines for the fingers. Redrawn from several sources and specimens approximately to scale. For more detailed accounts, see (43).

Growth on Pedicles, attachments to the skull

Antlers grow each year from pedicles, projections on the skull that are continuations of the frontal bone (Figure 5.3 A). A growth zone covered by skin with characteristic coarse hair inappropriately known as velvet lies at the tip of the pedicle (Figure 5.3 B, C). The size of these velvet knobs and the antlers that come from them increases each year as the deer mature. By the end of their first year the bone below the velvet of male red deer grows into a knob (70). These young stags are then known as "knobbers" (Figure 5.4). At the end of the second year, the knobs have become spikes that by the third year have two points each. A point is added in each subsequent year so that by six years a stag may be a full-grown six pointer, and by twelve years can be in his prime with a royal crown. Even in the largest antlers, growth only takes 4–5 months (117). Once the antler has reached full size, its peripheral blood supply is cut off, the stags rub off the remnants of the dried out velvet, leaving a clean, hard, bony surface ready for use in a rutting period lasting only a few weeks (5 in red deer). At this stage, the connection between antler and frontal skull bone is continuous, with little or no structural divide between antler and bone (Figure 5.3 E, F). After the rut in the spring, the antlers are shed, breaking between the coronet (Figure 5.3 G) and the frontal bone. This is not at a preexisting weak point, for the mature antler has continuous tough bone all the way from the thickened frontal bone through the beam (Figure 5.3 F). The break results from localized activation of osteoclasts that weaken a front in a characteristic rugose pattern below the coronet. Skin migrates in to create a new velvet surface from which the antler develops in the following year (71).

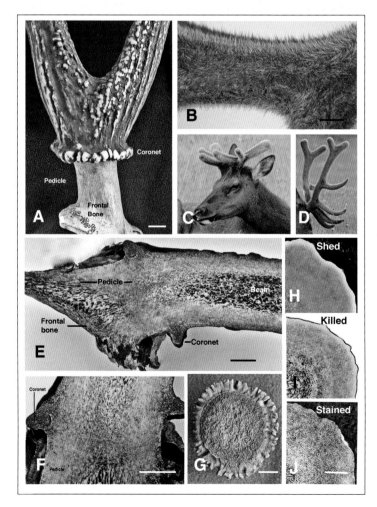

Figure 5.3. Antlers grow on pedicles, extensions from the frontal bone of the skull. A. The Pedicle is an extension of the frontal bone of the skull. The antler begins at the coronet. Not all deer have such a long pedicle as this Sambar buck. B. Velvet covered antlers growing out from the coronet in a white tailed deer buck in June. C. The early velvet covered antlers of an elk buck in June. D. Some blood remains in mature antlers before being shed. Very little blood remains after shedding, although staining shows the vascular compartments. Transverse profiles of shed, killed, and stained antler beam from white tailed deer. E, F. The bone is continuous from the antler to the frontal bone in a mature white tailed deer stag. G. A weak layer below the coronet develops at the end of the rutting season, allowing the antler to be shed. Basal surface of a shed white tailed deer antler.

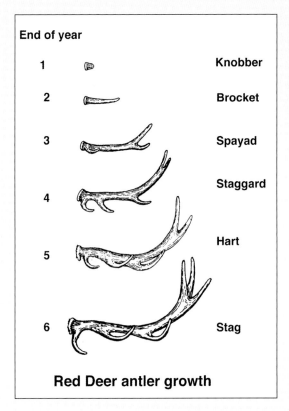

1   Knobber

2   Brocket

3   Spayad

4   Staggard

5   Hart

6   Stag

Red Deer antler growth

Figure 5.4. Antler growth in red deer. By the end of the first year, male deer are known as knobbers and have grown a pair of knobs from which the antlers arise in future years (20). After the first year, the antlers are shed and regrown every year.

Design of the Forks

Although antlers may seem to be like horns—both are just skeletal projections from the head—they are in fact quite different in their design and principles of development (126). Horns are axial rods limited in their growth by their cylindrical horn covering (see Chapters 3 and 7), whereas antlers are outspread surfaces limited only by the way that bone grows. At first glance, the flattened palmate racks (the collection of tines emerging from the beam constituting a whole paired set of antlers) of moose, Irish elk, fallow deer, and caribou seem to have little in common with the cylindrical structures creating three-dimensional racks in wapiti, red, white tailed, and other deer, but the difference can be reconciled in the following way. Deer have evolved antlers to

intimidate their opponents by tangling with them in head-on confrontations. There are two parts to the structure of their racks, short forward projections to protect the head from the opponent's antlers (except for sambar that bravely fight without head protectors) and long upwardly directed beams with tines to reach the opponent when the head is bent. Thinner and more fragile tines can be used when they are supported laterally as part of a surface. This gives tines on palmate antlers the advantage of support but tends to limit their position in space to one plane. To claim more space by becoming three-dimensional space fillers requires the crown of tines to separate from their lateral supports by extending out from the beam. This makes a more formidable armament, but at the expense of requiring more material. Figure 5.5 shows the relation between palmate and three-dimensional tined antlers and how those of a red deer might be derived from a palmate form. Moose themselves have both palmate and separately tined forms. Occasional moose like the "Monster of Matane," from Quebec in 2012, have more than sixty tines, rather than sixteen to twenty-eight. The developmental biology of antler patterning, the mechanism determining branching and extent of growth, has yet to be attempted. Goss (47) commented, "... the rewards for studying antlers are that practically everything that one finds out about

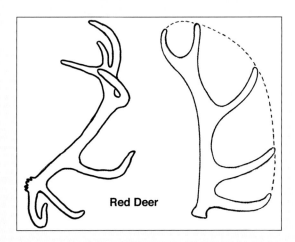

Red Deer

Figure 5.5. The three-dimensional array of tines (the rack) presented by the head of a deer can be derived from a flattened structure on a curved surface.

them is a new discovery (114)." I have found this statement to be true at every turn when trying to present a simplified account of antler structure.

Structure and Development

Overview

The structure of antlers is instructive in that the categories that conveniently describe bone—laminar, osteonic, and spongy—often overlap with one another, reinforcing the unifying description of bone as a compartment containing calcified collagen lamellae, the form of which is determined by the distortion of the compartment by the vascular pattern. Antler bone is primary bone, not exactly like laminae, osteons, or spongy skeletal bone or that resulting from endochondral ossification, but more like wound healing in having elements of each (70). Studies of the way that antlers grow help to understand these differences. Antler growth is like that for primary bone but from a stump rather than a flat surface. Growth occurs in a rounded end zone at the tip of the beam and at the tips of the tines as these arise (Figure 5.6).

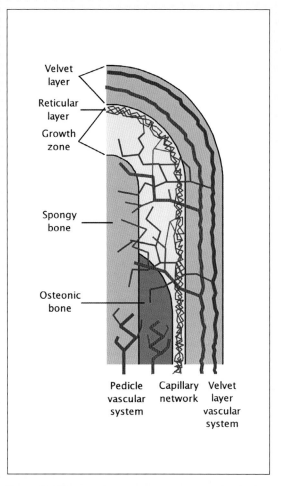

Figure 5.7. The vascular system in a growing antler. Antlers have two blood supplies. The blood vessels most important in growth come from the outside but penetrate to the core before supplying the superficial layers. Arteries from the velvet layer branch to arterioles supplying the interior osteons and spongy bone as well as the superficial capillary network contained in a reticular vascular compartment like that of laminar bone. This system is lost when the velvet layer is destroyed at maturity. The second system through the pedicle keeps the core of the antler hydrated enough to maintain its physical properties until shedding (114). Simplified after (133).

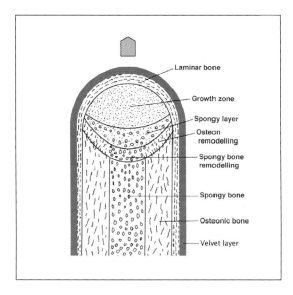

Figure 5.6. The width of a zone at the tip determines the diameter of an antler while its length depends on the distance that it has moved from the pedicle. The outer layer below the velvet resembles laminar bone with its reticular infolds containing capillary networks. Spongy and osteonic bone arise from the growth zone like regions of endochondral ossification at the ends of long bones. Spongy and osteonic bone are then progressively remodeled along the length of the antler similarly to growth in long bones.

Antler diameter is determined by the width of this growth zone, which enlarges from year to year. The base of the antler forms first, with the width beneath the growth zone remaining about the same as it moves away from the pedicle, tapering off slowly towards the points. Material for growth is transported to and from the zone by arteries and veins passing through the pedicle to the core and especially superficially in the velvet layer. As the antlers lengthen, the blood supply through the velvet layer becomes increasingly important until growth is complete. It then dies and is rubbed off with the velvet layer, leaving naked bone. This led to the view that the mature antler is dead, like the velvet layer above it. However, fallow deer antlers keep a functional vascular system with live bone cells incorporating calcium markers that allow bone remodeling long after velvet shedding (114). Antlers from killed stags can be recognized by the blood remaining in some of their blood vessels compared with the blank whiteness of shed antlers (Figure 5.3 D). The explanation is that antlers have a duplicate blood system (Figure 5.7). The blood vessels most important in growth lie superficially in the velvet layer from where they supply the interior osteons and spongy bone as well as the superficial capillary network in a reticular vascular compartment resembling laminar bone. This system is lost at maturity when the velvet layer is destroyed. The blood supply is reduced, but not entirely cut off, since the second system through the pedicle prevents desiccation and allows continued bone construction. Newly shed fallow deer antlers bleed profusely from cut branches (114). The survival of the blood supply up to and even past shedding allows antlers to remain hydrated when they are most functional, preserving their toughness and preventing them from becoming brittle (114, 133).

Structure

In general the structure resembles that of some long bones, but differs in characteristic details such as the three regions merging gradually rather than abruptly (see Table 5.2 and Figures 5.14–16). Most studies have focused on vascularization because the distribution of blood vessels makes it easy to recognize the structural form of the bone (Figure 5.9 K, L), but bone does not arise primarily around blood vessels. Bone is deposited in a compartment shaped by intruding reticular or tubular vascular spaces that blood vessels come to occupy.

The basic structure is shown in Figure 5.8. Below the shed velvet there is a shell of layers of reticular vascular spaces resembling laminar bone, characterized by its evenly spaced layers, but more intertwined and felt-like than the equivalent layer in long bones (Figure 5.9 A–D). This merges with the cortex of osteonic bone that is the main structural support of the antler (Figure 5.9 E–G). The cortical network of osteons is characterized by varied diameter, branching, and lack of precise longitudinal alignment unlike the parallel arrays of internal bones. This felt-like three-dimensional array of irregular cortical osteons merges into a core of spongy bone characterized by thick walls that tend not to be calcified (Figure 5.9 H–J). The walls are often so thick that they restrict the vascular spaces to narrow channels.

Variations on this general description of antler structure are described in Figure 5.10 for white tailed deer, Figure 5.11 for moose, Figure 5.12 for caribou and Figure 5.13 for elk.

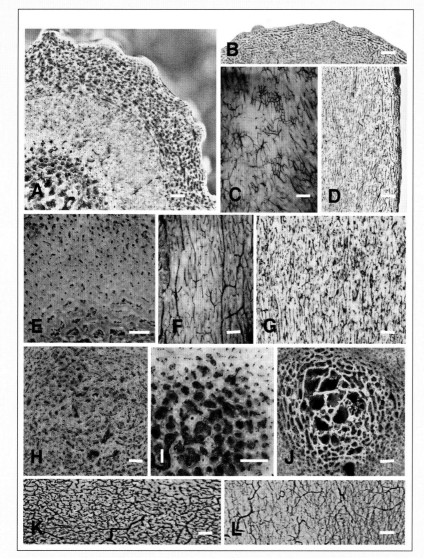

Figure 5.9. Antler structure. A. The three bone regions. The outer shell resembles laminar bone. It blends into a cortex of branched osteons that merges with a spongy bone core. Transverse profile of young white tailed deer beam. B. Transverse, C. Tangential, and D. Radial profiles of the laminar bone at the surface. In most antlers it is a narrower shell than in A. It has a coarser and less regular pattern than its counterpart in long bones, lacking the precise arrangement of laminae. E. Transverse, F. Tangential, and G. Radial profiles of the cortex. Osteons in the cortex range from thick-walled to narrow, with varied orientations, branching and lumen size. H., I., and J., Transverse profiles of the spongy core, with thick walls and varied spacing. These thick walls of spongy bone are less calcified than their counterparts in long bones and the osteons of the cortex around them. K. Transverse and L. Radial profiles showing blood vessels in the core with more tangled branching systems than in long bones as the vascular compartments suggest. The vascular compartments in A–J have been contrasted with black ink. Natural blood show the blood vessel pattern in K and L. B is from a moose antler, all others are white tailed deer. Scale bars = 1mm.

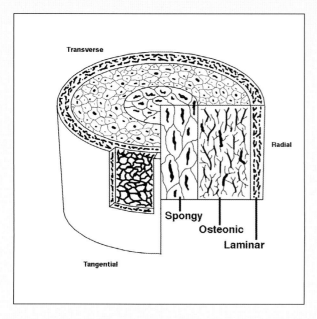

Figure 5.8. The general structure of antler bone interpreting the illustrations in Figure 5.9. During growth, the antlers are enclosed by a richly vascularized skin, the velvet layer. Below this, the bone is organized in three regions. On the outside, there is a shell of laminar bone recognized by the evenly spaced layers. Their reticular vascular spaces are more intertwined than the equivalent layer in long bones. These merge into a cortical network of osteons, characterized by their varied diameter, branching and lack of precise longitudinal alignment (Figure 5.9 F). The core is occupied by thick-walled spongy bone that is often uncalcified or only weakly calcified. The walls are often so thick that they restrict the central vascular compartment to a narrow channel. The layers merge with one another through intermediate structures more than is indicated in the diagram. There are many variations of this generalized structure.

Differences Between Bone and Antler

Bones are multifunctional and use their core for lipid storage and blood cell formation. Antlers have a single function—to resist the stresses imposed by opposing antlers. The structural differences between bone and antler reflect these different functions. Antler, like bone, has laminar, osteonic, and spongy structure. Although bones and antlers themselves vary greatly in structure, there are some general differences between them. Differences are summarized in Table 5.2 and Figures 5.14–16.

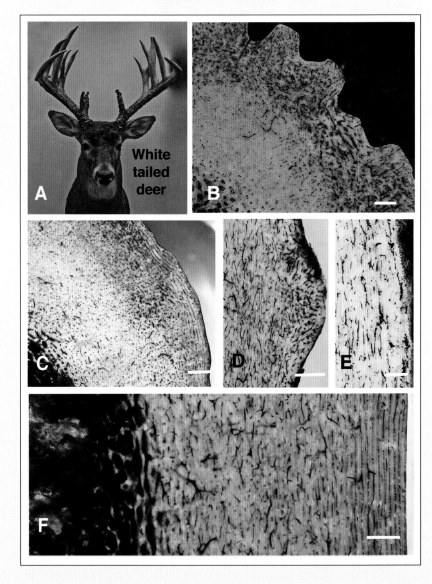

Figure 5.10. A. White tailed deer antler consists of a beam bearing forwardly projecting brow tines protecting the head and up to six crown tines. B. The beam has an outer shell of irregular laminae made more irregular by the surface granulation, a cortex of thick-walled osteons, and a core of thick-walled spongy bone. Transverse profile. C. Laminae of the outer shell become less regular as they merge with the osteons of the cortex. Oblique radial/tangential profile. D. The regularity of the laminar layer is interrupted by the surface granulation. Radial profile. E. Laminae of the shell are reduced to one or two layers in tines. Tangential/radial profile of a tine. F. The three layers differ in the size of their osteons. The shell has a few narrow parallel laminae. Osteons of the cortex are branched with thick walls but fine narrow blood vessels. The spongy core has even thicker walls, wider vascular spaces, and irregular orientation. Radial profile of a beam lacking rugosities and peripheral to B. Vascular compartments contrasted with black ink. Scale bars = 1mm.

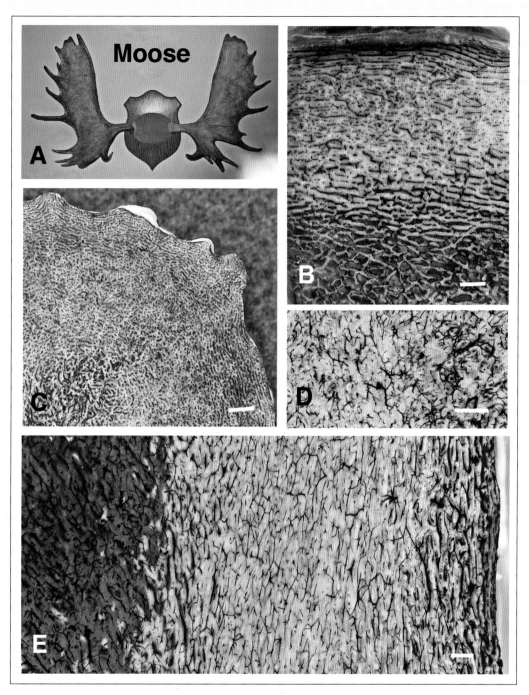

Figure 5.11. A. Moose typically have palmate antlers with tines supported on a flattened beam but some (strains or sub-species) have antlers with free tines. All regions have the typical layers—laminar shell, cortex of osteons, and spongy core. B. In palmate regions the laminar shell and cortex surround a wide core of thick-walled spongy bone. Transverse profile. C. The beam at the base is the densest of any antler, with thick walls around narrow vascular compartments in the laminar shell and cortical osteons. The spongy core has even been reduced by the thickened walls of the vascular spaces. Transverse profile of the beam below the palmate region. D. In the laminar shell and especially the cortex, the vascular spaces form a fine three-dimensional network. Tangential profile in a region near C. E. The core is much less calcified than the cortex. Glycerol infiltration leaves the core translucent while increasing the whiteness of the calcified regions. Radial profile of a beam peripheral to C. Vascular compartments contrasted with black ink. Scale bars = 1mm.

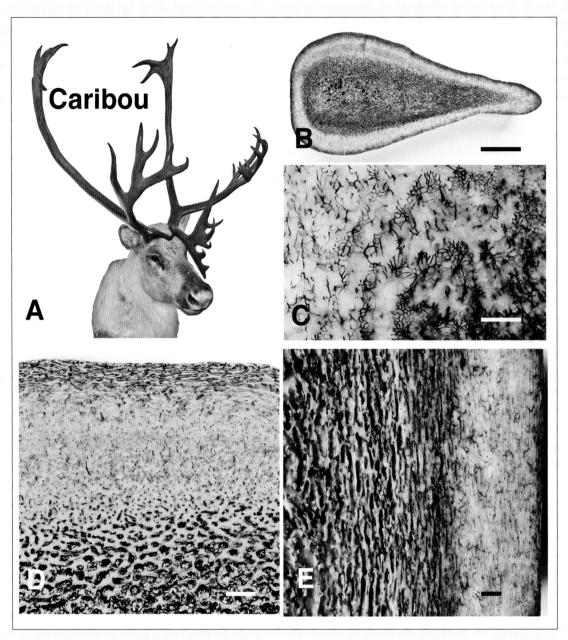

Figure 5.12. A. Caribou antlers share features with elk in that the cortex of osteons does not increase proportionally with the size of the antler. Their large antlers use more spongy bone to fill the central cavity, allowing lightness even with their length and size. Like moose, their beams are strengthened by flattening. B. The spongy core is wide relative to the shell and cortex. Transverse profile of a main beam. C. Tangential profile at the beam surface showing the very finely branched reticulum of the shell. D. Transverse profiles show the three layers—shell, cortex, and core. The reticulum of the shell consists of only a few interconnecting layers that merge fairly abruptly with the narrow branched longitudinal vascular spaces typical of calcified osteons in the cortex. The almost invisible osteons of the white cortical bone enlarge to form the spongy bone of the core. Transverse profile of the beam. E. Radial profile of the beam shows the three layers. Vascular compartments contrasted with black ink. Scales, B = 1cm, C–E = 1mm.

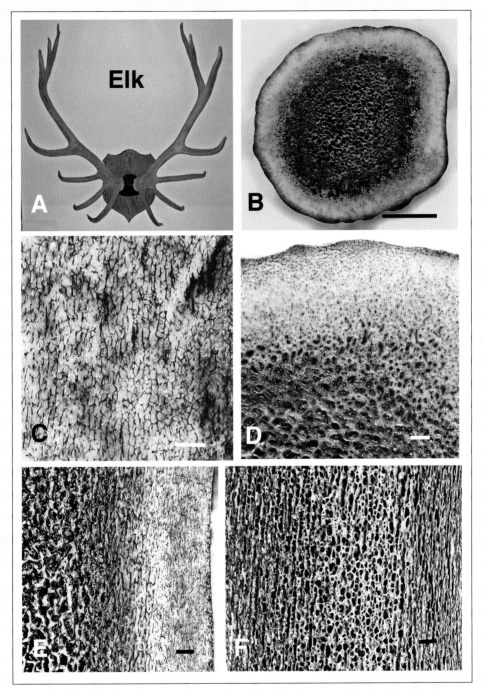

Figure 5.13. A. Elk antlers are among the largest, but their weight is not proportional to their size. Large antlers are not just scaled up versions of small ones. They remain relatively light, their greater thickness coming from a wider spongy core. B. The shell has a very fine reticulum of vascular infolds branching in three dimensions not in layers like laminar bone. Tangential profile at the surface of a beam. C. The cortex remains about the same thickness throughout the antler, the extra width coming from the increased spongy core. Transverse profile of a beam. D. Osteons of the cortex are mainly axial with a fine connecting meshwork forming a three-dimensional felt. Radial profile of a beam. E. Spaces in the core of spongy bone extend axially and are thinner and more calcified than in most other deer, more like that in long bones. Radial profile of the core of a beam. Vascular compartments contrasted with black ink. Scales, B = 1cm, C–F = 1mm.

Differences between bone and antler

	Bone	Antler
Outer surface	Smooth	Often rugose
Shell	1. Laminar bone of thin parallel sheets and few lamellae separated by reticular vascular spaces. Often form the whole thickness of the bone until replaced by secondary osteons. Few connections between laminae. 2. Primary osteons.	Few irregular laminae with wide lamellae and many connections between them form a felt-like meshwork merging with primary cortical osteons.
Cortex	1.Large secondary osteons with wide vascular spaces, some branching, mainly parallel to the axis with relics of laminae. With cement layers. 2. Primary osteons parallel to the axis.	All sizes of primary osteons not exactly aligned to the axis, many fine branches and almost occluded vascular spaces. No cement layers.
Inner surface	Smooth around marrow in long bones except at the ends. Spongy filling in bones such as ribs and digits.	Always filled with spongy bone, never smooth as in long bones.
Core	Marrow in long bones, spongy in others	Spongy bone
Core spongy bone	Thin calcified walls with large spaces and sometimes chambers and spicules oriented in response to stress.	Thick walled less calcified, often occluding chambers that tend to be symmetrical. Old specimens more likely to disintegrate.
General - colour	Opaque white due to even calcification	Sometimes yellow to brown with mottled tangential surface due to uneven calcification. Non-calcified spongy bone walls often translucent.

Table 5.2. Differences in structure between internal bone and antler. (See Figures 5.14, 15, 16). The most consistent difference is in the abrupt border between the cortex and core in internal bones compared with the gradual transition in antlers.

Unlike internal bone, antlers have to contend with extreme outside environments at their surface. In response, they have evolved a shell structured to resist surface cracking. The surface layers consist of bone lamellae around a reticular network of vascular spaces creating a skin with roughly uniform properties in the plane of the surface. It resembles laminar bone, but has more connections between layers, making it more like felt than stacks of laminae. The shell merges gradually with the cortex of osteons.

The structure of the cortex reflects the main function of antlers—to resist the stresses imposed by opposing antlers. Although there has been no statistical analysis of the shapes and sizes of osteons in antlers and bones, some general differences can be correlated with function. Bones tend to be built to resist stresses in particular directions and their osteon and spongy bone orientations reflect this (146). Antlers are built to resist torsion and bending in many different directions (23). The orientation of their osteons reflects this, being irregular, not in parallel array like the primary osteons of deer bone (Figure 4. 12). Osteonic bone consists of any branched or unbranched collection of cylindrical collagen lamellae surrounding tubular vascular spaces containing blood vessels. Osteons vary in diameter, thickness, and orientation. It has been claimed that typical osteons of antler are smaller than those of bone (100). This is partly true in that antlers have more branched vascular spaces and osteons. Whatever the size of antler osteons, their walls are frequently so wide that they almost obliterate the central vascular space. Internal bone is more often secondary, derived by erosion from laminar bone, and is coarser, straighter, and with wider vascular spaces.

The main shaft of a long bone has a core lacking structural components. The smooth surface on its inner face distinguishes it from antler. Spongy bone at the ends of such bones and in ribs, digits, and skull bones is easily distinguishable from antlers by their abrupt transition from the cortical structure.

In antlers, the gradual transition from the cortex to the core comes closest to being a key distinguishing feature. Other differences are the thin walls often oriented in spicules compared to antlers, where the spongy core tends to be thick-walled, even occluded, less calcified, and not oriented. Large antlers, such as those from elk, have a spongy core like that from long bones, but there is always a gradual transition from osteons of the cortex. If translucency rather than white opacity is an indication of lack of calcification, then antlers are less calcified than bone. Calcification in bone tends to be in layers, while that in antlers is often mottled. This is particularly obvious in immature antlers, which may appear translucent throughout. Lowered calcification may make an antler more elastic and less brittle, as well as being a calcium conservation measure.

Many of the structural differences can be traced to differences in development. Long bones grow in length at their ends but increase their diameter by progressive deposition of layers in the circumference. Each year antlers only grow in length from a base diameter that they increase in increments annually. The abrupt change from osteonic to spongy bone in the core of long bones is easily accomplished in a structure growing by the addition of layers. Antler growth is from the stump at right angles to this with all the different layers deposited at approximately the same time.

Observation techniques

All the procedures applied to bone (72) and ivory (73) can be used to study antler structure at low resolutions. Two different but related patterns stand out, the branching blood system and the reticular or tubular vascular space in which it lies. The branching blood system may be seen in killed antlers without staining, especially after decalcification or clearing by infiltration with glycerol. Informative preparations have been made of the blood supply of growing antlers by injecting black ink in newly killed specimens (133). The simplest procedure to show the vascular space is to paint the dry polished surface with a black marker pen and then remove the surplus ink with a swab of alcohol. This shows most clearly the pattern of the vascular infolds into the antler bone compartment. The image of an impregnated polished surface is similar to that of a section in that the impregnation does not penetrate deeply. The image of a stained surface cleared in glycerol, on the other hand, has depth and gives three-dimensional information like a whole mount. Glycerol also improves photography by reducing reflections from scratches and dust. A similar effect can be obtained by coating with crazy glue.

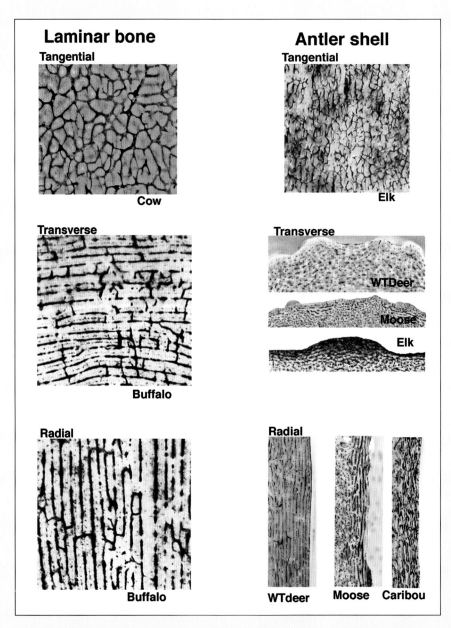

Figure 5.14. Bone, antler comparison—the Shell (See Table 5.2). The surface layers of antlers consist of bone lamellae around a reticular network of vascular spaces creating a skin with roughly uniform properties in the plane of the surface. It resembles laminar bone but with more connections between layers. Vascular spaces emphasized by staining.

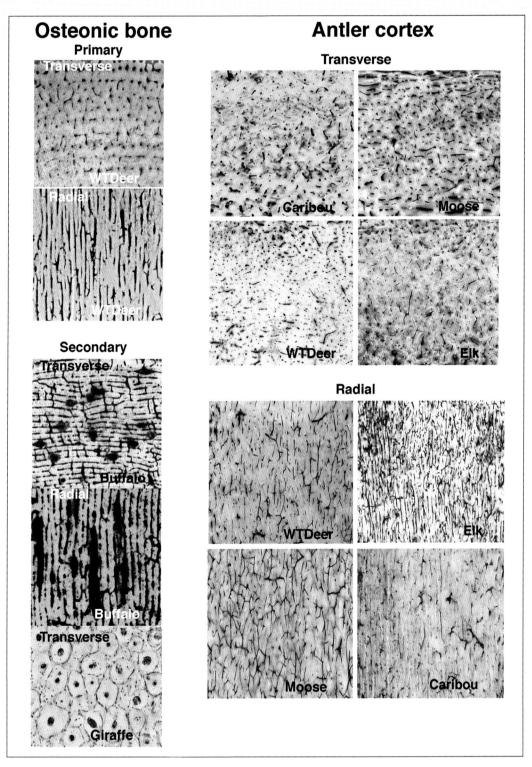

Figure 5.15. Bone, antler comparison—the Cortex (See Table 5.2). The shell merges with a wide cortex made from a meshwork of primary osteons, roughly longitudinal but branched in a three-dimensional network. The walls of these osteons are frequently so widened that they almost obliterate the central vascular space. Internal bone is more often secondary, derived by erosion from laminar bone, and is coarser, straighter, and with wider vascular spaces. Vascular spaces emphasized by staining.

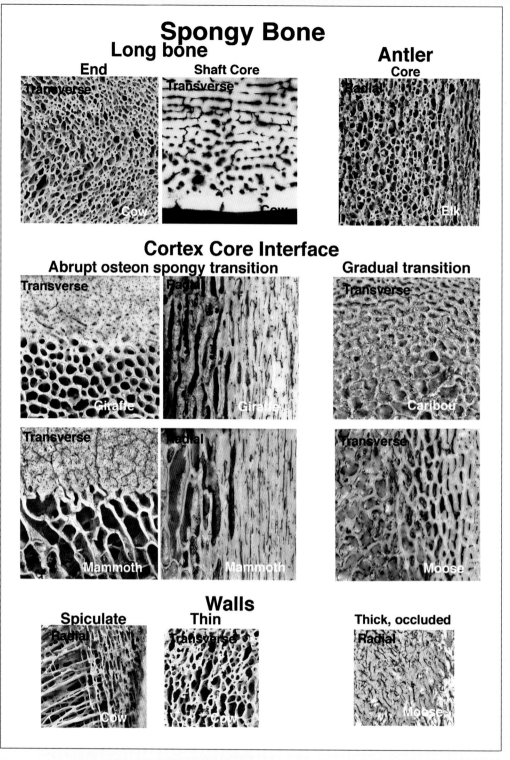

Figure 5.16. Bone, antler comparison—the Spongy Bone Core (See Table 5.2). Spongy bone is absent in the core of the main shaft of long bones that have a smooth surface like that figured. At the ends of such bones and in many others such as rib bones, the core is filled with spongy bone distinguished from that of antlers by the abrupt transition from the cortical structure, having thin walls and often oriented in spicules. Large antlers, such as those from elk, have a spongy core like that from long bones, but there is always a gradual transition from osteons of the cortex. The spongy core of antlers tends to be thick walled, even occluded, less calcified and not oriented. Vascular spaces emphasized by staining.

Chapter 6
Ivory
Teeth Large Enough to Trade

"The tooth of an olyfaunt is yuorye."
William Caxton, 1422–1491

6.1. Introduction

Ivory is the dentine from teeth and continuously growing tusks that are large enough for commercial use. Dentine, the main component, is secreted in layers from the forming face of the pulp cavity (Figure 6.1). The outer surface of most teeth is protected by enamel, but in most ivory (exceptions are some pig tusks, hippopotamus, fossil elephants like *Gomphotherium,* and the tips of juvenile elephants) enamel is replaced by cementum. Cementum is enamel that lacks a hard mineral component. Enamel and cementum form a continuous layer when they occur together in the same tooth. Cementum is added on the outside, unlike Dentine that is secreted at an epithelial surface from the inside. Below the line of the gum, the tooth is fixed through the cementum to the bone by a tissue called cement. The similarity of the two terms often creates confusion. Cementum is a layer secreted on the outside of the dentine below a surface epithelium; cement is a tissue between bone and tooth fixing it in the jaw.

Tusks are continuously growing teeth. Mammals have four kinds of teeth, incisors at the front of the mouth, followed by canines, premolars, and molars. A human adult has two incisors, one canine, two premolars, and three molars on each side in both upper and lower jaws. This is conveniently abbreviated into a dental formula of:

2 . 1 . 2 . 3
2 . 1 . 2 . 3

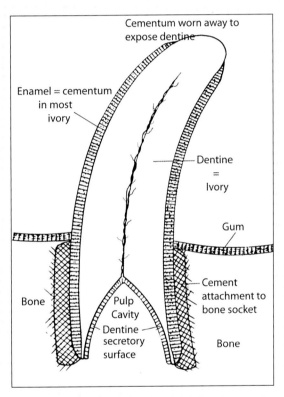

Figure 6.1. Ivory is the dentine of large, continuously growing tusks and teeth. It is secreted progressively from an inside epithelial surface lining the pulp cavity. The pulp cavity survives as a narrow eye containing blood vessels and nerves in the center of the core. Tusks are covered by a layer of modified enamel called cementum that is secreted from an epithelium on the outside, in the opposite direction from the dentine. Tusks are attached in a bone socket by a tissue called cement.

The mammals with tusks, most of which are sources of ivory.

Human	*Homo sapiens*	2 1 2 3 / 2 1 2 3
Proboscidea		
Elephant, African	*Loxodonta africana*, Blumenbach (and/or *L. cyclotis*, Roca et al., 2001)	1T 0 6-7* / 0 0 6-7
Elephant, Indian	*Elephas maximus*, L.	1T 0 6-7* / 0 0 6-7
Mastodon	*Mammut sp.*	1T 0 ?6-7* / 1T 0 ?6-7
Mammoth,	*Mammuthus sp.,*	1T 0 ?6-7* / 0 0 ?6-7
Cetartiodacytla, Artiodactyla, Suiformes, Suidae,		3 1T 4 3 / 3 1T 4 3
Wild boar	*Sus scrofa*, L. Europe, Asia. *Sus cristatus*, L. India, Ceylon, S.E.Asia	
Bushpig	*Potamochoerus porcus*, L. Africa	
Giant Forest Hog	*Hylochoerus meinertzhageni.* Africa	
Wart hog	*Phacocoerus africanus*, P. Africa	Record upper canines 60cms long.
Babirusa	*Babyrousa babyrussa*, Celebes.	Upper canines grow up and through the snout.
Tayassuidae	Tayassu angulatus, Peccary, Javelina. South America.	Smaller tusks than true pigs. Upper canines do not grow up and out.
Hippopotamidae		2 1 4 3 / 1T+1 1T 4 3
Hippopotamus	*Hippopotamus amphibius*, L.	
Pygmy hippopotamus	*Choeropsis liberiensis*, Morton.	
Ruminantia, Tragulidae		
Chevrotain Javan Mouse deer	*Tragulus meminna*, *Tragulus javanicus*,	1T
Cervidae		
Musk deer Muntjac, barking deer Chinese water deer	*Moschus moschiferus* *Muntiacus muntjak* *Hydropotes inermis*	1T
Pinnipedia, Odobaenidae		
Walrus	*Odobaenus rosmarus*, L.	1 1T 3 0 / 0 1 3 0
Cetacea, Odontoceti, Monodontidae		
Narwhal	*Monodon monoceros*, L.	Left 1T 0 0 0 usually male only / 0 0 0 0
Physeteridae		
Sperm Whale	*Physeter macrocephalus*, L.	Homodont, all teeth alike
Delphinidae		
Killer whale or Orca	*Orcinus orca*, L.	Homodont, all teeth alike
Sirenia, Dugongidae		
Dugong	*Dugong dugon*	1+1T 0 11 premolars and molars / 2 0 11 premolars and molars

* Elephants have tusk milk teeth at birth that are shed at about a year old when only 5cms long. A 4th molar (7th in line) is rare.

Table 6.1. Dental formulae for ivory bearing mammals. The formula gives the number of teeth occupying the positions of upper and lower incisor, canine, premolar, and molar teeth, with human dentition as a convenient reference. T marks tusks teeth, showing that ivory tusks have evolved several times from different kinds of tooth.

The dental formulae of ivory bearing mammals (Table 6.1) show that ivory tusks have evolved several times, arising from incisors and/or canines in both upper and lower jaws.

Overview

Ivory is made from dentine, the layer inside the enamel in all teeth and tusks. Dentine is said to be 20% organic and 80% inorganic by weight, but this gives a distorted representation of the composition, as the inorganic component is much denser than the organic and dentine in life is highly hydrated. The density of dentine lies between 1.7 and 1.98. If we take the density of apatite at 3.18 to represent the inorganic constituents and 1.0 to represent water and organic constituents, then Wright (143) calculates that with a composition of 80% inorganic and a specific gravity of 1.8 the inorganic and the organic parts would correspond approximately to 56 and 44 %, respectively by volume. Natural dentine is made less dense through hydration. Dry dentine is even less dense when water is replaced by air. This is the reason that ivory is so sensitive to cracking during drying out. The main inorganic component is hydroxylated calcium phosphate, hydroxyapatite, $(Ca_3OH)_2(PO_4)_6Ca_4)$ that has carbonate substituted to varying degrees for either the phosphate or hydroxyl sites to become the mineral Dahllite. From 4–6% by weight may be carbonate. Fluoride and many elements may be added to the mix so that the exact elemental composition becomes a signature for the origin of the ivory (38). Calcification, the deposition of such calcium salts, occurs on or near collagen fibers to give dentine its hardness of 2.5 on Moh's scale. About 90% of the organic component is the protein collagen. The remainder, forming the matrix around the calcified collagen, consists of other proteins and glycosaminoglycans. If calcification is like that in bone, complex polysaccharides interface between the proteins and minerals (112). Unlike horn, that is made from stable but dead keratins lying outside the body metabolic pool, dentine resembles bone, in that to some degree it can be resorbed and redeposited. This is demonstrated in a massive way when an abscess erodes a tusk base and new ivory is deposited in a grotesque pattern (Figure 6.27 I).

Structural components—dentinal tubules, spherites, and matrix

Dentine has a structure something like reinforced concrete on a microscopic scale (73) (Figure 6.2 A). Odontoblast cells of the secreting epithelium have tubular cellular extensions about 5mm in diameter (Figure 6. 2B). These dentinal tubules are often oriented as laminae with their alignment influencing mechanical properties (Figure 6. 2C). Dentine may replace cytoplasm in the lumen, or dentine matrix may build around the cell extensions to form a honeycomb-like structure. Up to 200 sheets of aligned tubules would be needed to make a stack 1mm thick. Spherites 5–20mm in diameter, often calcified to become calcospherites, are like the gravel filler in concrete, packing around but causing little distortion to the tubules. They are most noticeable as clear unstained masses standing out against a background of densely stained matrix. They should generally be called spherites since they are not all calcified but have the potential to become calcified. They are most abundant in marine ivory from walrus, narwhal, sperm whale, and orca. Early researchers, such as Kolliker, saw them as clear areas in the dentine of teeth that had been decalcified in acid to allow for sectioning. In elephants, they are noticeable in growth layers where they contrast with the more heavily stained matrix. In pigs they appear below the cementum. Difficulty in discerning them is probably due more to failure of the matrix to stain than their absence. Spherites near the forming face are 5–20mm in diameter and roughly spherical, becoming squeezed into polygonal shapes as they mature towards the periphery. A matrix equivalent to the cement in concrete binds the spherites together with the dentinal tubules. All ivory has this structure, varying in the proportions, stabilization, calcification, properties, distribution, and especially orientation of the components (Figure 6.2).

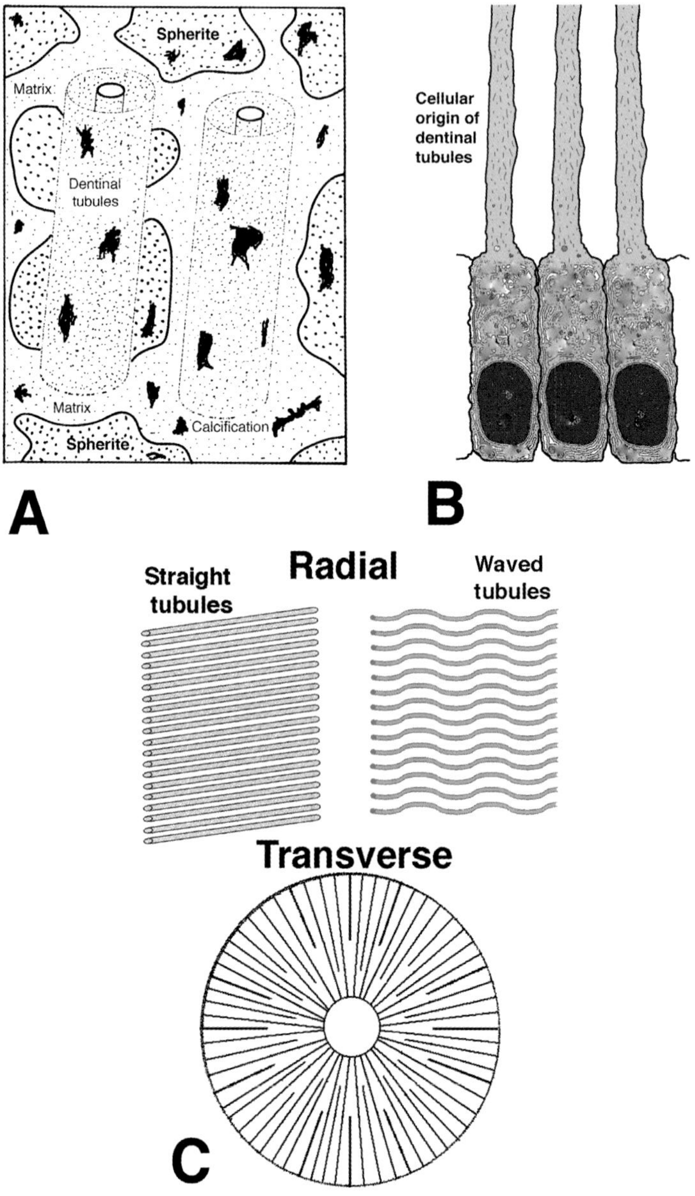

Figure 6.2. A. The dentine of ivory is composed of collagen, a protein, assembled around dentinal tubules about 5mm in diameter together with 5–20mm particles embedded in a matrix. All are made harder by calcification, the incorporation of calcium salts. The structure is like reinforced concrete on a microscopic scale, the particles being equivalent to pebbles cemented with the tubules in a matrix. B. The tubules arise around tubular plasma membrane extensions of odontoblast cells in the dentine secreting epithelium. (See (13), (68), (87)). C. The tubules are radially oriented and may be straight or waved.

Growth layers

Transverse tusk profiles almost always show alternating soft and hard layers that are in roughly symmetrical rings (Figure 6.3). Radial longitudinal profiles show the rings as cross sections of cones, confirming the interpretation of tusk structure as being like a stack of conical paper cups. The last formed layer is continuous above the growth zone and parallel to it, like the growth rings of a tree except that layers are added on the inside and growth in length occurs from the base. Growth layers may contain various ivory components deposited at the same time parallel to the forming face. Differences in composition of material deposited in particular positions at the forming face leads to the formation of bands that can be angled to growth layers as in hippos and pigs and the Schreger pattern in elephants.

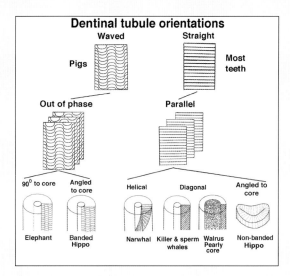

Figure 6.4. Each kind of ivory has its own characteristic arrangement of dentinal tubules aligned in sheets (laminae) that extend from the cementum to the core. They are straight in most teeth but in pigs they tend to curl into waves in the radial longitudinal plane with adjacent laminae having tubules with the same orientation. In elephants and hippos the waves are out of phase. Whales, walruses, and pigs all have their tubules angled to the axis. Narwhals are unique in having helical laminae spiraling in the opposite direction from their cementum. Walruses are distinguished by their pearly core.

Dentinal tubule patterns

The problem with many depictions of ivory in the literature is that they do not show microscope images of sections or profiles as parts of three-dimensional structures (see Figure 1.1). Dentinal tubules aligned into laminae are a common feature, but their shape, orientation, and positioning is characteristic for the dentine of each kind of ivory (Figure 6.4). Typically they extend from the forming face to below the cementum at the outer surface. When not in laminae, they can be straight, skeined (that is grouped together locally in their three-dimensional patterns), or curled (that is waved in several planes and therefore not in laminae). When in laminae, they are aligned side-by-side axially, most commonly in the radial/axial plane. Within the laminae, the dentinal tubules may be straight or curved in waves. Tubules may be parallel to one another and helical in the axis as in narwhals, angled to the forming face in whales, angled to a pulp cavity filled with pearl-like concretions in walruses, or

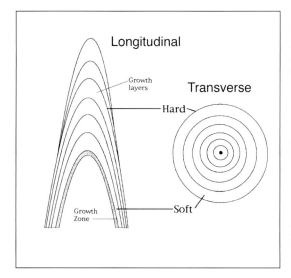

Figure 6.3. Tusks grow continuously from the base, where a growth zone deposits dentine in conical layers that alternate in hardness. The layers are seen as rings in transverse profile. The last formed layer is continuous above the growth zone and parallel to it. Each layer may contain different kinds of ivory. Growth bands in hippos and Schreger columns in elephants are deposited at an angle to the growth layers, showing that different ivory components can all be deposited at the same time.

angled to the forming face in non-banded hippos. Waving (that is curled in one plane) permits alignment in laminae. The patterns may be useful for identifying species, but their significance can only be understood by matching mechanical requirements with genetic and developmental limitations.

Observation techniques

The three-dimensional structure of ivory is easily studied using the techniques developed for bone (72). Three-dimensional interpretation has been hampered in the past by reliance on the tedious process of grinding and acid treatments of sections to be viewed by transmitted light. Polished surfaces viewed by incident light give more information with much less labor. Stains rapidly penetrate into the lumen of hollow dentinal tubules but give much slower staining of solid tubules and matrix. Silver impregnation, osmium, and metal sulfide staining all show dentinal tubules against a variably stained background, as do several conventional stains (coomassie blue, hematoxylin, toluidine blue, methylene blue). An instant method to show hollow dentinal tubules involves coating the dry polished surface with a marker pen and wiping off the surplus stain with alcohol. Stained polished surfaces easily cut with all orientations relative to the tusk axis can be viewed with epi-illumination to determine three-dimensional patterns (73). Natural, undercut, fractured, and cracked surface patterns viewed with a horizontal lateral light source also show the underlying structure, especially after accentuation by Indian ink or the scrimshaw artist's technique of smoking the specimen in a candle flame. Polishing with a soft pad causes undercutting that preferentially removes softer components. Hard parts, like some growth bands and tubules with particular orientations in the Schreger pattern then give an indication of underlying structures by projecting above the surface. Some crack patterns developed in old ivories give a striking but coarse indication of dentinal tubule orientation since they reflect the average orientation of underlying tubules.

Physeter and Orca

The ivory from most mammals comes from tusks, elongated teeth forming cylinders adapted to resist lateral stress. Ivory from the sperm whale (*Physeter macrocephalus*), also known as the cachalot in older literature, and the killer whale or orca (*Orcinus orca*), comes from large teeth that stop growing at maturity, unlike tusks that elongate continuously throughout life. Physeter is one of three members of the family Physeteridae, the others being the pygmy sperm whale, *Kogia breviceps*, and the dwarf sperm whale, *Kogia sima*, both of which have small pointed teeth. The killer whale is not a whale but a dolphin from the family Delphinidae; for this reason "orca" is more properly descriptive than "killer whale". Physeter, anglicized from the Latin *Physeter,* will be used here for brevity and to match the naming of orca.

Physeter

Male sperm whales (bulls) are from 16–20m long and weigh as much as 40,000Kg. Before whaling selectively removed them, the largest whales reached 50–80,000Kg. Their heads are a third of their body length and seem disproportionately large, as shown in Goodall's cheerful copy of Shaw's *Blunt Headed Cachalot* from about 1800. The females (cows) are smaller, 11m long, weighing about 14,000Kg. Sperm whales occur in all the world's oceans and have been hunted for blubber since the eighteenth century. The oily spermaceti wax and sperm oil in their head chambers gave them added value. Sperm whales also yielded ambergris, the partially digested squid remains from their stomachs used by industry to stabilize perfumes. In 1978, the market price for ambergris was more than 300£ [$400] per Kg. About a quarter of a million sperm whales were taken in the nineteenth century. More seriously for the whales, more than three quarters of a million were taken after the Second World War. International agreement for a moratorium on commercial whaling has protected them from massive exploitation since 1986. Japan's whale catch was then briefly zero, but a permit to kill for research allowed them to take 1,000 whales a year, giving them 3–4,000 tons of meat—as much as before the ban. Sperm whales have been targeted since 2000. The number surviving is unknown. The value of their teeth has not contributed much to their exploitation. Indeed, their ivory was so little esteemed that divers found teeth strewn on the seabed near whaling stations that had closed down in the 1970s. As other kinds of ivory disappeared, "whale teeth" were in demand, but strict laws around the world against the trading of teeth have prevented the development of a commercial market. However, many small teeth from female Physeter have come on the market in recent years.

Orca

Orca are big for dolphins, but dwarves relative to sperm whales. Males are 6–8m long and weigh up to 6,000Kg, females reach 5–7m and may weigh 3–4,000Kg. They occur in all the oceans worldwide, preferring cold water but penetrate the Mediterranean and have even been known to attack moose in the fresh water of river estuaries. They are the ocean's top predator, eating anything from herring to sea lions and the calves of the largest whales. There are several different races distinguished by their habits and food preferences. After commercial whalers depleted whale stocks, they took orca, but their small size made them an uneconomic catch. They are now threatened more by competition with other fisheries for food. The world population was estimated in 2010 to be about 50,000.

The teeth are too small to threaten orca by the creation of an ivory market, most being used for pendants or scrimshaw. It was a common practice in the 1970s for Russian sailors coming ashore on the Canadian West Coast to sell orca and small Physeter teeth for pocket money. Many of the teeth now marketed may come from similar sources.

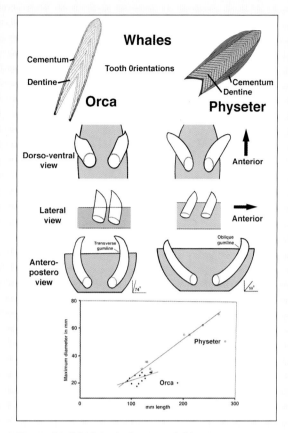

Figure 6.5. Whale ivory has a tooth-like structure, except that enamel is replaced by cementum. Only 20–30% of the length is exposed above the gum line where the tip is worn down to expose the dentine. Orca are more elongated and tusk-like than Physeter that have a broad waist from a wide layer of cementum that locks the tooth firmly in the bone. Dentine is laid down as stacks of conical growth layers at about 450 to the axis with tubules at about 900 to the growth layers. Changes in width vary with the extent of lateral growth while growth in length comes from the addition of new growth layers. Orca are thinner than Physeter in relation to length (graph), but small teeth are hard to distinguish from one another. However, Orca and Physeter teeth differ in the angle at which they are set in the jaw. Orca point at ~ 740 (~ transverse to the gumline) compared to ~ 500 (oblique to the gumline) in the vertical plane transverse to the jaw.

Tooth structure

The teeth. Whale and orca ivory is from teeth with a limited lifespan rather than continuously growing tusks (Figure 6.5). Both orca and Physeter are homodont, that is, their teeth are all alike rather than being identifiable as incisors, canines, and molars. While Physeter has teeth with a maximum width to length to ratios of ~1:2.7, orca are more tusk-like, ~1:5.7, as befits their dolphin ancestry adapted as predators capable of tearing up many different kinds of prey (Figure 6.5). Mature male Physeter teeth weigh from 500–1,000gms, but may have reached almost twice that in the large whales from the early days of whaling. Fossil teeth from the Miocene raptorial sperm whale *Leviathan melvillei* found in Peru were even larger (65). Female Physeter teeth weigh much less, overlapping with orca in size. Orca teeth rarely exceed 100gms and tend to be parallel-sided (Figure 6.7 H, J) rather than conical and convex like Physeter (Figures 6.6 D; 6.7 A–F). Mature teeth narrow from the mid-point towards the base and have an irregular lumpy pulp cavity, often containing pearly concretions (Figure 6.6 E, 6.7 J). Most of a tooth is locked in the jaw with only 25–30% of the length of a mature tooth exposed above the gumline. Their structure is appropriate for resistance to axial compression rather than lateral stress as in tusks.

Growth. Growth is not continuous. Immature teeth have cone-shaped pulp cavities (Figures 6.6 C; 6.7 I,) with a flared base half as wide in orca as in male Physeter of similar length (Figures 6.6 B, 7 H). In mature teeth, the pulp cavity becomes obtuse and almost sealed off (Figures 6.6 E, 6.7 C). Large male Physeter teeth are easily distinguished from orca by their size (Figure 6.5. Graph) but female Physeter are smaller and overlap with orca in size. Several features can be used to distinguish them.

Abrasion at occlusion surfaces. Physeter has teeth only in the lower jaw, twenty to twenty-six on each side (Figure 6.6 A). Lacking upper teeth to rub against, the exposed surfaces of Physeter are rounded, presumable from contact with prey, although their function remains controversial (Fig. 6.6 D, F). In contrast, orca have upper and lower teeth, ten to fourteen on each side, that grind where they meet to create flat occlusal surfaces angled to the length of the tooth (Figure 6.7 E–G). In older animals the abrasions may cut diagonally across, leaving both teeth with sharp points. The polish on these occlusal surfaces is finer than the smooth but matt surfaces produced by abrasion from food. Occlusal surfaces easily distinguish older orca from Physeter teeth, but they are not helpful for identifying young ones. Ten cms of tooth may be below the gumline before the 2–3cms of emerging tooth can begin to abrade with its opposite number in orca (Fig. 6.7 G) or round the surface in Physeter (Figure 6.7 A). Abrasion from feeding may indicate the type of food preferred by the race of orca. Those eating sharks and rays, for example, may be worn flat by the hard, sharp denticles in the skin of their prey.

Tooth orientation (Figure 6.5). The angles at which the teeth are set vary along the length of the jaw, but in both orca and Physeter they tend to angle forward and outward while curving backward and inward, orientations maximizing grasp while guiding prey into the gullet. Orca and Physeter differ significantly in their orientation. In particular, a prey's eye view from the front of Physeter (an antero-postero view) shows teeth more splayed out to the sides (50.1^0 sd 3.8^0 to the vertical) while orca teeth are more vertically arranged (73.6^0 sd 4.2^0 to the vertical). This is easy to see in whole skulls, but the researcher is usually presented with single teeth. Fortunately, each tooth carries its orientation history in the angle made with the gumline. It tends to be transverse to the main tooth axis in orca and oblique in Physeter.

Enamel and cementum. A detailed and authoritative report of a whaling commission (102) introduced confusion by using a figure (Figure 9) of a tooth with labeling inappropriate for ivory. It refers to cementum as enamel and cement as cementum. Most whale teeth have cementum but no enamel. Reports of enamel at the tips of Physeter teeth are probably in error, although they might be difficult to find if they are like the evanescent caps to newly formed teeth (elephants). The idea that orca have enamel is also made more plausible from the whiteness of the cementum and the outer layers of dentine. However,

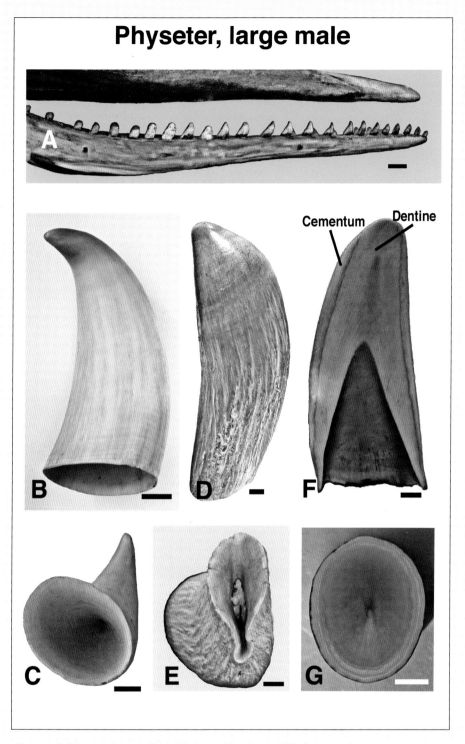

Physeter, large male

Cementum   **Dentine**

Figure 6.6. Physeter, large male. A. Upper and lower jaws. The lower jaw has twenty to twenty-six teeth on each side. The upper jaw has none. Photograph of part of the Physeter skull from the Tring Museum by kind permission of the Natural History Museum, South Kensington. B. Immature tooth has a base twice as wide as that of an Orca of similar length (see Fig. 6.7 H–K). Weight 80gms [3 oz.]. C. Immature teeth have cone shaped pulp cavities. The deep cone-shaped pulp cavity of B seen from the base. D. Mature tooth narrows from the mid-point towards the base. Seventy percent of the tooth lies below the gumline. Weight 920gms [32 oz.]. E. The closed pulp cavity of D seen from the base. The lumpy center consists of pearly concretions often found in older teeth. Saggital F. and transverse profile G. show a thick cementum layer. The gumline is oblique to the main tooth axis and tips are worn evenly into rounded domes. Scale bars, A = 10cms, B–G = 1cm.

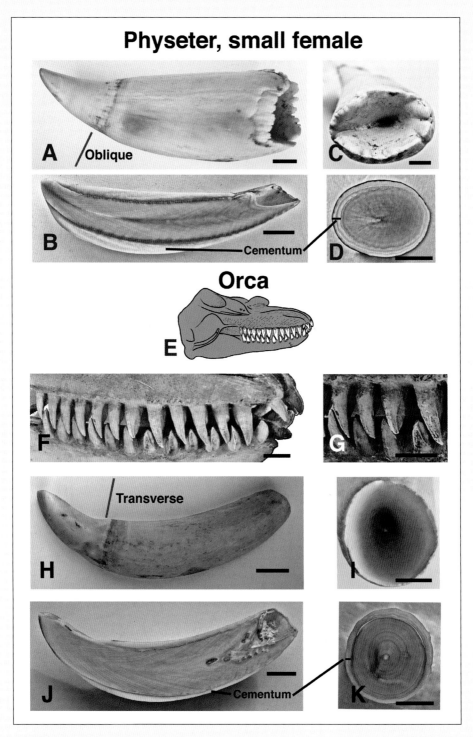

Physeter, small female

Orca

Figure 6.7. Physeter, small female. A. Teeth narrow from the mid point towards the base with 75% below a gumline that is oblique to the main tooth axis. C. End view of A with occluded pulp cavity showing that growth has been completed. B. Saggital profile showing the thin cementum near the root and the tip with a bulge in the middle locking it firmly in the jawbone. The gumline is oblique to the main tooth axis and the tip is worn evenly into rounded domes. D. Transverse profile from the middle of a tooth showing the thick cementum. Orca. E, F, G. Skulls have teeth in both upper and lower jaws that interlock, resulting in older teeth having flattened occlusal surfaces where they have worn against one another (62). The teeth are oriented closer to vertical than in the Physeter. H. Tusk-like tooth similar in length to the immature sperm whale in Fig. 6.6 B but almost cylindrical and only half its diameter. The gumline is transverse to the main tooth axis and the tip has a flattened occlusal surface. Weight 75gms. I. The incomplete conical growth cone of C viewed from the base. J. Saggital profile of H showing the thin layer of cementum and the cone-shaped pulp cavity of a tooth that is still growing. K. Transverse profile of a tooth like H showing the mostly narrow cementum made variable by position along the length and plane of profile. Scale bars, F, G = 5cm, others = 1cm.

enamel and cementum, its mineral reduced equivalent, are easily distinguished by their hardness. A steel needle scratches cementum and exposed dentine easily and equally but leaves real enamel on a test tooth, such as a hippo, unmarked.

For an understanding of ivory structure, it is essential to remember that cementum is a **layer** that lacks mineral hardening but is continuous with enamel and secreted by the same ectodermal epithelium. Cement is the **tissue** that fixes the tooth in the bone. By calling cementum enamel, the commission buried the question why teeth from so many marine mammals (orca, Physeter, walrus, narwhal [beluga, apart from the tip]) have cementum rather than enamel. Perhaps permanent large teeth require reduced mineralization to be free from chipping. The small replaceable teeth of sharks and crocodiles are heavily enameled.

Much of the thickness of the teeth comes from layers of cementum giving mature teeth a broad waist around a narrower conical or cylindrical core of dentine. The dentine, being secreted from the inside, can only increase in length. The cementum, being on the outside has no such restriction and can increase the width of the root as well as covering the growing length. The layers are laid down progressively from the outside front to back at a slight angle ($\sim5^{0}$) to the interface with the dentine, which joins at $\sim15^{0}$, making an asymmetrical herringbone pattern in longitudinal profile (Figure 6.8 A). Thin layers begin at the tip, thicken towards the middle to lock the tooth firmly in the bone, and thin again at the root (Figure 6.6 F, 6.7 B, J). The thickness of the cementum has been used to identify artifacts made of orca ivory from those of Physeter. In general, orca cementum is thinner than Physeter (145) (102). Problems arise from single observations of the thickness since it changes along the length of the tooth (Figure 6.7 B, J) and around the circumference (Figure 6.7 K). The perceived thickness also changes with the tooth curvature and the plane of the profile.

Cementum dentine interface. The interface reflects the surface pattern of the cementum at the time of deposition. It is a record of the external surface pattern that tends to be ridged longitudinally in Physeter and smooth in orca. This results in a wavy pattern in transverse profiles of Physeter and a smooth interface in orca (Figure 6.8 B–D).

Microscopic structure. Sperm whale and orca teeth resemble one another in their microscopic structure. Their dentine has many spherites, especially in the growth layers (Figure 6.8 E, F). An excess of spherites might be expected in structures where resistance to axial compression is more important than stiffness and resistance to cracking in bending. The dentine is laid down as stacks of conical growth layers at about 45^{0} to the axis (Figure 6.8 A, D). In spite of irregularity due to the abundant spherites, dentinal tubules are aligned in laminae (Figure 6.8 G, H). The tubules lie at approximately 90^{0} to the forming face, becoming thinner and irregular in the bands (Figure 6.8 F). Growth in width is accomplished by lateral extension of the growth layers and the addition of a thicker layer of cement, and in length by the addition of new layers. Nerve channels are not conspicuous as they are in tusks presumed to be sensory—elephants, hippos, upper boar canines, and narwhal.

Similarities and differences between Physeter and orca are summarized in Table 6.2.

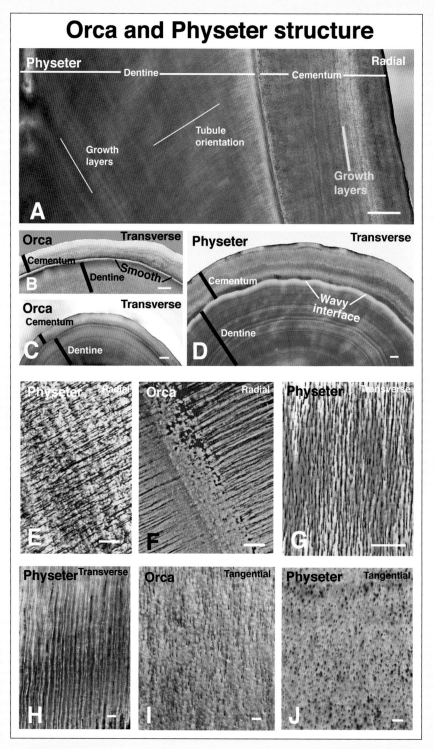

Orca and Physeter structure

Figure 6.8. Orca and Physeter tooth structure. A. Dentinal tubules lie at approximately 900 to growth layers parallel to the forming face and angled to the cementum. The interface with cementum is dense and often white or light colored before staining. The thick cementum has many layers at an acute angle to the interface. B, C. Transverse profiles show the cementum/dentine interface tends to be narrow and smooth in Orca and wide and wavy in Physeter, D, reflecting the ridged or smooth surface patterns of the cementum. Dentine below the interface is light colored. E. and F. Abundant spherites separate the tubules, especially in growth layers where the tubules become narrower. G. Tubules are cut into short lengths as expected from their approximately 450 angle to the transverse plane. H. In spite of the irregularity due to the abundant particles, unstained transverse profiles show regular laminae in which the tubules are embedded like stacks of corrugated cardboard. I. and J. Tangential profiles show orderly tubules in laminae between the bands. Tubules are less regular in the bands where particles are more abundant. Scale bars, A–D = 1mm, E–G = 100mm, H–J = 10mm.

Comparison of Orca and Physeter teeth.		
	Orca	Physeter
Number of teeth	10 - 14 each side upper and lower jaws.	20 - 26 each side lower jaw only.
Tooth separation at gumline in relation to tooth diameter	0.25 - 0.5.	0.5 –2.25.
Length at maturity (pulp cavity is short and obtuse).	~ 12cms.	~ 25cms. Up to 33cms have been recorded {Hanak V., 1979 #231}.
Mature tooth shape and orientation. Variable but Orca more tusk-like. All teeth are angled forwards and outwards and curve backwards and inwards. Angle with gumline transverse in Orca, oblique in Physeter.		
Tooth orientation significantly different. Angle subtended with vertical in the antero/postero plane seen in frontal view.	73.6^0 sd 4.2^0	50.1^0 sd 3.8^0
Immature tooth shape. In teeth of similar length Physeter are much more widely flared at the base.	Immature 12cm long	Immature 12cm long
Shape in cross section at position of greatest breadth. Approximately elliptical. Difference barely significant.	Ratio short/long = 0.86 sd 0.06. Short. Long. May become almost rectangular in the close packed root.	Ratio short/long = 0.78 sd 0.04. Short. Long.
Pearly concretions in core.	Common	Occasional
Tooth wear.	Uneven. Flats on occlusal surfaces from teeth in opposing jaw. Very old teeth may be reduced to sharp spikes.	Uniform. Rounded conical tops that may become flattened in very old teeth. Occasional terminal chips are unlike Orca occlusal flats.
Mature weight.	70 - 100gms.	Male. 500 - 900gms. Up to 1,900gms reported {Hanak V., 1979 #231}. Female smaller like large Orca.
Microscopic structure similar.	Axial radial microlaminae. Abundant spherites particularly in growth layers. Dentinal tubules at about 45^0 to the axis.	Axial radial microlaminae. Abundant spherites particularly in growth layers. Dentinal tubules at about 45^0 to the axis. May have pearly concretions in core.
Colour. {Meinke, 1964 Chart #232}	Dentine core Orange Yellowish Brown. 73. p.OY. Cementum and nearby tip dentine whitish.	Dentine core Yellow Olive Brown. 89. p.Y. Cementum and nearby tip dentine whitish.
Cementum thickness. Measurements vary around the circumference, along the length and with the angle of the profile .	Thinner than Physeter in most teeth. 1 – 2mm.	Thicker than Orca in the mid region especially in large teeth. {Yates, 2006 #235}. 3 – 5mm.
Cementum surface	Smooth with faint longitudinal ridges.	Broad longitudinal ridges.
Cementum/dentine interface	Smooth in transverse profile reflecting the surface pattern.	Wavy in transverse profile reflecting the surface pattern.

Table. 6.2. Orca and Physeter teeth compared. Numerical conclusions based on small numbers are guides to experiments using larger samples.

Before printing, Europe depended upon word of mouth, or at best, hand copying of manuscripts, both of which conveyed information about as well as the parlor game of "Rumor." Early printing did no better, often propagating the errors: Konrad Gesner had never seen the narwhal, unicorn of the seas, when he figured it with a horn on its head. It took more than 200 years before accurate depictions like the Sherwood illustration, 1812. Myths depended upon such strange depictions and the magical attributes that antiquity gave to both horns and animals. There are two related myths, one concerning the animal and the other the tusks, joined through that other single horned creature, the rhinoceros, by conflation of its horn with mammoth ivory. The myth concerning the animal itself came from a literary error in the Bible backed by the real life presence of the *unicornum falsum* (false alicorn), ivory tusks of the narwhal, and gave rise to the legend of the elegant, horselike creature, protector of virgins, or at least maidens, figured above by Gesner (69). The second set of myths grew from the supposed magical properties of the tusks of the *unicornum verum* (true alicorn), mammoth tusks dug from the earth.

Myths related to the animal began with the many references to unicorns, including the King James Bible, while modern translations refer to wild ox rather than unicorns:—*"Will the unicorn be willing to serve thee, or abide by thy crib? Canst thou bind the unicorn with his band in the furrow? Or will he harrow the valleys after thee?"* Job 39:9–10.

"Save me .... Also from the horns of the unicorns." Psalms XXII 20.

"Save me from the lion's mouth for thou hast heard me from the horns of the unicorns." Psalms 22:21.

"He maketh them also to skip like a ... young unicorn." Psalms 29:5.

The Old Testament was written in Hebrew. In the third century B.C. the high priest Eleazar sent seventy-two translators from Jerusalem to Alexandria, one of the largest cities in the world with a population estimated at 300,000, to begin the task of translating it into Greek, creating what became known as LXX or the Septuagint. An awesome but poorly described animal mentioned seven times in the Hebrew version was the *Re'em*. The translators were Alexandrian "townies," who rendered *Re'em* as *monokeros*, Greek for one horn. They knew nothing of the plough and green fields or they would have realized that the *Re'em* were oxen or perhaps the extinct Aurochs, *Bos primigenius* (76). Perhaps they recalled travelers' gossip of the fearsome one horned beasts from Africa, or Babylonian bas-reliefs showing only one horn in side view depictions of the Aurochs or other wild cattle ancestors. Thus was the legend of the unicorn born (69). It was a publicist's dream, mentioned in a book that became the most widely read in history and one that had to be believed. The reality of this unicorn animal was assumed to be confirmed when narwhal tusks (*unicornum falsum)* were brought to Europe by Norse traders.

These tusks were not the *unicornum verum* that could cure diseases and counteract poisons. Such properties were first attached to rhinoceros horn. In the fourth century BC the Greek historian Ctesias, physician to the king of Persia Artaxerxes II, came back from India with the knowledge that potions made from powdered rhino horn were an antidote to poisons. Knowledge of the potency of rhino horn probably came from China, where its value as a medicine survives so strongly today that it is the single highest risk factor for rhinoceros survival. *A Barefoot Doctor's Manual* (1977) informs us: "His-chiao (Shui-niu Chiao), Scientific name *Rhinoceros indicus*. Properties and action: Has han (cooling properties), bitter, sour, and salty to taste. Clears fevers, cools the blood, detoxifies, controls convulsive spasms. Conditions most used for: Low and high grade fevers, restlessness and great thirst, cracked lips and parched tongue, delirium, epistaxis and hematuria, quinsy sore throat, fatigue, boils and abscesses. Preparation: For each dose, 2 to 8 fen, in decoction." Similar properties were ascribed to the *unicornum verum*, or true alicorn in medieval Europe. It was thought to be a most potent cure for the plague (63). In one Portuguese recipe from 1430, blood, liver, and teeth from a badger that had been decapitated after being plied with wine, camphor, gold, coral, and pearls, was mixed with cinnamon, pepper, ginger, verbena, cloves, myrrh, aloes, and unicorn horn. The proportions of one part of horn to 380 of the other ingredients attested to the belief in its potency. Cups made from *unicornum verum* were thought to confer resistance to epilepsy and evil drugs. Tomás de Torquemada (1420–1498), the Inquisitor General of Spain, was so afraid of assassination that he traveled with a retinue of 50 mounted guards and 200 foot soldiers. To protect himself from poisoning he never dined without his "unicorn's horn" at table (101). This may have been a rhinoceros horn, but it was more likely made from ivory.

Unicornum verum may have been rhinoceros horn originally but its magic was probably transferred to cups made of mammoth ivory. This may seem surprising, as a European savant 4–500 years ago would have known about elephant and hippo ivory carvings of people, triptychs and religious themes, often at first hand, and would not have confused their ivory with cups made of rhino horn. But he would have heard traveler's tales of animals from Africa or the Orient that had single horns on their heads, and he knew of cups with the shape of a rhino horn made from that of the magical unicorn, the *Unicornum verum*, dug from the ground and known as a remedy for all kinds of sickness. Strangely, this ivory came from the north through Russia. The finding that "unicorn tusks" (= rhinoceros horns) known to be common in the Orient, came to Europe through northern waters was viewed as strong evidence for a north-eastern sea route to the East. In 1611, Josias Logan returned to London with the tusk of an "elephant" (69). The remarkable thing was that he was returning from Russia, not from Africa or Asia. The tusk was bought from Samoyed tribesmen near the shores of the Arctic Ocean. Mammoth ivory dug from the frozen Siberian tundra had been exploited as a trading commodity for millennia, becoming known in Russian as *mamontova-kostji*. The explanation for cups made from *unicornum verum* is probably that they were made from such ivory. In old, poorly preserved mammoth tusks, the collagen may be lost preferentially from the softer layers, allowing a tusk to separate into several conical sections (see Figure 6.30 A for the arrangement in elephants). I have seen tusks fall apart like stacks of paper cups, ready made drinking vessels shaped like the slightly curved cones of a rhinoceros horn but made of ivory. The similarity in shape between Asian rhino horns and sections near the base of very old mammoth tusks may therefore be the origin of the early tales of unicorns coming from the frozen north of Russia where mammoth tusks were dug and traded with nations further south. Ivory as *unicornum verum* has another thing going for it, survival. Horn is eaten by beetles or moth caterpillars and rarely survives for long.

Not all narwhal tusk myths are as favorable as the unicorn, protector of virgins. One of Hogarth's "Marriage a la mode" etchings portrays a Viscount and his mistress with a narwhal tusk symbolizing her venereal disease.

6.3 Narwhal

Introduction

The word narwhal comes from the old Norse word *nar*, meaning corpse, from their mottled grey color said to resemble the flesh of sailors long dead in the sea, and *hval*, whale. Males weighing up to 1,600Kg and females 1,000Kg live together in groups of five to fifteen offshore in the Canadian Arctic and Greenland in seas North of latitude 65^0

North. They feed, often under pack ice, on benthic halibut, cod, shrimp and squid at depths of 800m but are known to dive to 1,500m, the greatest depth of any marine mammals. This specialized habitat-related diet may be the reason that they do not survive in captivity. The world population was estimated in 2008 to be about 75,000 and in the "near threatened" class. They are vulnerable more from sale of their tusks as curiosities and trophies rather than useful ivory, the market for which is small, mostly for knife handles. As trophies they are valuable. A tusk 6.7 ft. [2.05m] long was for sale for the equivalent of $6,500 in Portobello market, London, in 2001. Lopez gives a fine account of much narwhal lore (76).

Unicorn mythology

No material described in this book is more bound up in mythology than the unicorn. The single horn came from the head as in a rhinoceros, but it was made of ivory like an elephant tusk.

Tusk structure

Tusk size and shape. Narwhal have two upper teeth but only the left one emerges from the skull and that only in males, giving them their characteristic single long tusk, shown to be the canine (96A). Ward lists a record tusk of 2.86m in 1907 (135) but tusks up to 3m long and weighing as much as 10Kg have been found since then. Narwhal tusks are unique in being straight, those from all other mammals are curved or helical (Figure 6.9 A). Although there was much earlier speculation about their use, narwhal do little with them other than to battle one another in ritualized "sword fights" showing them to be secondary sexual features as Darwin noted (26). Narwhal tusks seem to be out of proportion to the body length of 4–5m, as are many secondary sexual characteristics (peacocks tails, Irish elk antlers). Narwhal tusks have a very short root (15% of the length compared to 40–75% in all others (73)). Tusk clashes are buffered,

(Opposite page)
Figure 6.9. Narwhal tusks. A. This mature Narwhal tusk is 3.8m long and weighs 7.3 Kg. B. The angle made by the cementum ridges relative to transverse is inversely related to diameter. The angle decreases from the base to the apex. Immature tusks lack the base of about 50cm embedded in the skull that does not increase in diameter with length. Mean values from two mature tusks. C. The cementum has ridges making a left-handed counterclockwise helix. Surface view with ridging emphasized by ink. Viewed from the outside, the ridges run from bottom right to top left. D. The tusks are hollow, except at the tip. The base is almost occluded by dentine when mature. Transverse profile showing the cementum on the outside and the wide dentine below. Methylene blue stained. E. The forming face has much finer ridges that reflect the shape of the secreting epithelium. They form a right-handed clockwise helix opposite to that in the cementum. Although these images have the same rotation from bottom right to top left as the cementum in A, they are being viewed in the opposite direction, from the inside to the outside. If both inside and outside could be viewed in the same direction through an invisible dentine as in G, they would appear as crossed helices. This explains the counterintuitive sense that C and E can be crossed helices. F. The skull has a greatly enlarged left socket to hold the tusk. The right socket contains a short tooth primordium that fails to erupt. H. Occasionally both left and right primordia erupt to make two tusks. Scale bars, A, F = 5cm, C-E = 1cm, H = 10cm.

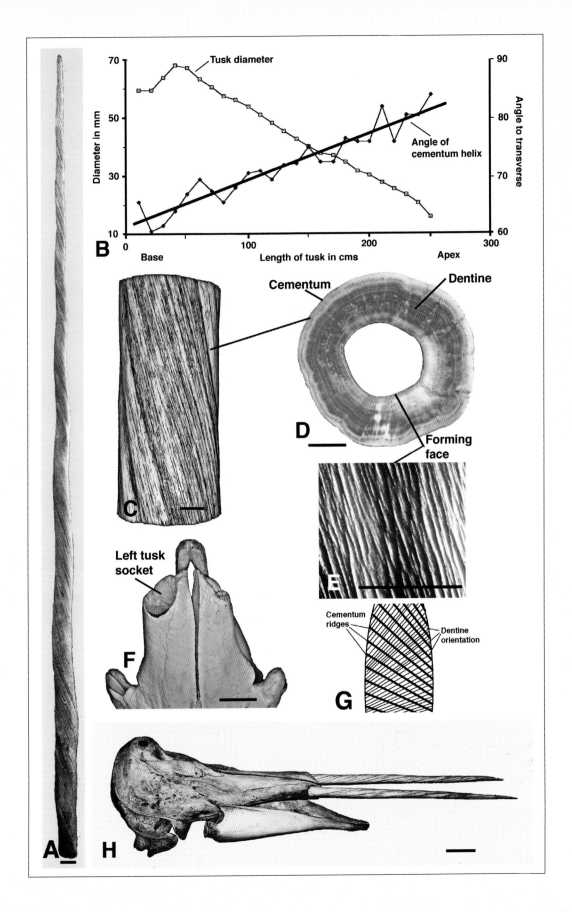

B Tusk diameter

Diameter in mm

Angle to transverse

Angle of cementum helix

Base   Length of tusk in cms   Apex

Cementum   Dentine

D

Forming face

C

E

Left tusk socket

F

Cementum ridges   Dentine orientation

G

A   **H**

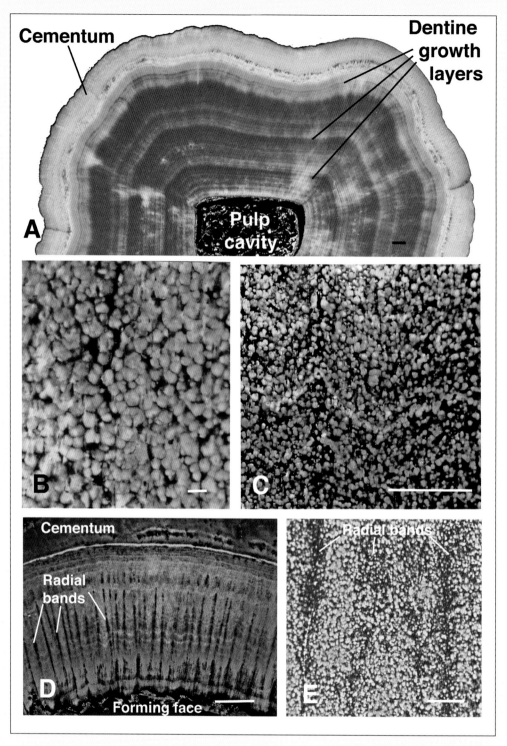

Figure 6.10. Narwhal growth layers, matrix, and radial/longitudinal bands. A. Well defined growth layers, probably annual, are made from layers of particles and matrix in which they are embedded. The pulp cavity contains nerves and blood vessels. Transverse profile methylene blue stained. B. The abundance of lightly stained spherical particles and the density of the matrix around them is a characteristic feature of narwhal ivory. C. Growth layers composed of these characteristic particles embedded in densely stained matrix retain the ridge outlines from their forming face. D. Particles in dense matrix also concentrate in characteristic longitudinal radially oriented bands appearing like spokes originating at the base of the ridges on the forming face. B, C, D, transverse profiles mercury sulfide stained. E. The radially oriented bands consist of densely stained matrix around densely packed particles. Methylene blue stained transverse profile. Scale bars, A, D = 1mm, B = 10mm, C, E = 100mm.

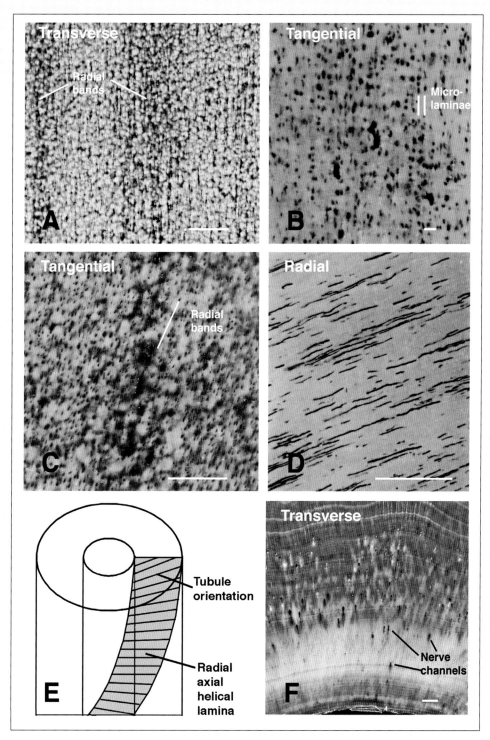

Figure 6.11. A. Narwhal dentinal tubules are radially oriented like the bands, but profiles are cut into short lengths as would be expected if they are angled axially rather than being exactly transverse. Methylene blue stained. B. Tangential profiles below the cementum show the tubules in axial laminae having the same orientation as ridges on the forming face at the base of the tusk. Marker pen stained. C. Tangential profiles in the mid-region show that both bands and tubules have twisted diagonally. Trypan blue stained. D. Radial profiles show tubules with a diagonal orientation as expected from A. Marker pen stained. E. Tubule orientations in A–D are explained if they are arranged in helical laminae within which they are diagonal to transverse. F. Nerve channels are much larger than the tubules but have the same orientations, radiating diagonally forward from the pulp cavity suggesting that the tusks are sensory. Transverse profile marker pen and methylene blue stained. Scale bars, A, C, D = 100mm, B = 10mm, F = 1mm.

making a longer root unnecessary since their body is relatively small and floating in the water rather than being fixed to the ground by gravity, unlike elephants, where the tusk is so firmly fixed that the animal's weight can be safely used to transmit enough force to uproot trees. The tusks are probably also sensory (Figure 6.11 F).

The right socket contains a 20cm long undeveloped primordial tooth that occasionally develops (1 in 500), giving such males two tusks (Figure 6. 9H). Females rarely have a tusk, but there is a record of one with two. The tusk itself is a shell of cementum and dentine around a wide pulp cavity of blood vessels and nerves narrowing to a solid tip about 20cms long (Figure 6.9 D). In growing tusks, the diameter increases continuously from the tip to the base where the pulp cavity is wide open. At maturity, the base embedded in the skull diminishes in diameter while the dentine thickens, reducing the wide pulp cavity to a narrow channel (Figure 6.9 A, B).

Cementum distribution. The tusks have no enamel, but cementum extending as a layer about 1mm thick at the tip to about 5mm at the base. It has characteristic ridges 1–2mm wide over broader 1–2cm waves (Figure 6.9 A, C). The ridges at the tip are acutely angled to the length, becoming more obtuse as the tusk widens in direct proportion to the diameter, that is, the frequency of the helix is constant per unit length but the amplitude increases with diameter (Figure 6.9 B). The cementum forms a left handed anticlockwise helix. The structure of the whole tusk is not so simple. The outer layer of cementum is helical with one continuously varying pitch, but the dentine layers below have a helical pitch opposite to that of the cementum reflected by the orientation of grooves in the surface of the forming face (Figure 6.9 E, G). These grooves begin parallel to the long axis at the base of the tusk where dentine is deposited directly below the cementum and twist clockwise as more layers are added in thicker parts of the tusk (73).

Growth layers, matrix and spherites. Tusk profiles show broad, well defined growth layers (Figure 6.10 A). A most striking feature is the way that the abundance of spherites and the density of the matrix in which they are embedded define these growth layers (Figure 6.10 B, C). The layers retain the grooved outline of the face where they formed. Spherites in matrix are evident in most other ivories below the cementum and in growth layers, but in narwhal they are the major component throughout, appearing as unstained spheres deformed by compression against one another in a densely stained matrix. The dominance of spherites agrees with Currey's findings that narwhal tusks are of low stiffness but very tough (16). The packing of the spherites also outlines a characteristic feature of narwhal ivory: in transverse profiles oriented bands arise like spokes from the forming face (Figure 6.10 D, E).

Dentinal tubule and lamina orientation. Narwhal ivory has dentinal tubules oriented in laminae packed between the dense aggregations of spherites. Transverse profiles show tubules radially oriented parallel to the radially oriented bands but cut into short lengths as would be expected if they are radial but oblique axially rather than exactly transverse (Figure 6.11 A). Radial profiles confirm their oblique axial orientation (Figure 6.11 D). Tangential profiles show the tubules lie in laminae with their own orientation (Figure 6.11 B, C). The orientation of the laminae changes from axial just below the cementum (B) where they had been deposited parallel to the axial grooves of the forming face at the base of the tusk, to oblique (C), corresponding to the oblique grooves of the forming face in most of the tusk. The structure of narwhal dentine is like multiple winding staircases twisting clockwise with the steps of the floor sloping inwards to the center indicating the tubule orientation (Figure 6.11 E). The conclusion that narwhal tusks are crossed helices of cementum and enamel (Figure 6.9 G) confirms the results of Currey (16, 25), who measured the fracture directions at various depths in mechanically stressed tusks.

Darcy Thompson correlated the straightness of narwhal tusks with their helical cementum (126). Coiled springs tend to straightness, but this solves only half the problem. Helical springs may be straight at rest but they are very floppy, easily deformed. The addition of a structure coiled in the opposite direction adds stiffness. A sheet of material made from parallel fibers bends easily one way and is stiff in the other. Two sheets with opposing fiber orientations make a board that is stiff in both directions. A narwhal tusk is like a cylindrical board made from two such sheets with opposing fiber orientations.

Growth. There is a reduction of units from the periphery to the core to allow for transverse growth since their separation is constant. Some tubules at the periphery must lose their connections with the forming face as longitudinal helical matrix bands become closer together and fuse or disappear as they approach the core. The helical pattern might suggest that narwhal tusks rotate as they increase in length. However, the wear at the tip is asymmetrical as would be expected for a tooth in a constant position and the connective tissue cement prevents rotation. The deposition of cementum and dentine within the socket in helical form allows the tusk to be extruded from the base without rotation.

Nerve channels. Like the lower incisors of hippos, the upper canines of pigs, and the tusks of elephants (Figure 6.45 **F**), narwhal tusks have nerve channels radiating out diagonally from the pulp cavity to the cementum, easily stained with a black marker pen in dry ivory (Figure 6.11 **F**). The channels are so abundant in some regions that very small samples might be mistaken for bone. The general role of some tusks as sensors is a field waiting to be explored.

6. 4. Pearly Concretions—Ivory "Pearls"

Concentric pearl-like concretions occur occasionally in the core of many teeth, especially the tusks of hippos, pigs, orca, and sperm whales. They may lie freely in the pulp cavity as in the lower canines of hippos (Figure 6.12 **A, B**), in depressions on the forming face, or be firmly embedded in the core dentine as in hippo upper incisors (Figure 6.12 **C, D**). Some are spindle-shaped or like stalactites rather than spheres. Their growth layers are deposited from the inside to the outside like pearls rather than from the outside inwards like geodes. Some also have concentric banding (Figure 6.12 **E, F**). Most have radial dentinal tubules, but some are like the cores of walrus teeth, lacking tubules and banding (Figure 6.12 **G**, 18 **A, B, C**). Both tusks and teeth of the walrus have a core of many small clear pearls as a characteristic feature, giving them a unique translucent "frog spawn-like" appearance (Figure 6.12 **H**).

6. 5. Walrus
Introduction

"A loaf of bread, the Walrus said, Is what we chiefly need: ... Now if you're ready Oysters dear, We can begin to feed."
The Walrus and the Carpenter
Lewis Carroll. 1832–1898

Walrus is a corruption of the Norse word *"Valross"* meaning whale-horse, an apt name for a 2,000Kg animal that both swims in the sea (elegantly) and runs on ice and land (floppily). Morse, an old word derived from *"Morsa,"* the Lappish word for walrus, is now rarely used.

Walrus are exclusive to the Arctic. There are two species and a subspecies, (or two subspecies and a race). The Pacific walrus, *Odobaenus rosmarus divergens* L. 1758

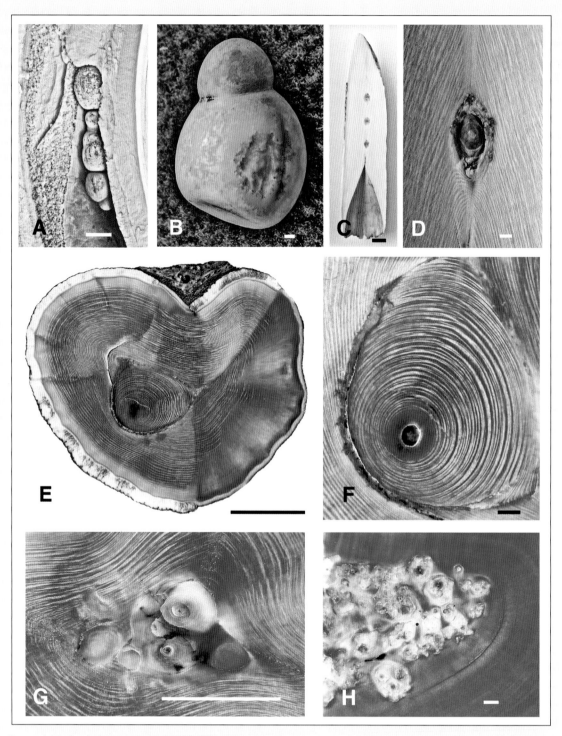

Figure 6.12. Pearl-like concretions in Ivory. A. Hippo lower canine broken to show pearls in the lumen. B. loose pearl from A. C, D. Longitudinal profile of hippo upper first incisor with "pearls" lacking dentinal tubules embedded in the core. E. Transverse profiles of hippo upper canine with transverse profile of a spindle shaped pearl. F. The pearl in E has concentric bands and dentinal tubules. G. Transverse profile showing several pearls in the center of an upper canine from the Giant forest hog that resemble the core of a walrus tusk except that they have dentinal tubules. H. The core ivory of walrus teeth and tusks is made up of many small pearls. Transverse profile of tusk. A–D unstained. E–H methylene blue stained. Scale bars. A, C, E, G = 1cm, B, D, F, H = 1mm.

(= *O. robesus*) is larger than the Atlantic walrus *Odobaenus r. rosmarus* Illiger, 1815. *Odobaenus rosmarus laptevi* Chapskii, 1940, is a race from the Laptev Sea in the Russian Arctic. Pacific walrus extend from the Russian and Alaskan coasts east and west of Wrangel Island in the north through the straights south into the Bering Sea. Atlantic walrus are more split up, extending from the shores of Baffin Island to Greenland to Svalbard, the Barents Sea, Novaya Zemlya, and the Kara Sea (61). The evolutionary history of walruses parallels that of mammoths, which died out in Siberia only to be repopulated from North America. Ancestral walrus once lived throughout the northern Arctic but died out in the Pacific, which was later recolonized by the Atlantic population (61).

All walruses have suffered from commercial exploitation of their ivory, oil from blubber, meat, bones, and skins in the nineteenth and early twentieth centuries. Commercial walrus hunting is now illegal, but native populations are still allowed to kill small numbers regulated by their countries resource managers (U.S., Russia, Canada, Denmark). Populations rebounded as ivory became walrus' only valuable contribution to modern economies. However, the scarcity of ivory due to the decline in elephant populations from the mid-nineteenth century led to more Atlantic walrus being hunted for their tusks. At least 100,000 were killed between 1870 and 1880 for their ivory. Since global trade in ivory was restricted by a CITES 3 listing, they may have fared better, but they now number less than 20,000, split among eight subpopulations. The Laptev race is down to 5–10,000. Pacific walrus have fared the best, numbering perhaps 200,000. Neme gives a good account of the problems besetting walrus (95).

The former habitat of walruses was on shelving coastal beaches, feeding on bottom living shellfish at depths of less than 300 feet [ninety meters]. As a result of human predation, they took to spending more time on nearby ice floes, helped by the functions of their tusks as aids to climbing onto the ice and as picks to create and enlarge breathing holes. Bulls also use them to fight rivals. Less certain is their role in disturbing bivalves from the sea bottom. Global warming is a new threat. The disappearance of coastal ice is forcing them further out onto floes over water too deep for easy fishing.

Tusk structure

Tusk size and shape. The canine tusks of both bulls and cows curve down and slightly inwards (Figure 6.13 A). They lie forward and outside the other teeth, incisors and three somewhat smaller premolars (Figure 6.13 B). The lower jaw has canines and three premolars. Bulls have the larger tusks, with record lengths of 60–80cms for Atlantic walrus and 80–90cms for the longer but more slender Pacific tusks. Those from cows are smaller, 40–50cms. Record tusks may weigh 4–5Kg (135) but 2–3Kg is a more common weight for a contemporary 60–80cm tusk.

Enamel/cementum distribution. Both teeth and tusks are covered with cementum that varies in thickness, wearing to a thin layer in older tusks (Figure 6.13 E) but up to 2cms wide in teeth and some tusks (Figure 6.13 C, D). Both upper and lower teeth (incisor and premolars) have a very thick cementum extending over the sides, sealing off the pulp cavity, leaving the teeth rootless, like small pebbles that become progressively shorter with wear. The pearly core is harder than cementum and dentine, causing it to project above the flattened crown as it wears down. Sealed off teeth also occur in Odontoceti such as the beluga whale (*Delphinapterus leucas*) and deserve further study.

Dentine and the pearly core. Dentine between the cementum and the pearly core consists of radial dentinal tubules angled at about 900 to the growth layers, giving them a forward slant pointing towards the tusk tip. The tubules are branched just below the cementum (Figure 6.14 B). New layers are added at the base, causing growth in length rather than widening. The matrix around tubules is often pearly white due to

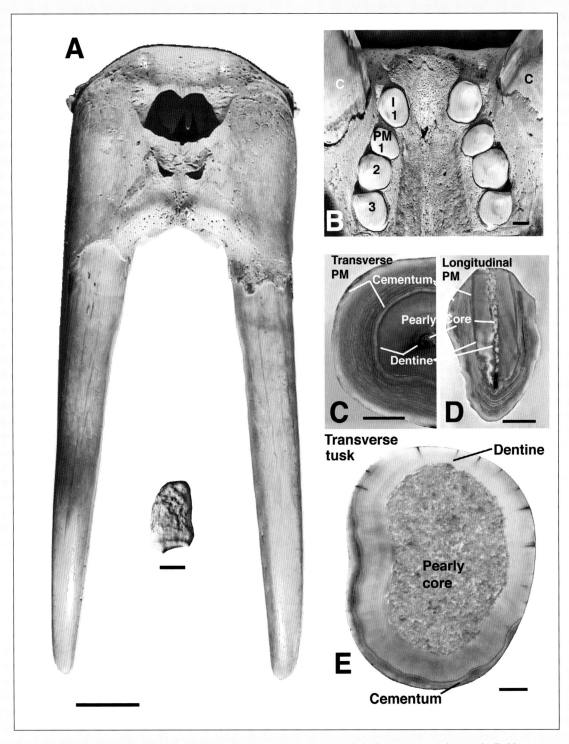

Figure 6.13. Walrus tusks and teeth. A. Atlantic walrus canine tusks and skull. Inset, premolar tooth. B. Upper jaw viewed from below. C = Canine tusks, I = incisor, PM = premolar. C, D. Premolars. All the teeth have a very thick cementum, wider than the dentine layer and a characteristic pearly core. In mature teeth, the crown is worn down to expose the pearly core. The cementum may cover over the pulp cavity. Methylene blue stain. E. Transverse profile of canine tusk showing cementum outside the rather thin layer of dentine and the extensive pearly core characteristic of walrus termed secondary dentine by (35). Unstained natural colors of old ivory. Scale bars. A, = 5cms, inset 1cm. B, C, E. = 1cm. D. = 1mm.

an abundance of calcospherites (Figure 6.14 D). This has an effect like that in pigs, causing the tubules to be grouped into skeins rather than laminae (Figure 6.14 C, E). The dentine continues as a thin layer about 1 cm wide below the cementum (Figure 6.13 A, 14 E). Teeth as well as tusks have the characteristic, unique walrus pearly core conventionally termed secondary dentine (35). However, the pearly core is not secondary in the sense that secondary is distinct from primary in bone development. Secondary bone is a replacement for primary bone but the pearly core is a structure in its own right, deposited in the core at a particular stage of development. The tip of a walrus tusk below the cementum has dentine or dentine with only a string-like pearly core for about 20 cms, after which the pulp cavity fills with the pearly concretions that may come to occupy 60–80% of the diameter (Figure 6.13 E). Most of the concretions are concentric spheres, appearing with similar profiles in transverse, radial and tangential orientations, but a few are cylindrical, mixed with blood vessels typical of pulp cavities (Figure 6.14 F, G). Most are translucent and lack dentinal tubules, but some large ones have concentric calcified bands. They are embedded in sheaves of tubules curving around them, mixed with large calcospherites, often separated by air spaces. The reflections from calcification and air spaces create a peculiar whiteness.

The core of spheres in matrix sheathed by a cylinder of dentine may allow toughness by minimizing potential fracture planes. The core of dentine spheres in matrix, and dentinal tubules with calcospherites in matrix, may be thought of as two levels of miniaturization of reinforced concrete-like structures.

6.6. Pigs, Suidae

"How d'you explain the Indian Hog?" He cried. How d'you account for its two bent teeth, more than a yard long, growing upwards from its upper jaw?"
"To defend itself?"

"No young man, it has two tusks for that purpose issuing from its lower jaw like those of a common boar. ... No, the answer is that the animal sleeps standing up and, in order to support its head, it hooks its upper tusks on the branches of trees...for the Designer of the World has given thought even to the hog's slumbers!"
J.G.Farrel's 1973 portrait of a Paley trained divine in The Siege of Krishnapur.

Introduction
On first reading, this description of hog's teeth has little truth, being merely succor for Paley's followers or contemporary creationists. Could its tusks really be a yard long? In Indo-Pacific regions hogs were bred for their long lower tusks and reared to prevent their tips from wearing away in foraging. The tusks then grew back on themselves to make a closed circle that could make a bracelet about 4 inches in diameter or a ring strong enough to hang a hog or a very heavy curtain (Figure 6.16). The most prized were those that continued their growth to make two or three tusk circles. About two and a half turns would be almost a yard long. This was the kind of bracelet that Luther bought from Bloody Mary—"Say, is that a boar's tooth bracelet on your wrist?"—in the song from Rodgers and Hammerstein's South Pacific.

Wild boars (Sus scrofa) are natives from Europe and North Africa to the Pacific with a separate species (Sus cristatus) in India, Ceylon, and Burma, along with numerous subspecies. Their domestic descendants and feral offspring are now worldwide. All have lower tusks longer than upper tusks. Bushpigs (Potamochoerus porcus) and warthogs (Phacochoerus africanus and P. eotheopicus) occupy similar ecological niches in Africa south of the Sahara. Tusks are present in most pigs only in males, but both sexes have them in warthogs. Their upper tusks are larger than lower ones and are those most commonly used for stick or corkscrew handles. None of these pigs is threatened with immediate extinction. The giant forest hog (Hylochoerus meinertzhageni) was only discovered in 1904, but is widespread in tropical equatorial forests from Kenya to Liberia. Unlike other pigs, its upper tusks have enamel as well as cementum. Both its upper and lower tusks are massive, the uppers weighing as much as 500 gms.

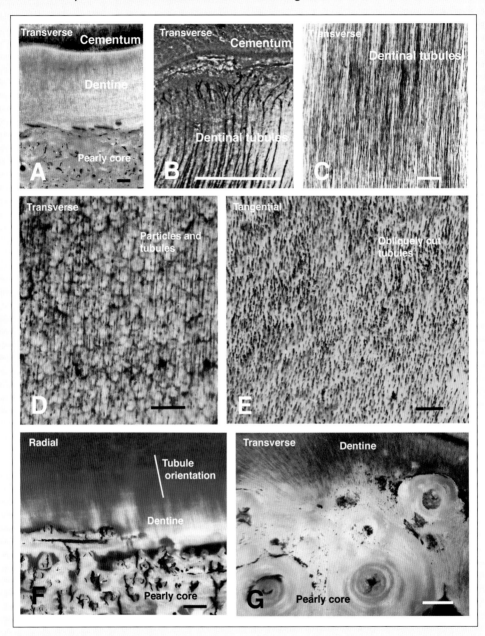

Figure 6.14. The structure of a walrus tusk. A. The tusk consists of cementum, dentine, and a pearly core. B. The dentinal tubules are branched at the junction with the cementum. C. Transverse profiles cut the dentinal tubules into lengths as expected for an orientation angled to transverse. D. Granules are abundant and strongly calcified in some regions causing the tubules to be skeined as in pigs. E. Tangential profiles of dentine cut the tubules obliquely, confirming their orientation angled to transverse. The tubules are clumped in skeins rather than aligned in laminae. F. A few "pearls" are profiles of cylinders, but most are approximately spherical. They are translucent or calcified, resistant to staining that shows up dentine and tubules. Marker pen staining penetrates local cracks through the calcified pearls that fail to propagate. G. Pearls in the core are surrounded by swirls of dentinal tubules. Staining fills the air pockets around the calcified particles as well as tubules. Scale bars. A, F, G = 1mm. B, C, D, E = 100⌈m.

Although their small size and curved structure limits their use, the wide distribution of pigs, both native species (Table 6.1) and many feral descendants of domestic varieties, has ensured the use of their tusks in many cultures around the world. Species differ in size, weight, thickness, shape of cross sections, and the relative tusk sizes, but are similar in many fundamental features (Table 6. 3). Cross sections of the lower tusks are triangular while the uppers are rounded rectangles with a waist that becomes more obvious with increasing size. The upper and lower tusks differ in their curvature, their shape and enamel/cement distribution, and in the tubule patterns of their dentine. Their dentine is characterized by having many spherites, forcing the tubules into irregular skeins and curls, suggesting a step to the waved tubules of hippos and elephants.

Record Tusk sizes of Hippos and Pigs (cms)

Suidae	Upper canines	Lower canines
Wild boar *Sus scrofa*, L.		33
Crested Wild boar, *Sus cristatus*, L.		**37.5**
Bushpig, *Potamochoerus porcus*, L.	8.9	16.5
Giant Forest Hog, *Hylochoerus meinertzhageni.*	26.7	22.9
Wart hog, *Phacocoerus africanus*,	68.6	24.1
Babirusa, *Babyrousa babyrussa*,	43.2	34.3
Hippopotamidae	Lower incisor	Lower canine
Hippopotamus, *Hippopotamus amphibius*, L.	54.6	163.8
Pygmy hippopotamus, *Choeropsis liberiensis*,		73.7

Table. 6.3. Pig and hippo records.

Tusk type	Straight	Straight	Curved	Curved helical Left Right
Profile transverse to tusk	Circular	Elliptical	Elongate elliptical	Skewed elongate elliptical
Profile transverse to tusk axis	‖	‖	More elongate	More skewed, elongate and elliptical
Symmetry	Symmetrical	4 - fold	Bilateral	Assymetric to tusk center
Column orientation	Transverse	Transverse	Transverse and oblique	Transverse oblique and skewed

Table 6.4. The influence of tusk shape on pattern symmetry. The table illustrates the complexity introduced in the changes from circular cross section to elliptical cross section, elliptical cross sections increased by tusk curvature, to elliptical cross section with a helical twist. Proboscidean tusks are all to some degree in the latter category, although the helix may not be pronounced. These tusk differences all affect measurements of ridge frequency, column dimensions, Schreger angles and ellipse dimensions. Most such measurements require positional provenance for them to become reliable discriminators between Proboscidean taxa.

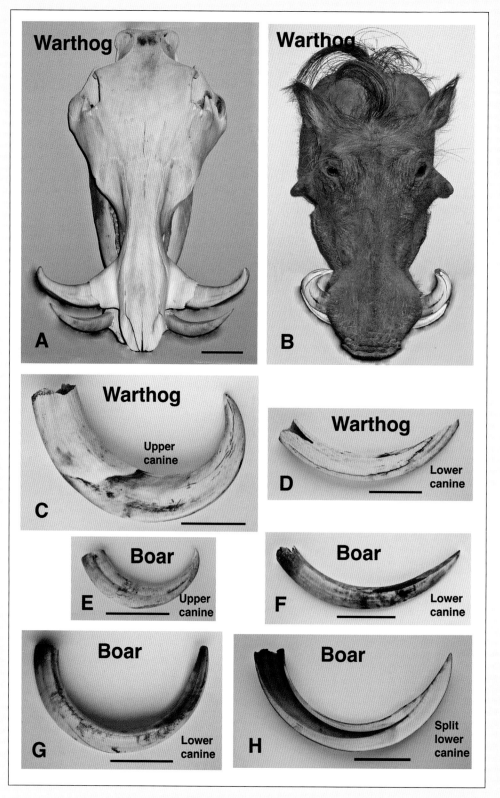

Figure 6.15. The ivory of pigs comes from upper and lower canine tusks. A. Warthog skull and B. Warthog head. C. Warthog left upper canine. D. Warthog left lower canine. The lower canines are much smaller than the upper ones. E. Wild boar, right upper canine. F, G. Wild boar, right lower canine. In boars, the lower canines are much longer than the upper ones. H. Wild boar, natural longitudinal fracture showing the extent of the pulp cavity. Scale bars = 5 cms.

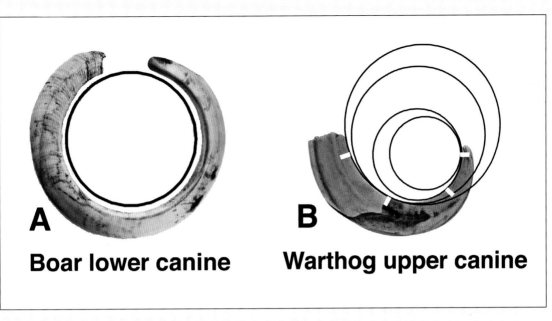

A

Boar lower canine

B

Warthog upper canine

Figure 6.16. The upper and lower canines of pigs differ in their growth. A. Boar lower left canine. Lower canines grow upwards and outwards in a closed circular path with a diameter constant for each tusk but varying in diameter in different species and races. Growth is in a flat plane. The almost complete absence of a twist ensures that if they are prevented from wearing down at the tips they will grow in complete circles or even several circles. Right side view. B. Warthog right upper canine. The upper canines grow upwards and outwards but in an open circular path the diameter of which increases with age. Positions matching the curvature of four circles of increasing diameter are marked on the curved tusk. Growth is in a spiral, with a right handed clockwise twist on right side tusks and a left handed counterclockwise twist on left side tusks. Right side view.

Curvature and tusk growth

The lower canines grow upwards and outwards from the massive lower jaws adapted to hold them (Figure 6.15, 16). Depending on wear at the tip, half the tusk may be below the gumline. They grow continuously in an almost exact circle in the same plane, species and races differing in the diameter of the circle. The constant curvature and the almost complete absence of a twist ensures that If basal growth is not compensated by wear at the tip the tusks will curl back on themselves in a flat helix like Luther's bracelet.

The upper canines also grow upwards and outwards but they follow an elliptical path with age as if following circles progressively increasing in diameter (Figure 6.16). Growth also differs from that in the lower canines in not being in one plane but helical, with a right-handed clockwise twist on right side tusks and a left-handed counterclockwise twist on left side tusks. The result is a loose open curve pointing the tusk up and away from the head.

The lower canines

Tusk shape and enamel/cementum distribution. The lower tusks are formidable sharp spikes weighing up to 150 gms but with a lighter construction than the upper ones. They are economical with their dentine, which forms a shell rarely more than 1 cm thick around a pulp cavity that occupies as much as 4/5th of the tusk length (Figure 6.15 H). The cross-section is triangular with the wider rounded surface innermost and the other two shorter sides outermost (Figure 6.17 A). In this they resemble hippopotamus', with an open V-shaped forming face accommodating the triangular profile of the tusk. The outer very flat surface is in line with the jaw and the third occlusal face is on the inner curve. All three faces have a covering barely 0.5 mm thick (enamel or cementum), much thinner than that of the upper canines. Enamel on two faces takes a high polish and often shows growth increments. The concave side of the curved tusk is covered with cementum as in hippo lower canines (Fig. 6.17 A). In transverse profile the enamel layer has a characteristic rounded edge that curves below the cementum in both upper and lower canines (Figures 6.17 A insert and 6.18 D). The enamel surfaces are prone to fracture longitudinally, carrying a layer of dentine with them (Figure 6.15 H).

Growth layers. Growth layers in boars and warthogs are about 40 mm wide, parallel to the forming face (Figure 6.17 A insert), and often grouped together into broader layers that probably record seasonal growth. The layers may be calcified but there are no irregular broad bands like those in the lower canines and hippos.

Dentinal tubule orientation patterns. The basic orientation of pig dentinal tubules is like that in many teeth, including whales, radial with a forward slant from the forming face towards the tusk tip. The tubules are not in ordered laminar arrays like those in hippos and elephants (Figures 6.22 D, 6.30 B) but in skeins (Figure 6.17 E, F). A characteristic of pigs is that their dentine matrix contains many spherites that force the tubules into irregular paths bundled together into skeins, especially just below the cementum/enamel layer. The skeins are oriented radial/diagonal to the tusk axis from the core to the cementum as in a series of funnels stacked one above the other, except for the distortion introduced by the triangular cross-section (Figure 6.17 D). Transverse profiles in the middle of the V-shaped forming face (Figure 6.17 C) cut the skeins into short overlapping sections oriented at about 90^0 to both the forming face and the enamel/cementum. The distortion from the V rather than the O shape in transverse profile results in these overlapping skein sections fanning out at the tips of the triangles (Figure 6.17 B, C). Axial profiles show the tubules curving forward to make an acute angle with the surface (Figure 6.17 D).

(Opposite page)
Figure 6.17. Pig lower canines. A. Like most pigs, boar lower canines have a triangular cross section and a very thin coat of cementum covering the concave face of the curved tusk with enamel on the other two sides. The forming face is a wide V shape with few nerve spaces penetrating a dentine that has growth layers but lacks calcified bands. A, C. Tubules extend at about 900 from the forming face to the surface in the middle of the triangle, fanning out and curving to make more acute angles with the surface towards the tips of the triangles. Inset, growth bands are about 40 mm wide. Scale bar = 100 mm. B. Tubules make an acute angle with the forming face at the tips of the triangles where they are embedded with many particles that separate the tubules into skeins. Transverse profiles of boar lower canines. D. Longitudinal profiles show that the tubules also fan out axially. E. In tangential views the skeins appear as clusters of transversely cut tubules bundled together and in rings around the particles, unlike the ordered laminar arrays in elephant ivory portrayed in Figure 6.16 B. F. Transverse profiles cut tubule bundles obliquely. Marker pen and methylene blue stain. Scales A = 1 cm. B = 1 mm, E, F = 100 mm.

Pig lower canines

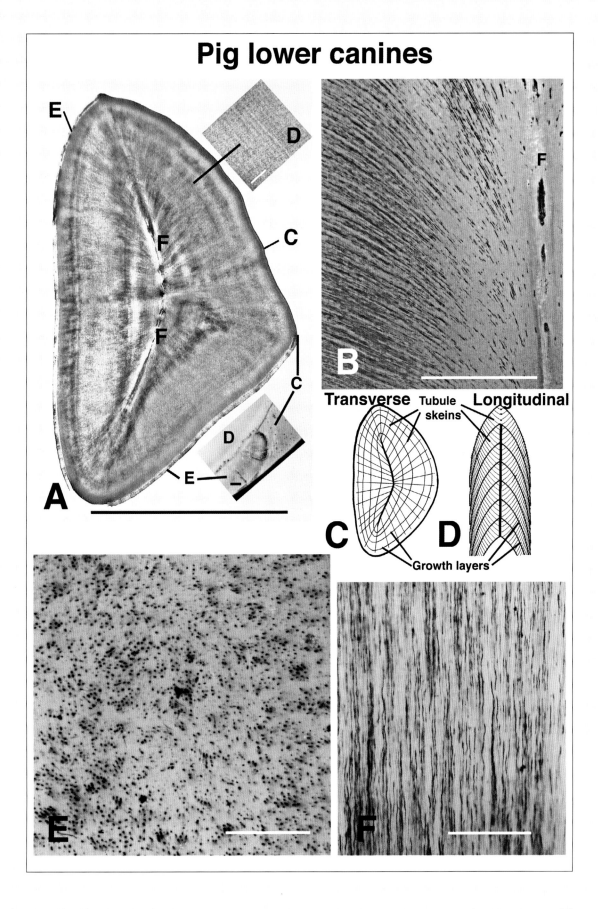

Transverse — Tubule skeins — Longitudinal

Growth layers

The upper canines

Tusk shape. The upper canines are robust, weighing about 500 gms in a giant forest hog, giving a curved ivory block up to 4 cms across. Warthogs are smaller, weighing 150 gms and 3 cms across. Most boars, even trophies, are smaller still. They have a polygonal cross section with a pulp cavity half the tusk length. Nerve channels extend from the forming face into the dentine below each of the lobes, especially in the giant forest hog, suggesting that the upper canines may be sensory. The thick cementum of the upper canines is a marked contrast to the thin layer in lower canines. Boars and warthogs only have cementum (Figure 6.18 A). The giant forest hog differs from boars and warthogs in having enamel (Figure 6.18 B, C, D). The rounded edge of the enamel layer curves below the cementum in the same characteristic way as it does in the lower canines. The big differences in gross structure between upper and lower canines may be related to their use, the uppers needing strength for rooting and the lowers long rapier-like points for defense.

Growth layers and banding. Pigs are like hippos in having growth layers and bands. In boars and warthogs, **growth layers** are narrow and deposited synchronously at the forming face as they are in the lower canines. **Bands** are deposited asynchronously, angled to the forming face like those of hippos. They are wider, less regular than growth layers, fusing and separating from one another (Figures 6.18 C, E; 6.19 C).

Curly tubules. Setting the dentinal tubules in a granular matrix favors their tendency to skein. Such an amorphous matrix may also give the tubules the three-dimensional freedom to form curls, as happens more in the upper than the lower tusks and more in the series boar—warthog—giant forest hog. The curls are smaller and much less regular than the waves of hippos. Although the tubules are approximately radial, the planes in which their direction changes are transverse as well as radial, making them curls rather than waves (Figure 6.19 C). The small size of the curls allows some of them to be resolved as continuously curving tubules (Figure 6.19 D). These curls are not composite images created by overlapping short lengths with different orientations. Tangential profiles of curly tubules appear as spots with tails pointing in various directions. The curls do not line up in laminae, as in hippos and elephants, but appear as swirls in tangential profiles (Figure 6.19 E).

Calcification. As in hippos, shining banded regions of calcification correspond with waves and bands positioned independently of growth layers (Figure 6.19 A, F, G, H). Calcification occurs especially in and around the dentinal tubules preferentially at particular positions in relation to the waves, giving rise to the banding pattern. Understanding the difference between growth layers and bands illuminates a general principle of ivory growth. Layering from an epithelium is a uniform process across the surface. Spatial and temporal differences in the material laid down result in characteristic structures such as bands, Schreger patterns and sheets of calcification.

The small curls shown by pig tubules suggest how the more complex patterns in hippos and elephants might have evolved in a series beginning with straight radial transverse (human), straight radial diagonal

(Opposite page)
Figure 6.18. Pig upper canines. A. Upper canines of boars and warthogs are more robust, with a thick cementum but no enamel. Nerve channels extend from the forming face into the dentine below each of the lobes. Calcified bands occur in the inner half. Warthog transverse profile. B, C, The upper canines of the giant forest hog are even more robust, with very thick cementum or enamel. Nerve spaces are more pronounced than in warthogs, suggesting that the upper canines may be sensory. Calcified bands occur through most of the thickness, but especially towards the core that often contains "pearls." D. The rounded edge of the enamel layer curves below the cementum in a characteristic way. Transverse profile of the junction between the thick enamel and cementum layers in a giant forest hog. E. Narrow parallel growth layers below the cementum become wider and more calcified towards the core, replaced by less regular growth bands. Radial profile of giant forest hog. Methylene blue and black marker pen stain. Scale bars A–C = 1 cm, D – 1 mm. E = 2 mm.

Pig upper canines

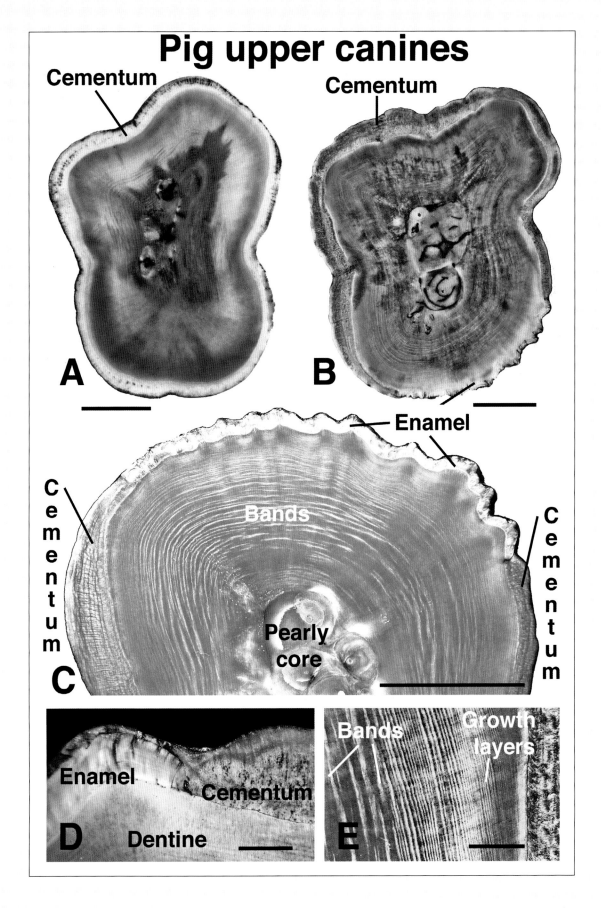

Cementum

Cementum

Enamel

Cementum

Cementum

Bands

Pearly
core

Enamel

Cementum

Dentine

Bands

Growth
layers

A

B

C

D

E

Waved tubules and bands in Pig ivory

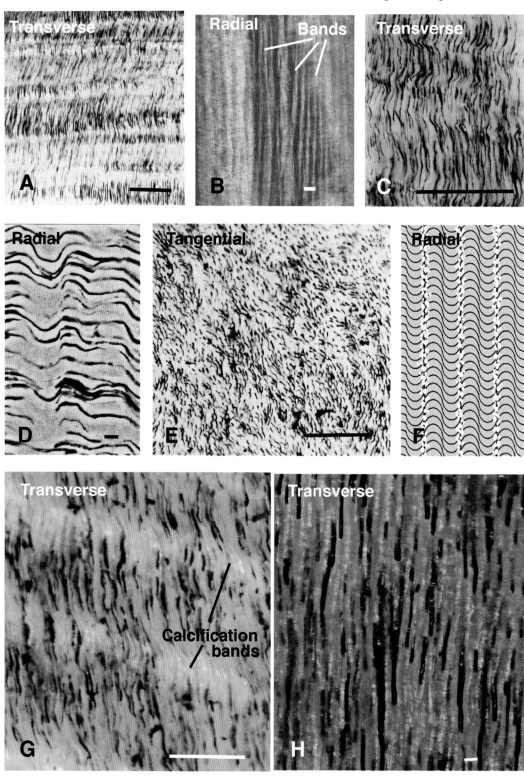

(orca), irregular radial diagonal (pigs), curly radial diagonal (pigs), parallel axial/wavy radial diagonal (pigs), enlarged wavy (hippo), out of phase waves (elephants). This is not an evolutionary series but illustrates how tubules might have appeared in their evolution from straight rods to out of phase waves in laminae.

6.7. Hippopotamus

There are two kinds of hippo, the pygmy hippo, *Choeropsis liberiensis*, Morton and the commoner one, *Hippopotamus amphibius*, L. The pygmy hippo is now rare, living singly or in pairs in West African wet forests. Its decline is probably from hunting for bush meat and habitat loss due to human encroachment on its wet forest habitat, as it is not known for its ivory. The common hippo is aquatic, leaving rivers to forage for vegetation at night. It lives in large groups where clusters of males surround the females and young. It used to be much more abundant, stretching in historical

(Opposite page)
Figure 6.19. Dentinal tubule arrangement and banding in pig upper canines. A, B. Calcified bands occur preferentially at particular positions in relation to tubule waves. Regions of calcification and denser staining seen as bands in transverse (A. Giant forest hog), and radial profiles (B. Warthog), correspond to waves in dentinal tubules and are much wider than growth layers (insert in Figure 6.38 A). Bands are angled to the forming face and separate and rejoin with one another. C. Waves are smaller and much less regular than those in hippos. Although the tubules are radial, the plane of the wave varies, allowing waves to appear in transverse as well as radial profiles—giant forest hog. D. The small size of the waves allows them to be seen as continuously curving tubules and not from composite overlapping short lengths as in hippos—warthog. E. Transverse profiles of wavy tubules appear as spots with tails having many different orientations. The waves do not line up in laminae as in hippos and elephants, but appear as swirls in tangential profiles—giant forest hog. G. Calcified bands result from deposition at similar positions on the tubule waves—giant forest hog. F. Diagrammatic interpretation of the relation between calcification and tubule waves in giant forest hog. Calcification occurs especially in and around the dentinal tubules—warthog. Methylene blue and black marker pen stain. Scales bars D, H = 10 mm, others 100 mm.

times from Palestine down the Nile to most large rivers south of the Sahara to the Cape. It was worked and traded from prehistoric times in Greece (64) and Egypt (55). Now, it is a vulnerable species on the IUCN Red List, restricted to river systems across central Africa from Southern Sudan in the north to the Zambesi in the south with an estimated population in 2006 of 125,000 to 150,000.

Hippos have a mouthful of ivory, but the largest pieces come from the lower second incisors and the upper and lower canines (Figure 6.20). Most of the teeth/tusks have broad longitudinal strips of enamel continuous with the cementum over the rest of the surface. The pattern of enamel/cementum is approximately, but not exactly, the same for each kind of tusk. For example, the lower first incisor always lacks enamel, the upper canine only has cementum on the inner lingual surface, while a strip of enamel may be present or absent on the upper second incisor. The arrangement of these enamel strips is interesting in that it correlates with the kind of ivory below. Ivory below enamel is banded. Below cementum, there are only growth layers at first, bands appearing later towards the core. The enamel is hard, giving rise to a common myth that hippo ivory can be used to create sparks when struck sharply with an iron tool. The real ivory below the enamel is, of course, as soft and easy to work with metal tools as other ivories. The smaller teeth have a thin cementum layer only 0.5–1 mm thick with an enamel layer up to twice as wide raised above the surface. Some have a helical twist. Larger tusks have thicker enamel (1.5–2 mm) raised above the surface of the even thicker cementum (2–3 mm). Raised enamel surfaces, like the strip on the second upper incisor, are not just due to wear on the softer cementum since they occur even below the gumline. As happens in many herbivores, the leading enamel edges becomes like sharp knives as the teeth wear down. Longitudinal profiles show the enamel in units probably correlated with daily growth layer increments of the dentine. The canines and incisors differ from one another in many ways. The canines

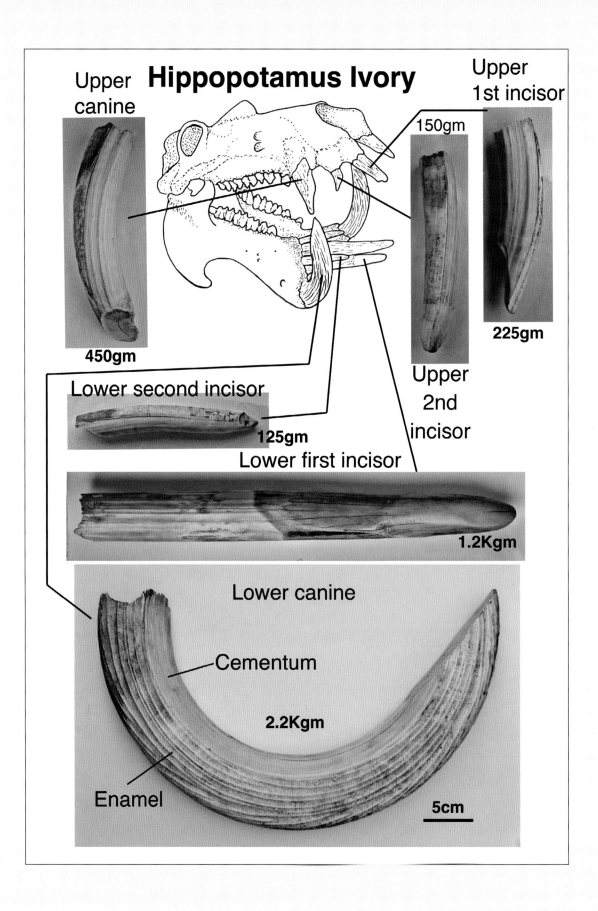

Hippopotamus Ivory

Upper canine

450gm

Upper 1st incisor

150gm

225gm

Lower second incisor

125gm

Upper 2nd incisor

Lower first incisor

1.2Kgm

Lower canine

Cementum

2.2Kgm

Enamel

5cm

(known in the trade as "lowers") are curved almost in a circle that commonly grow to 70 cms long (outside edge) and 7.5 x 5.5 cms wide with a strongly patterned enamel surface on two outer sides of their triangular cross-sections. Record tusks measure up to 165 cms (135). They are prone to longitudinal cracking. Their ivory has strong bands set off by shining white calcification throughout, except for a layer about 3 mm wide below the cementum on the shorter inner face. These bands were called growth bands (73), an inappropriate term for the reasons given below. Here they will be called bands to distinguish them from the much fainter growth layers that have a different distribution. The first incisors ("straights") are almost straight, with ridged cementum but no enamel. They may grow to be 50 cms long and 6 cms in diameter, looking like straight elephant or walrus tusks. They are unique among the hippo tusks in having easily resolved holes, presumably containing nerve endings radiating from the pulp cavity. Unlike the other tusks, they point forward rather than form an occlusive surface with their upper counterparts, also suggesting that they are sensory. Near the surface their ivory is white and almost featureless, with calcified bands only deposited towards the core. Hippo ivory is interesting in that its bands are not growth layers and that its dentinal tubules have both waves (correlated with bands) and simple arrangements (correlated with growth layers and a lack of bands).

The basic structures of hippo ivory

Like most ivory, that of hippos is a composite of three basic architectures: synchronously deposited layers mark cycles of growth, dentinal tubules have characteristic

orientation patterns, and calcified bands are deposited asynchronously from the growth layers. The nature of these three architectures and the way they interact give rise to two different kinds of ivory. The dentinal tubules may be 1) Simply oriented, often skeined, with poorly discernible growth layers and no bands, or 2) Waved with banding obscuring growth layers. The two kinds of ivory correlate with the overlying enamel or cementum. Simple layers lacking bands lie below cementum and banded waved regions lie below enamel (Figure 6.22 A).

Growth layers

The common features in all ivory are dentinal tubules, spherites, and matrix (Figure 6.2). These components are deposited synchronously at a growth zone, leaving layers parallel to the forming face in a series of conical shells, like a record of tree rings. In hippos, this ring structure is not easily discernible. Faint layers having little structural differentiation occur below the cementum for about one third of the distance to the center of the lower incisor tusk (Figure 6.21 A, B, C). Radial profiles show layers 40–100 ⌈m wide parallel to the forming face comparable to the daily growth layers in elephant ivory. Artifacts made from tusks of this kind can be difficult to identify as ivory because they are almost featureless.

Dentinal tubule orientation—Simple non-banded ivory

In most teeth, such as the human molar in Figure 6.22 B, dentinal tubules extend from below the enamel to the forming face in almost straight radial paths. There are some variations. They are often radial but angled forward in the axis from the forming face to the outer surface; when not close packed, individual tubules have room to depart somewhat from straight paths or to clump together in skeins. In simple, non-banded hippo ivory below cementum (Figure 6.22 A), profiles cut with various orientations all show tubules oriented at about 90^0 to the surface

Figure 6.20. Hippo tusks. Most hippo ivory comes from the lower canine (known in the trade as "lowers"), the lower incisors ("straights"), and the upper canines ("uppers"), but the other tusks are also used. The weights of the tusks figured give an idea of their relative importance. Except for the lower incisors, they are all covered by strips of enamel on the leading and outer edges, separated by strips of cementum. Wear on the dentine leaves a sharp enamel cutting edge.

(Figure 6.22 C–F). Tangential views show fields of dots representing transversely cut tubules (C) that may be skeined, like those in pigs or stacked into laminae in some regions. The forming face has longitudinal striations and lacks the patterns characteristic of tusks with banded ivory. Transverse (D) and radial profiles (E–F) both show lengths of tubule in side view. This, then, is the basic structure of simple hippo tusks or parts of tusks—cylinders of matrix reinforced by radial dentinal tubules.

The forming face below non-banded ivory is relatively smooth with no particular pattern. In contrast, the natural surface forming banded ivory, such as that at the base of the lower canine, shows dentinal tubules with the characteristic wavy pattern (Figure 6.23 A, B) similar to the forming face in elephants. Dentinal tubules in banded ivory are aligned in waves within planes of axial laminae.

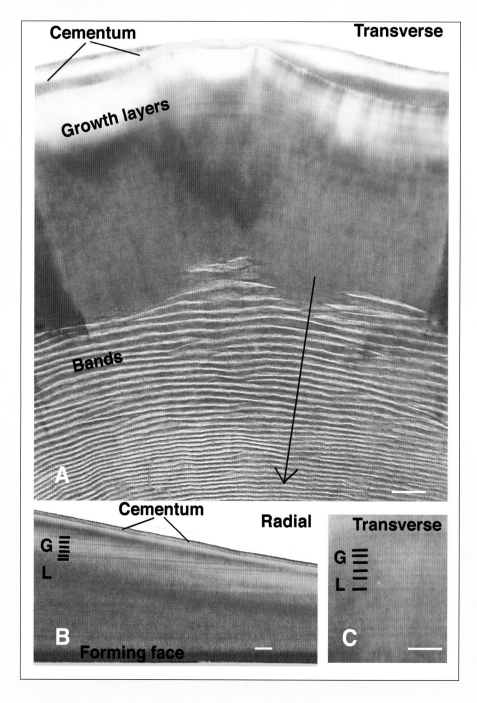

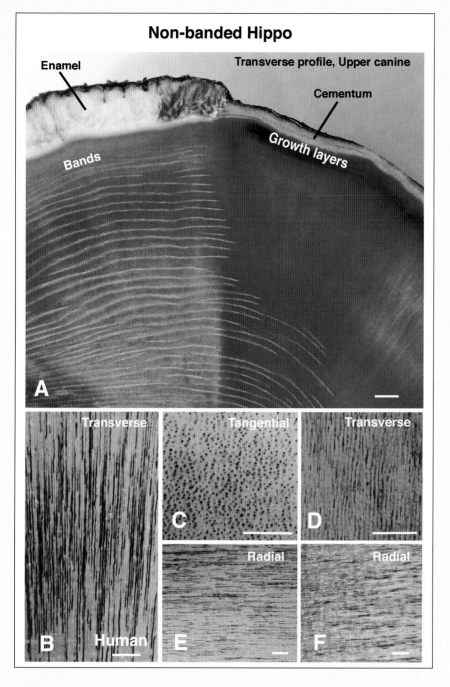

Non-banded Hippo

Enamel

Transverse profile, Upper canine

Cementum

Growth layers

Bands

A

Transverse

Tangential

Transverse

C

D

Radial

Radial

B   Human   E   F

Figure 6.22. Dentinal tubules are straight in non-banded hippo ivory. In non-banded regions below the cementum in the upper canine (A) or in the first lower incisor (C, D, E, F), dentinal tubules follow almost straight radial paths at about 900 to the surface. In this they resemble many teeth such as the human molar (B). A. Methylene blue stained transverse profile of an upper canine showing the two kinds of ivory. B–F. Marker pen staining to show the dentinal tubules. Scale bars = A = 1 mm, others = 100 mm.

(Opposite page)
Figure 6.21. Growth layers in hippo ivory. Growth layers are only resolvable below the cementum. Elsewhere, they are obscured by wide calcified bands at various angles to the forming face. A. The lower first incisor has cementum with no enamel. Bands appear late in development in the core, leaving growth layers visible in the outer cortex. The bands in the inner cortex become progressively narrower (arrow). Methylene blue stained transverse profile of a lower first incisor. B. Tusk diameter increases with the addition of new layers angled to the cementum and parallel to the forming face. Radial profile at the base of a lower first incisor. C. Faint layers 40–100 mm apart are probably daily growth increments. Occasional wider layers may record seasonal changes. Methylene blue stained transverse profile of a lower first incisor. Scale bars, A = 1 mm, others = 100 mm.

Banded Hippo

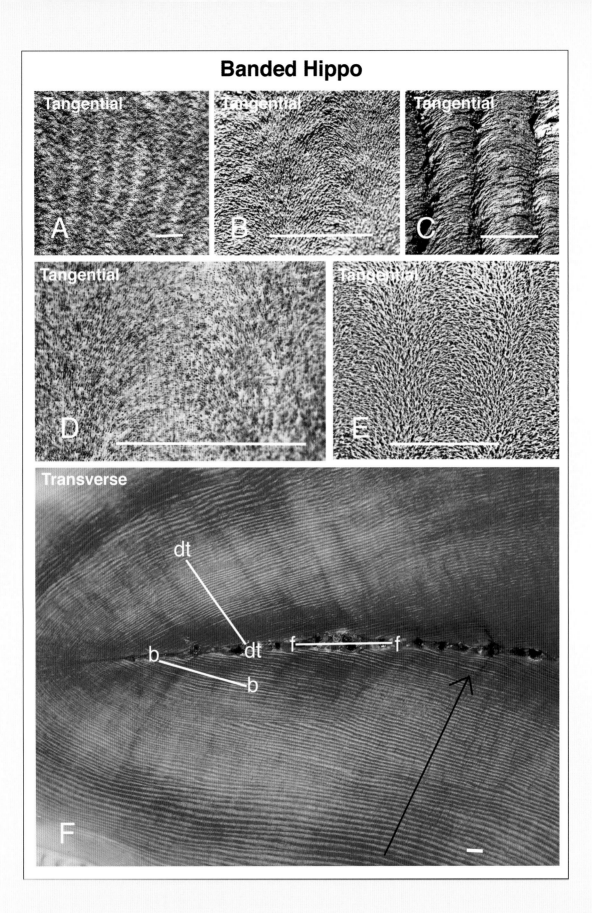

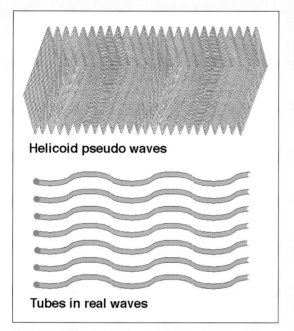

Helicoid pseudo waves

Tubes in real waves

Figure 6. 24. A, B. Helicoidal architecture is the structure achieved when parallel fibers form sheets that stack above one another in such a way that the orientation of the fibers changes in a regular manner from sheet to sheet, rotating through 1800 or 3600. Overlapping images of straight line profiles of the laminar components create profiles with characteristic curved patterns, such as chitin in insect cuticle and keratin in hooves (75). C. The waved patterns of tubules in hippo and proboscidean ivory do not result from helicoidal arrangements (131) but from waved tubules.

(Opposite page)

Figure 6.23. Dentinal tubules are waved in banded hippo ivory from the first lower canine. A, B. The natural forming surface at the base of the lower canine has the characteristic pattern expected to result from waved tubules. Surface irregularity contrasted by ink. C. Surface from a lower canine fractured tangentially shows patterns similar to those seen on the forming face. Ink contrasted. D. Stained tangential profiles have the characteristic curved patterns due to overlapping short lengths of curved dentinal tubules. Marker pen stain. E. Reflection image of an undercut tangential profile similar to D. F. In transverse profiles of lower canine tusks the forming face (f-f), dentinal tubules in laminae (m-m), and bands (b-b) lie at different angles. Laminae lie at about 450 to the forming face, allowing the orientation of their dentinal tubules to show the pattern seen in the forming face (A, B) and in tangential profiles (C, D, E). Methylene blue stained. Scale bars = 1 mm.

Dentinal tubule orientation— Helicoids vs. Waves in banded ivory Helicoids

Promising ideas, more often than not, lead nowhere. That's the nature of scientific research.

The Fabric of the Cosmos, 2004
Brian Greene

Helicoidal architecture is the structure achieved when parallel fibers form sheets that stack above one another in such a way that the orientation of the fibers changes in a regular manner from sheet to sheet to achieve a rotation through 180^0 (Figure 6.24). Many profiles of structures with helicoidal architecture, such as chitin in insect cuticle and keratin in hooves, show curved patterns from overlapping images of straight line profiles of laminar components changing in their trajectory (75). It was proposed incorrectly (73) that the waved patterns in hippo and proboscidean ivory resulted from such helicoidal arrangements of dentinal tubules. Virag (131) building on the work of Raubenheimer (109, 110) has shown that proboscidean ivory is indeed made from waved tubules. The description below reinterprets the description of hippo and proboscidean ivory as due to waved tubules aligned in laminae.

Waves

Tangentially fractured surfaces show similar waves to those on the forming face (Figure 6.23 C). In tangential profiles, the dentinal tubules in banded ivory have the typical waved arrangement described below for elephants. Stained tubules show how their orientation gives rise to the characteristic curved waved pattern (Figure 6.23 D). Reflection images of the surface show the same pattern caused by undercutting of the surface around the tubules (Figure 6.23 E). The plane of the laminae in banded hippo ivory is often as much as 45^0 to the forming face (Figure 6.33 D), creating oblique profiles that emphasize the waved pattern (Figure 6.23

F), unlike elephants, where tangential profiles are close to 90⁰ to the radial direction, causing wave profiles to appear as lines in edge view (Figure 6.33 A).

We may conclude that the tubules in banded hippo ivory are in a waved pattern angled to the core (Figure 6.4) with tubules in adjacent laminae out of phase relative to a perfect radial profile.

Banding—the structural reinforcement around dentinal tubules in waved patterns

Bands are functional reinforcements longitudinal to the axis but angled to the growth zone and not parallel to the growth layers (Figure 6.25 C). Bands are not deposited synchronously. The forming face cuts across the bands in the same way that the forming face in elephants cuts across components of the Schreger pattern (Figure 6.25 A). Bands are correlated with the waved arrangement of tubules. In waved arrangements (see below for elephants), the adjacent tubules are in phase with one, giving rise to the characteristic pattern.

In some regions, short radial stacks of dentinal tubules group together in skeins (Figure 6.25 E). Other skeins form ragged waves intermediate in structure with the precise waves forming the banding pattern. Edges of the band sheets start, stop, and fuse together as if their component tubules are aligned in waves that change their height. (Figure 6.25 D, H). Bands in hippo ivory are repeating units in the same sense that the Schreger columns of elephants are repeating units. Calcification occurs fairly evenly in all components in most ivory, but in hippos the bands are preferentially calcified, giving the bright shining whiteness characteristic of hippo ivory (Figure 6.25 B, G, H). For a visualization of the band structure in three dimensions, imagine a cylinder wrapped in stacks of shallow, elongated platters that represent the bands. Now think of some of the platters with ghostly properties that allow them to merge into one another at their edges

to create VVV and XXX profiles where they fuse (Figure 6.25 B, D, F). Sims has pointed out that particular profiles of such fused bands can sometimes resemble VVV or XXX Schreger patterns, potentially causing species misidentification for customs authorities (118).

In hippos, as with any cylindrical structure secreted from the outside to the inside, the forming face gets progressively smaller. The number of dentinal tubules must therefore be progressively reduced from the periphery to the forming face. Hippos compensate for the reduced area of the forming face by narrowing the bands and reducing their number, some disappear and others fuse together (Figures 6.21 A and 6.23 F).

(Opposite page)
Figure 6.25. Bands in hippo ivory are correlated with wavy patterned dentinal tubules. A. In elephant ivory, the Schreger columns lie at an angle to the growth layers, showing that different columns and parts of columns can be deposited at the same time. Radial profile near the base of a tusk. B, C. Bands in hippo ivory lie at various angles to the tubules and the forming face, intersecting with growth layers (ends marked I), showing that their various components can all be deposited synchronously. D. Edges of the band sheets start, stop, and fuse together as if their component tubules are aligned in waves that change their height. Radial profile reflection image. E. In some regions, short radial stacks of dentinal tubules group together in skeins that form more ragged patterns. Tangential profile marker pen stained. F. The edges of bands may fuse or cross one another, creating VVV or XXX patterns in profile. Methylene blue stained transverse profile. G. The wave pattern is made from overlapping images of variously curved tubules in agreement with the interpretation in Figure 6.35. White speckles show calcification. Marker pen stained transverse profile. H. Bands consist of lighter regions containing spots of calcification alternating with denser regions having longer sections of tubules set at an angle. This pattern is consistent with a staggered wave pattern of tubules. Radial profile stained with trypan blue. Scale bars A, B, F = 1 mm, all others = 100 ʃm.

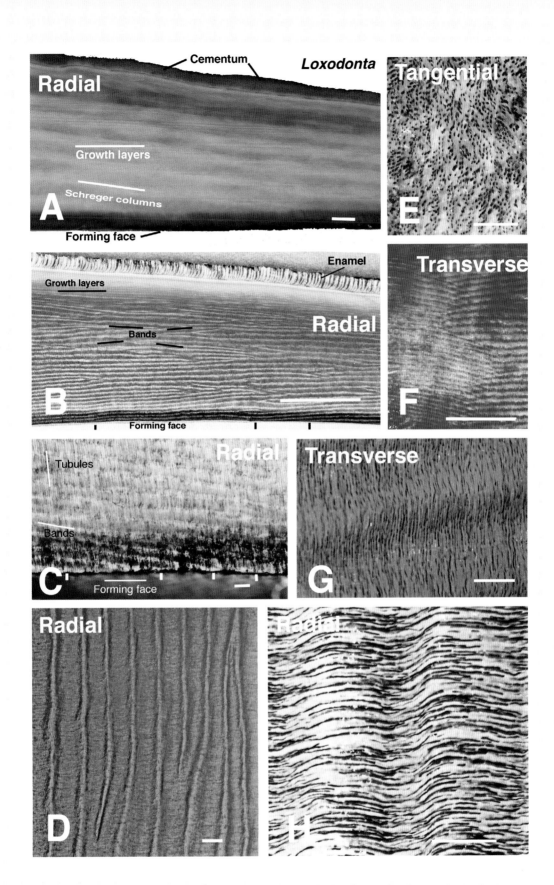

A Radial — *Loxodonta* — Cementum · Growth layers · Schreger columns · Forming face

E Tangential

B Radial — Growth layers · Enamel · Bands · Forming face

F Transverse

C Radial — Tubules · Bands · Forming face

G Transverse

D Radial

H Radial

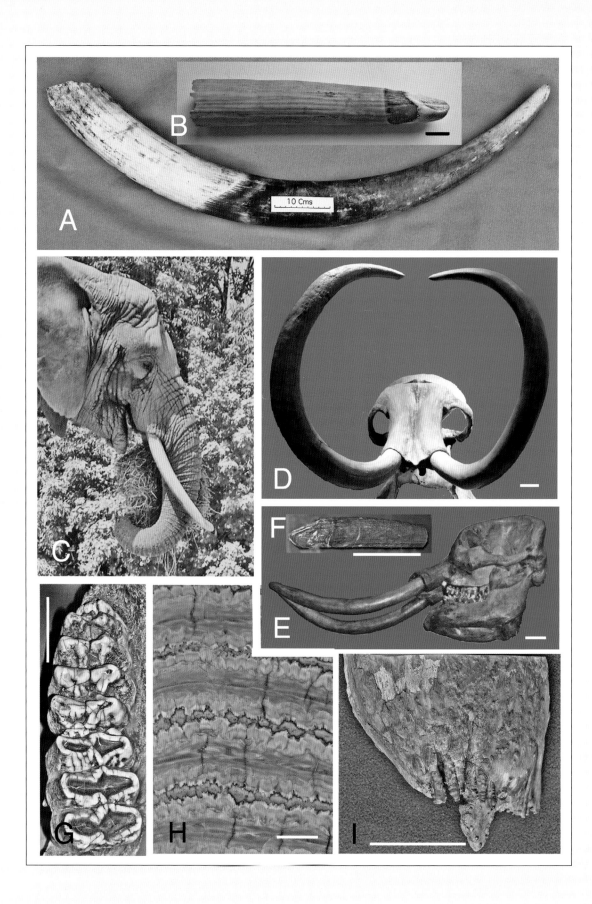

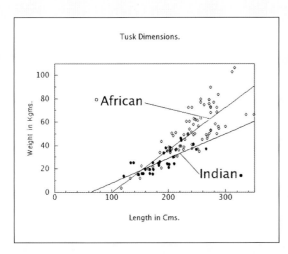

Tusk Dimensions.

Figure 6.27. Tusks from Asian elephants (*Elephas*) are smaller than those from African elephants (*Loxodonta*). Tusk weight is roughly correlated with length. Data from trophy tusks shot in the nineteenth century (135).

(Opposite page)
Figure 6.26. Tusks and teeth of Proboscidea. A, B, C. African elephant, *Loxodonta africana*, about 40% of the tusk is below the gumline. B. The emerging first tusk of an African elephant has a coat of enamel instead of cementum at its tip. An irregularly shaped milk tusk about half this size lies beside it at this stage. D. Mammoth, *Mammuthus sp*. E. Mastodon, *Mammut sp*. Upper and F, small tusks from lower jaw. G. A Mastodon molar tooth surface does not wear down like that in other elephants. It has a pattern most like that of an African elephant, with hard enamel standing proud of the cement and cementum. H. Polished surface of an Indian elephant molar, see Figure 6.9. I. The base of an abscessed mammoth tusk has eroded and been resecreted as a bulbous concretion, a massive example of dentine resorption and deposition. Scale = 10 cms except H = 1 cm.

6.8. Elephants, Mammoths and Mastodons

African Elephants

The commonest ivory in commercial use comes from elephants, mostly from Africa (Figure 6.26 A, C). African elephants have larger tusks than Indian elephants (Figure 6.27) and both sexes have large tusks. Even exports from Bombay were African ivory brought from the Congo through Mozambique and Zanzibar by slave and ivory traders like Tippoo Tib. The two species of African elephant diverged from a common ancestor about 2.6 million years ago. The savanna elephant *Loxodonta africana* is larger, with thicker and more curved tusks. Until tusk exploitation in the Industrial Revolution, it occupied all except the heavily forested areas of Africa. Fossil evidence suggests that it expanded its range at the end of the Pleistocene about 10,000 years ago, when its major competitor *Elephas iolensis* became extinct. (Was this due to human predation like the extinction of mammoths and mastodons at about the same time?) The smaller forest elephant *Loxodonta cyclotis* has straighter and thinner tusks. Although unequivocal genetic evidence for the two species only came to light in 2001 (113), the trade had long recognized that ivory from West Africa was harder, darker, and more translucent, while that from the east was softer, whiter, and less likely to crack. Perhaps for this reason nineteenth century ivory workers preferred Egyptian ivory coming from the Sudan.

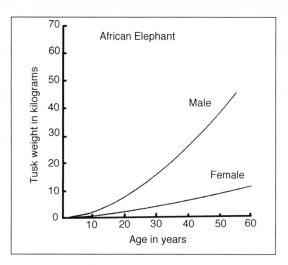

Figure 6.28. African (*Loxodonta*) male (bull) elephants have larger tusks than females (cows). (Data from 105).

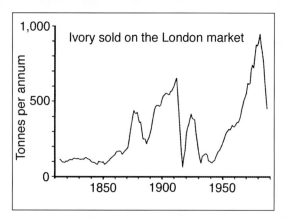

Figure 6.29. The weight of ivory sold each year on the London market in the nineteenth and twentieth centuries. Major increases in the export of African elephant ivory occurred in the mid-nineteenth century, largely to meet the demand of English cutlery makers, and in the twentieth century after the Second World War, to supply the Asian carving trade. (Data from 91).

Tusk size and life span

Tusk lengths are measured along the outer curve and circumference at the widest point. In African elephants, both bulls and cows have tusks. Bulls have the largest, commonly over 50 lbs (Figure 6.28) (105). There is a rough correlation between tusk weight and length. Record African elephant tusks include one presented to the future George 5th in 1893 that was 8' 7" long, 22 3/4" in circumference and weighed 165 lbs. Ward records twenty-eight tusks longer and heavier than this, the record being 11' 5" long. A pair sold in Zanzibar in 1898 weighed more than 450 lbs (135). One of these is in the Natural History Museum in South Kensington, London, and the other in the Rodgers collection at Sheffield. Rodgers cutlery was probably the world's largest consumer of ivory in the nineteenth century. Small milk teeth are shed early in life, before the main tusks can emerge. It is claimed that tusks can grow as fast as 6–7" per year, but the average rate must be much less since an elephant's life span approaches sixty years. Allowing ten years for childhood, a growth of 3" a year would still allow a thirty-year-old bull to have 5' tusks. Their life span is limited by the number of molar teeth that are worn down and replaced in sets. They die of starvation after their sixth and last set wears down. The sixth set does not appear until about age thirty, allowing for life spans almost as long as humans. Selection pressure caused by killing animals with large tusks for the ivory market has almost halved the average tusk size since the major exploitation of the mid-nineteenth century. However, tuskless strains have also evolved due to random gene loss in small isolated populations (139).

Distribution. African elephants originally roamed over most of the African continent. Until the early fifteenth century ivory was a rare commodity, coming from East Africa and India mainly through Egypt. Then in 1415, King Joao I of Portugal sent an expedition across to Ceuta from Gibraltar. The expedition included his son Henrique, later to become Henry the Navigator. World navigation began with these Portuguese voyages to the East around the west coast of Africa, bringing back ivory as well as precious cargos of slaves and spices. Thus began the European demand for ivory that became insatiable, climaxing in the Industrial Revolution of the nineteenth century, when machine carving replaced careful medieval craftsmanship. Although many authors euphemistically referred to the imports as "dead ivory" collected from animals dying naturally, the enormous tonnages shipped to London and other carving centers in the nineteenth century probably came from elephants killed for their tusks. The London Board of Trade records 150 tons of ivory imported from Africa in 1827, 400 in 1850, 718 in 1890, 546 in 1895, 499 in 1900, and 453 tons in 1904. An average of 500 tons a year would be a reasonable estimate for African elephant ivory imports in the latter part of the nineteenth century (Figure 6.29). If the tusks from these elephants averaged 30 lbs a pair, then almost 40,000 died each year or nearly 2,000,000 over the fifty years up to 1900. (This death rate at more than 100 elephants a day for fifty years dwarfs the horrific display put on by the Roman Consul Metellus in the Circus Maximus in 251 BC. To celebrate his victory over the Carthaginians he slaughtered 140 captured elephants by shooting them with bows and arrows. These probably came from a now extinct race of elephants in the Atlas Mountains. Perhaps it was their mountain origins that enabled Hannibal to take them over the Alps to attack Rome.) Ivory was also exported to Germany, France, the United States, Portugal, and especially Belgium. After 1865, when Belgium under King Leopold II (1835–1909) was involved in ivory export from West Africa, Antwerp became as important as London. Although hunting for ivory contributed to their decline in numbers, habitat loss was probably more important in the nineteenth century (91). The more recent reduction in elephant populations in the twentieth century began as China and Japan turned to African ivory, having used up that from Asia. China

had traded for African ivory from the first millennium AD, but only in small quantities compared with that in the twentieth century. It is a sad fact that in the latter part of the twentieth century the exceptional traditional skills of Chinese and Japanese carvers was used to make cheap tourist trash, rather than beautiful figures or okimono. Although ivory is banned as an international trading commodity, elephants remain threatened by poaching and human overpopulation. The best estimate for the population of wild elephants in Africa in 2003 was 400,000 to 660,000, down from 1.3 million in 1979 and several million estimated at the beginning of the nineteenth century. They are now restricted to many small enclaves scattered through their former domain, but some local populations are recovering. In 2008, South Africa reintroduced elephant culling to control the rise in population from 8,000 to 20,000 in the previous decade. This recovery itself presents a problem. The periodic release of "legal" ivory for sale from these culls makes it hard to determine provenance once it has dispersed on the market. In 2008, raw ivory was available on the Internet for $900 per kg. Such a valuable commodity is irresistible to poachers and warlords. Ninety-two illegal shipments were intercepted every month in Africa in 2006. Many more tons were seized after reaching their Asian destinations (95). Laurel Neme gives a very readable account of the problem and what is being done about it.

Mammoths and Mastodons

Until about 12,000 years ago, mammoths (*Mammuthus* sp.) and mastodons (*Mammut* sp.) roamed over most of the northern hemisphere with a few isolated mammoth populations surviving in Siberia as recently as 3,700 years BP (Figure 6. 26 D, E). These mammoths were probably a different species from an earlier Siberian population that died out about 40,000 years BP. DNA samples from mammoths in Siberia, Yukon, and Alaska show that the recent Siberian mammoths descended from North American immigrants moving in along the Beringia land bridge before the last ice age (28). The final decline at the end of the last ice age coincided with the spread of humans into their habitat of peat bogs, where cold, humic acids and tannins preserved many of them. The tusks were particularly resistant to decay and have since been dug up throughout their range, but especially in Northern Russia. Their survival may also have been helped by their very thick covering of cementum, much thicker than in modern elephants. Some mammoth tusks were very large. One of a pair dug up at Dungeness in Kent, England, was twelve feet long and weighed 200 lbs. This is probably the one in the Rothschild collection at Tring (135). Tusks reached Europe from Russia in small quantities from the Middle Ages and by the ton in the nineteenth century. Lots of 10–20 tons were common on the London market up to 1900, but the quality could not compete with that from Africa and the market declined in the twentieth century. With the threatened extinction of elephants and the strict restrictions on illegal ivory imports, the end of the twentieth century has seen a revival in the use of mammoth ivory in small quantities, mostly from Siberia, but also from Northern Canada and Alaska. This has helped the craftsmen skilled in ivory carving to survive in parts of China and especially Java, which has produced some exquisite naturalistic carvings of animals.

Mastodons differ from mammoths in their Schreger pattern (see the following) and also in having a pair of very small tusks not more than 5 cms in diameter and 25 cms long derived from incisors in the lower jaw (Figure 6.26 E, F).

Asian Elephants

"... the Indian elephant fights in a different manner according to the position and curvature of his tusks. When they are directed forward and upward he is able to fling a tiger to a great distance—it is said to even thirty feet; when they are short and turned downward he endeavors suddenly to pin the tiger to the ground, and in consequence, is dangerous to the rider who is liable to be jerked off the howdah."

quoted by Charles Darwin in *The Descent of Man*

Asian and African elephants diverged from a common ancestor about five million years ago. Asian elephants (*Elephas maximus*) once roamed over a wide area from Iraq through India to Ceylon, Burma, Assam, Thailand, China, the Malay peninsula, Sumatra, and Borneo. Their tusks are smaller than those from Africa, the record from Assam being 8' 9" and weighing 81 lbs. Female tusks known as tushes are short, not projecting beyond the jaw. Ceylonese elephants have the smallest tusks, the record being 5' 3" long and weighing 42 lbs. Except for a small population of about 250 that still survives in the forested valleys of tropical Yunnan, Chinese elephants died out in the Sung dynasty (960–1279 AD). By this time Asian junks were trading for African ivory along the west coast of Africa. Asian elephants have been endangered since the 1970s, declining from as many as a million in 1900 to 30–50,000 in the wild and 15,000 in captivity by 2000. They are now threatened more by competition with humans for habitat than for their ivory. Even so, smaller tusks and even tuskless strains, notably in Ceylon, have evolved in response to selection of those with tusks for an early death.

Elephant molar teeth

Although not commercially important, the beauty of sliced and polished elephant molar teeth merits their study (Figure 6.26 H). They have been used as display bases, cutlery handles, and to make very elegant boxes. In India they are also powdered and taken as medicine. The jaw holds only four of these massive grinding tools at a time, upper and lower, right and left. Each tooth moves forward in the jaw as it wears down and is replaced by one from behind. The teeth are stacks of hard enamel plates embedded in the softer dentine and cement. Wear at the surface of the stack exposes the enamel as ridges standing like blunt knives above the eroded dentine and cement surface. This cement is not the "soft enamel" cementum that extends over the dentine in continuity with enamel in ivory, it is the tissue outside the enamel in which teeth are embedded. The pattern made by the enamel ridges is different for each species. In Indian elephants and mammoths the ridges are transverse; in African elephants the transverse ridges are broader, each one making an X shape with its neighbor (Figure 6.30). The pattern in Mastodons is like that in African elephants but with their enamel resisting abrasion and remaining as broad raised mounds (Figure 6.26 G).

The structure of elephant ivory

Lord Rutherford once said that if you understand a hypothesis, it should be possible to explain it successfully to the local barmaid. This is the challenge: to explain the three-dimensional architecture of elephant ivory to the non-specialist. It will not be easy. We will first describe the three components, then the three architectural patterns that these components make together. Finally, we shall put these three interlocking architectures together to make the complete structure. Although an elephant has one of the most complex of ivory structures it will serve as a base for understanding those of all the others. Once the principles of the structure are understood, complexity dissolves into simplicity. The description below builds on the outline of ivory structure in the introduction and the progressively more complicated structures of the species described, especially that of hippos, which resemble elephants in having a waved dentinal tubule architecture.

Three components

The emerging first tusk of an African elephant has a coat of enamel instead of cementum at its tip (Figure 6.26 B). An irregularly shaped milk tusk about half this size lies beside it at this stage. However, the tip enamel is soon lost, leaving only a thin coat

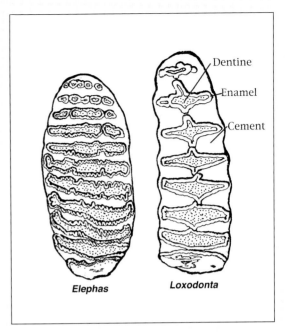

Figure 6.30. Grinding surfaces of African (*Loxodonta*) and Indian (*Elephas*) elephant molar teeth are distinguished by the patterns made by their enamel, cement, and dentine. The enamel is harder than the other components and projects above the surface as sharp ridges. It has a smooth face apposing the dentine, which is like that in other teeth with variably oriented dentinal tubules. The outer surface of the enamel has a rough surface apposing the cement, a tissue with blood vessels visible with a hand lens. (Mnemonic—I for Indian, X for African—*Loxodonta*. The pattern in Indian elephants is like a stack of Is on their sides; in African elephants the enamel is oblique like a stack of Xs. *Loxodonta* comes from the Greek *loxos* meaning oblique). See Figures 6.5 G, H.

of cementum around a cylinder of dentine, the ivory of commerce. All ivory is made from dentine, the layer inside the enamel or cementum of teeth and tusks (Figure 6.1). By light microscopy dentine looks like reinforced concrete on a microscopic scale. There are three components (Figure 6.2). 1. **Dentinal tubules** about 5 mm in diameter with a spacing of 10–20 mm can be sharply defined by stains that leak into their hollow cores. 2. **Spherites,** 5–20 mm in diameter, that may be calcified to become calcospherites, are readily seen in narwhal dentine, but although present in all ivory are easily overlooked because of their weak staining. Near their forming face, the spherites are roughly spherical. As they mature towards the periphery they become squeezed into polygonal shapes with little distortion to the dentinal tubules.

3. **Matrix** in which the tubules and spherites are embedded is featureless at the level of light microscopy. In the concrete model, the matrix corresponds to cement, the spherites are the pebbles, and the dentinal tubules the reinforcing rods. All are made of proteins, mainly collagen, hydrated and variably calcified. This calcified three-part composite structure is the generality for the dentine of all ivory. Different kinds of ivory vary in the way these components are put together, especially in the frequency of spherites, the chemistry of the matrix, and dentinal tubule orientation (Figure 6. 4).

Three architectural patterns

1. Layering in growth cycles

The most easily observed structure is that resulting from growth cycles. Soft layers alternate with hard layers that tend to exclude stain and stand proud above a polished surface. The bands result from properties of the matrix causing differences in staining, the packing of spherites around the dentinal tubules, and the angle at which the waved tubules are transected. The main layers, 1–5 mm wide, probably correspond to annual cycles (Figure 6.31 A, B). Within them there are narrower bands, perhaps secreted daily, having a more constant width of about 100 ⌠m. They appear as concentric rings transversely (Figure 6.31 C, D, E). In axial longitudinal profiles angled to the radius short sections of the radial tubules appear as axial columns (Figure 6.31 F). Growth in length is from the base, where the growth zone deposits dentine in discrete layers. A consequence of this layered growth is a tusk made from a stack of elongated cones that are almost cylindrical like the leaves in a greatly elongated onion* (Figure 6.31 A). In most tusks, the last formed growth cone is more elliptical than the outside one preceding it. For example, the main growth layers seen in longitudinal profile in Figure 6.31 A form a series of ellipses in transverse profile starting on the outside with the nearly circular ratio of 1:1.06 changing in successive rings to 1:1.27, 1:1.31, 1:1.40, and 1:1.80. The circular cross section without belies the progressively elliptical cross section within, perhaps formed in response to the main direction of stress from using the tusk as a lever.

(Opposite page)

Figure 6.31. Growth layers result from differences in the matrix and packing of particles around the dentinal tubules. A. Conical growth layers in proboscidean tusks become increasingly obtuse with age. Mammoth tusks sometimes separate along these growth layers freeing basal cones shaped like rhinoceros horns, perhaps giving rise to one of the unicorn myths. Diagrammatic longitudinal profile. B. Widely spaced bands several mm apart in transverse profile probably represent annual growth layers. Silver stained mammoth ivory. Scale = 1 cm. C–E. Fine bands tens of m apart in transverse profile probably represent daily growth increments. C. Very small particles separate tubules in growth layers. Silver stained. D. Particles and/or matrix stains differently in these layers. Mercury sulfide stain. E. Some tubules seem to disappear in lighter parts of the bands, perhaps because they end (see Figures 6.12 and 6.18) or more probably because they fail to stain. Mercury sulfide stain. F. Radial profiles always show the growth bands in parallel array. Methylene blue and black marker pen stained. C–F. Scales = 100 mm.

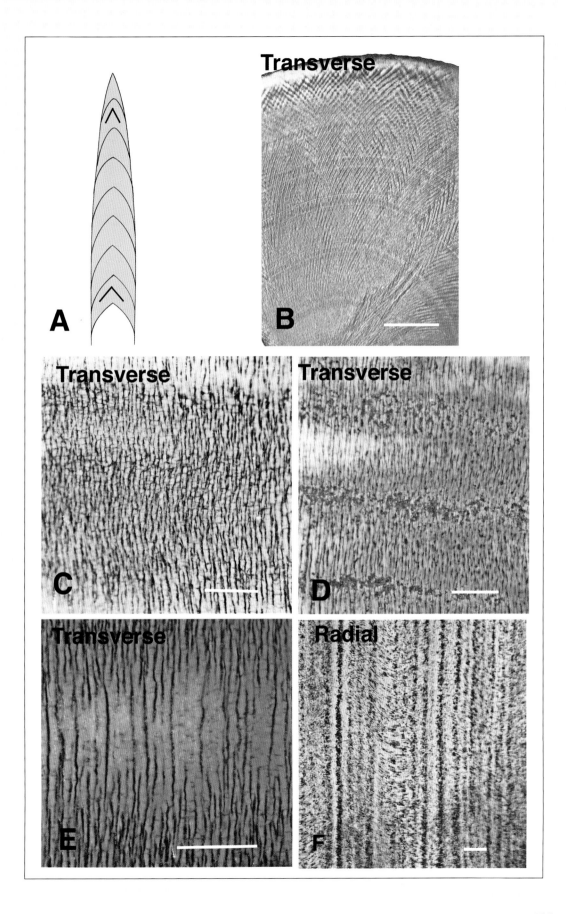

A

B
Transverse

C
Transverse

D
Transverse

E
Transverse

F
Radial

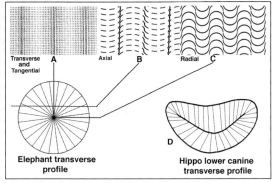

Figure 6.33. The pattern due to the changing orientations of dentinal tubules in adjacent laminae of a proboscidean tusk depends upon the angle made with the wavy tubules. In exact transverse and tangential profiles of two segments, the image would appear as in A. The image would be made from cutting the wave into short (transverse to the wave where it is ascending or descending in the axis) and longer sections (longitudinal to the wave where the curve extends radially). A real ivory image would contain 70–150 sheets of tubules as in Figure 6.34 B, C, D. In B, axial profiles would stretch curved patterns due to overlapping images of longer lengths of waved tubules. C. Exact radial profiles delineate complete wavy tubules. D. In hippo ivory the laminae are cut so obliquely that most "radial" profiles have a waved pattern as in B, C, and Figure 6.23 A–E.

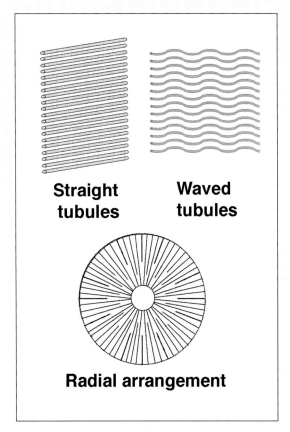

Figure 6.32. Dentinal tubules aligned in radial laminae in the length are either straight or wavy in their path from the forming face to the cementum. The tubules are about 5 mm in diameter and of indefinite length. Since the center to center separation of the tubules remains constant from the outside to the inside, few laminae extend all the way from the periphery to the forming face. In a 10 cm diameter elephant tusk there would be space for 56–120 x 103 laminae, only 10% of which would reach as far as a 1 cm diameter core.

2. Dentinal tubule arrangement

Dentinal tubules are arranged in a very simple way. They stack side-by-side in the length of the tusk to form **radial laminae** (Figures 6.31, 32). At the periphery of an idealized 10 cm diameter elephant tusk (circumference D = 314 mm = 314,000 mm) there is enough space for 31,400 radial laminae 10 ⌠m wide, made from 5 ⌠m dentinal tubules. The reason for thinking of them as laminae is a descriptive convenience, they tend to align one above the other axially. It does not necessarily mean that they are bonded together in this way, falling apart preferentially as sheets. In tangential profiles crack patterns (Figure 6.34 F) follow the V shape of tubule orientations (Figure 6.34 D).

Radial laminae are grouped together into **segments** about 1 mm wide.

The segments are subdivided radially into blocks to create the **Schreger pattern.**

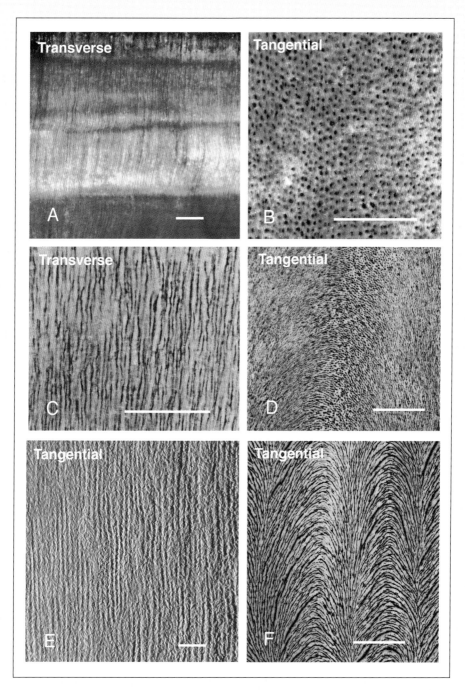

Figure 6.34. Dentinal tubule arrangement in proboscidean ivory. A. Transverse profiles of unstained ivory show radially arranged laminae as in Figure 6.32. Osmium fixation. B. Stained tangential profiles show cross-sections of dentinal tubules stacked up radially as in Figure 6.14 A to form the laminae in A. Black marker pen stain. C. Stained transverse profiles show dentinal tubules in short lengths as would be expected if they are oriented radially but mostly at angles to the transverse-plane. Black marker pen stain. D. Tangential profiles as in B show stacks of radially out of phase wavy tubules cut transversely at the top and bottom of a waves and longitudinally in between create the C patterns expected. E. The segments depicted in D repeat hundreds of time in the circumference of a tusk. Poorly preserved mammoth ivory often flakes into sheets along the growth layers exposing the many segments seen here. Natural unstained surface. F. Crack patterns in tangentially cut old elephant ivory confirm the radial helicoidal architecture. The cracks develop with orientations corresponding to the average orientation of the dentinal tubules below. Most of the segments appear wider than those exposed in E because they are on a plane cut across curved cylindrical surface layers corresponding to those in the mammoth.

3. Waved tubules appear as longitudinal Schreger columns in transverse profile.

The billiard sharp ... plays extravagant matches, ...With a twisted cue And elliptical billiard balls.

The Mikado, Libretto by W.S. Gilbert

Ivory patterns are indeed twisted extravagantly and the tusk cross sections are elliptical. Stacks of laminae can be glued together to create plywoods: ivory is a radial plywood that in elephants is subdivided radially into segmented longitudinal columns. The German anatomist Bernhard Gottlieb Schreger (1766–1825) was the first to describe the radial checkered patterns of these columns (Figure 6.42). The best way to think of them is that they mark the bonding that has evolved in proboscideans to make their plywoods more resistant to radial cracking. According to Virag, the checker patterns are due to differences in staining between transverse and longitudinal tubule presentation (131). This may be true, but there is more to ivory structure than tubules. Variations in the matrix and the concentration of spherites may also contribute to different densities of staining. Transverse profiles of Schreger columns show that the finest (possibly daily) growth layers vary in the intensity of their staining independently of the tubule orientation (Figure 6.36 B). Whatever the relative contributions of tubule orientation vs spherite/matrix density and stainability to the contrast giving rise to the Schreger pattern, it is still convenient to consider the pattern as if it were in longitudinal columns.

Transverse profiles show that the Schreger patterns correspond to soft stainable regions boxed in by harder, less stainable walls, while radial and tangential profiles show the boxes to be of indefinite length. These long boxes have two radial walls outlining the segments and two circumferential walls subdividing the segments into columns. The sides are like radial longitudinal curtains separating

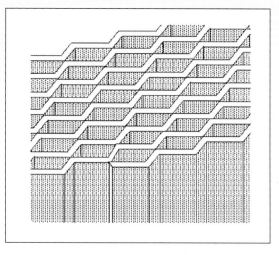

Figure 6.35. The Schreger patterns of elephant ivory result from the division of segments into longitudinal columns by walls of harder material. The walls are like radial longitudinal curtains with folds at about 900 separating radial dentine segments into box-like columns. The columns may be square, rectangular, or hexagonal in cross section (Figure 6.36 B, C), or the circumferential, or diagonal folds may dominate and the radial sides may be incomplete.

segments with 90^0 bends in the circumference that divide the segments into columns, further reinforcing the radial plywood (Figure 6.35). The translucent yellow to brown walls are like the hard parts of growth layers in appearance, giving the characteristic off-white tone of ivory (Figure 6.36 A, B, C). Dentinal tubules tend to stain less as they pass through the walls but change little in their orientation. Growth layers also cross column walls without interruption. The walls are lost towards the core and the box arrangement disappears in a process discussed in more detail below under Schreger patterns. The columns themselves change in shape in the length of the tusk. As they progress from the periphery to the center they change from a roughly symmetrical transverse profile to a thin radial sliver (Figure 6.43).

These longitudinal columns can be thought of as basic repeating units. With columns measuring 1 mm radially and circumferentially an idealized 10 cm diameter tusk could contain about 50 columns from the cementum to the core and about 314 columns around the periphery.

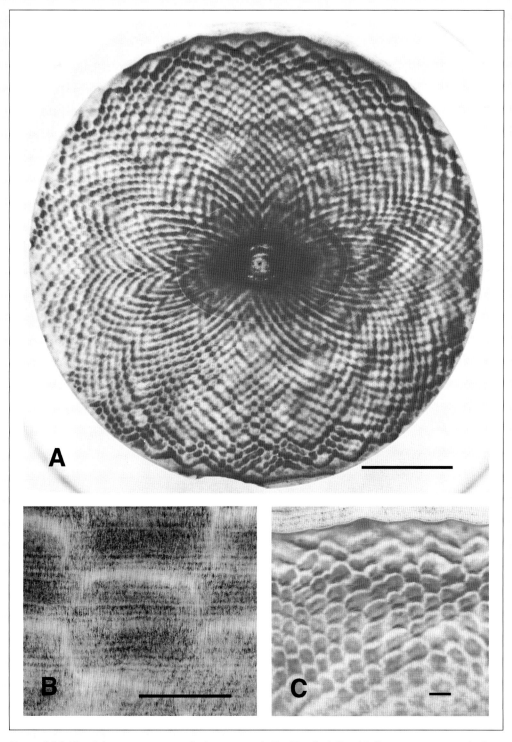

Figure 6.36. The Schreger pattern in elephant ivory. A. Profile of a billiard ball cut transverse to the long axis of the tusk. Each longitudinally stacked segment of a Schreger column is offset to those on each side, creating the V patterns. The pattern is emphasized in two quarters because the curved elliptical tusk cross-section causes slightly overlapping images of the columns at the top and bottom of this figure. The curve also induces a slight asymmetry at 900 restricting the pattern to bilateral symmctry as in Table 2. Methylene blue stained. B, C. Transverse profile of columns just below the cementum. Material within the columns stains more than the harder column walls and growth bands. B. Silver; C. methylene blue stained. See Figure 6.23. Scales, A = 1 cm, B, C = 1 mm.

The complete elephant ivory structure

The complete elephant ivory structure can now be assembled from the three interlocking substructures—dentinal tubules, growth layers, and Schreger columns. Components (dentinal tubules, spherites, matrix, and column walls) are deposited in conical layers. At right angles to the growth layers, waved dentinal tubules align parallel to one another in longitudinal radial segments of laminae. The phase of tubule waves changes by a small amount from one lamina to the next. Reversal of the direction of the phase difference creates VVV radial segments. Different staining properties of tubules according to their presentation in transverse profiles cuts these segments radially and circumferentially into columns, making the Schreger pattern. Cylindrical growth layers and laminae of waved dentinal tubules (and perhaps longitudinal Schreger columns, depending on whether their dense staining is due to reinforcement or merely tubule orientation) are interlocking three-dimensional patterns of structural organization.

Tangential and transverse profiles of out of phase tubule waves appear as feather patterns

Creating a rod from radially arranged laminae presents a problem. A flat surface is easily made thicker by stacking sheets one on top of another, but radial alignment in segments requires that the number or size of the segments must decline in the progression from the periphery to the center. Some dentinal tubules may extend all the way from the cementum-dentine interface to the forming face, but most must end, since the dentinal tubule separation of about 10 mm remains constant in the radial direction even though the area of the forming face declines. In the progress from the cementum-dentine interface of a 10 cm diameter tusk (circumference = 314 mm = 314,000 mm = 31,400 radial laminae 10 mm wide) to a pulp cavity 1 cm across (= 31 mm = 3,140 radial laminae 10 mm wide) some 28,000 laminae must disappear. Similarly, about 314 Schreger columns might occur at the forming face of a 10 cm diameter tusk. Some 280 of them will have disappeared by the time that the pulp cavity has declined to 1 cm across. The loss is accomplished both by reduction in the number of laminae per segment and by loss of complete segments (Figure 6.37). Below the cementum segments are wider and contain more laminae than those nearer the center (Figure 6.42). Closer to the core the columns continue to lose laminae, but also lose complete columns (Figure 6.37). The change from s to the VVVV feather pattern corresponds to a change in the wave shape from deep, just below the cementum, to much shallower in core ivory with its feather pattern (Figure 6.36, 41). This interpretation of the "feather pattern" is confirmed by the appearance of radial profiles where dentinal tubules form a more gentle wave at the core than at the periphery (Figure 6.40).

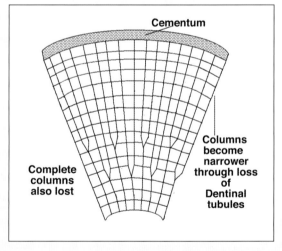

Figure 6.37. Dentinal tubules are lost from the periphery to the forming face (Figure 6.32) in two stages. In a profile of a 10 cm diameter elephant tusk there would be about 800 columns in the ring just below the cementum. These outer Schreger columns become narrower through the loss of tubules. The inner regions also lose complete columns (Figure 6.24C).

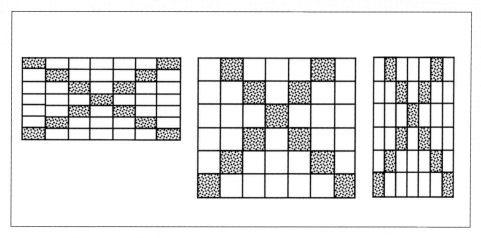

Figure 6.38. Transverse profiles of columns stacked as flat sheets show that the angles made by diagonals depend on the dimensions of the columns. The angles become more acute as the ratio of circumferential to radial dimensions declines. Wide columns give obtuse angles, narrow columns result in more acute angles. The nature of the diagonals is a little more complicated than portrayed in this simplified diagram. See Figure 6.23.

These dentinal tubule arrangements are presumably a response to a need to maximize resistance to bending while reducing the risk of deep cracking originating from the surface.

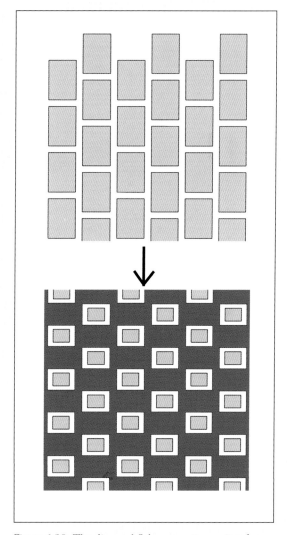

Figure 6.39. The diagonal Schreger pattern arises from a staggering of the columns. The outer columns below the cementum are aligned in a staggered array. Darker and more densely stained material comes between the columns as their walls separate, forming the diagonal array of the Schreger pattern.

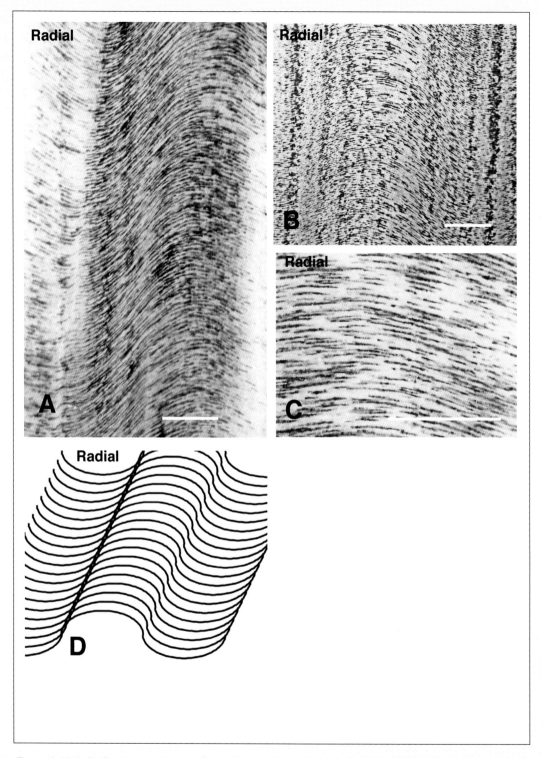

Figure 6.40 A, B. Overlapping images of waved dentinal tubules give the illusion of broader waves in radial profiles of elephant ivory. C. Higher magnification and better resolution from shallower staining show the overlapping giving the illusion of a curve. D. An interpretation of the waved tubule pattern. Toluidine blue and black marker pen stain. B, C black marker pen. Scales = 100 ſm.

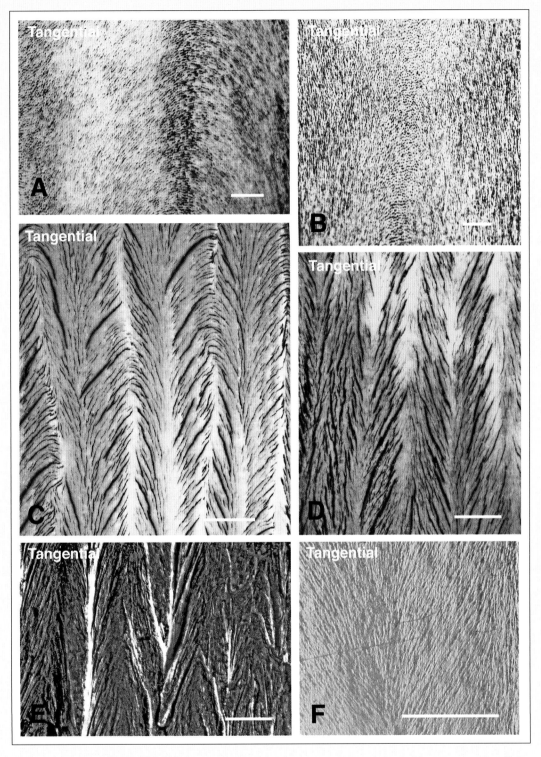

Figure 6.41. Dentinal tubules in core ivory display a feather pattern in tangential profile. A. One cm below the cementum the proportion of radially oriented dentinal tubules is reduced from the almost complete helicoid nearer the surface (compare with Figure 6.15 D). B. In the core ivory the radial and near radial tubules are further reduced. C, D. The increased proportion of axially oriented tubules is reflected in the crack patterns that change from shapes to VVV shapes. C. The same position as A. D. Core ivory. E. Mammoth ivory fractures along VVV shaped planes as predicted from the crack patterns in elephant ivory. F. Reflection image of polished tangential surface of elephant ivory shows both the axial orientation of the laminae and the VVV pattern. A, B marker pen stained. C, D surface crack pattern on tangential profiles of old ivory emphasized with ink. E, natural surface of tangentially fractured mammoth ivory. Scales, A, B = 100 mm. C–F = 1 mm

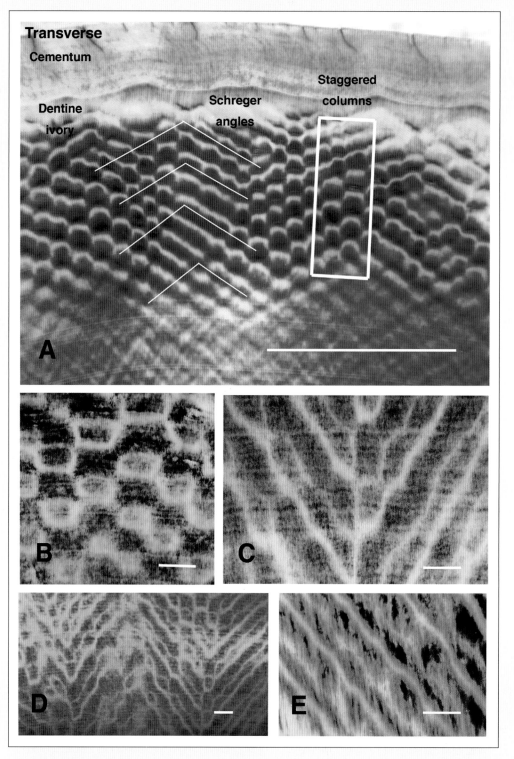

Figure 6.42. The origin of the Schreger pattern. The walls of the Schreger columns become less distinct in the progress from periphery to the core. Transverse profiles of elephant ivory. A. Below the cementum the staggered columns form clear ∧∧∧ arrays emphasized by their position on the least convex surface of the elliptical cross section. B. Below the region in A the column walls enclose narrower columns leaving unenclosed darkly stained material that also emphasizes the ∧∧∧ pattern. C, D, E. Columns become increasingly indistinct as they lose circumferential walls and then some diagonals. Staining: A, D. Methylene blue. B. mercury sulfide. C. Silver. E. Lead sulfide. Scales, A = 1 cm, B–D – 1 mm.

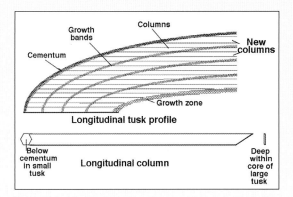

Figure 6.43. The origin and fate of Schreger columns. The growth zone and the layers deposited from it cut across the columns. As a tusk increases in diameter, new ridges and columns are added below the cementum. These columns are covered in turn by more new columns, further increasing the diameter. From the position where the columns are first deposited, their radial dimensions (about 1.3 mm in elephants, 0.8 mm in mammoths) decline progressively as they are buried under the new columns until they disappear in the core center.

The Schreger pattern

Schreger patterns for the identification of different kinds of elephant. Transverse views of whole tusks show columns arranged in Schreger patterns. These are so characteristic of the tusks of elephants, mammoths, mastodons, and their allies in the group Proboscidea that the great anatomist Richard Owen (98) defined ivory as tusks having such patterns. We now define ivory more broadly as the dentine from any teeth large enough to be commercially valuable. However, with the need to protect endangered species, Schreger patterns have become of interest because they may allow the identification of ivories that were formerly accepted in international trade but are now illegal (35, 36). In particular Schreger angles differentiate between modern elephants and extinct mammoths and mastodons (130).

The Schreger pattern seen in transverse profile comes about because the columns are staggered and color or stain differently in diagonals. The reason for the staggering is that the starting points of tubules are also staggered. They arise at the dentine/cementum interface that is shaped into waves at the circumference due to the longitudinal ridges (Figure 6.37 B, 6.44 A, and 6.46). The Schreger angle is defined as the outer angle made by the diagonal formed by these columns. The value of the angle depends upon the dimensions of the columns (Figure 6.40). Wide columns result in larger angles than narrow columns. The angles are species specific (35, 36, 130). Transverse tusk profiles of African elephants, Indian elephants, mammoths, and mastodons all differ in the angles made by the diagonal Schreger columns. Average values for Schreger angles of mammoth ivory are 73°, distinguishable from elephant ivory with angles of 124° (35). Statistical analysis of angle measurements can distinguish African from Indian elephants, "fossil" from "modern" tusks, and mammoths from mastodons (130). However, the Schreger angles made by the diagonals vary with position (Figure 6.47), such as distance from the cementum to the core (Figure 6.44 F), with position around the circumference (Figure 6.45 E), and with diameter and position along the length of a tusk (Figure 6.44 G), so that measurements for reliable inter-species comparisons must take many factors into account. Measurements may distinguish different proboscidean ivories taken from known positions on large, carefully oriented samples, but they are less helpful in practice since fragments or small polished artifacts are rarely conveniently oriented. However, some simple underlying causes of the pattern may help as taxonomic discriminators.

Factors influencing the Schreger angle

There are two main determinants of the Schreger pattern, the frequency of starting points at the periphery and the decline in lateral dimensions of the columns from the periphery to the core. Before discussing these it is necessary to understand the origin of the diagonals in the Schreger pattern.

The origin of the diagonals. The pattern depends upon the way that the wavy tubules divide the tusk into radial segments and the circumferential subdivision of these segments into longitudinal columns. Transverse profiles of columns just below the cementum are aligned side-by-side in a staggered array in the circumference (Figure 6.39). Closer to the core, the walls become narrower (Figure 6.42 B, C). Single, curtain-like walls only enclose one column, leaving alternate columns and gaps without walls continuous with one another. These connected "gap columns," tend to be darker colored or more heavily stained, and are perceived as the diagonals making the Schreger pattern (Figure 6.42 D, E). Some arms of the columns making the angle tend to appear linked together due to overlapping of the column profiles, as surfaces cannot be cut exactly normal to all the components in a curved tusk. The position of the outer columns in the staggered arrays determine the initiation points of the $\wedge$ Gothic arches forming the Schreger angles.

The frequency of starting points. If the interface at the surface between dentine and cementum were flat, then the tubule waves would start in phase with one another. Schreger columns would be aligned side-by-side in equally flat sheets like those in Figures 6.37 and 38. However, the surface of the dentine below the cementum has longitudinal ridges 2–5 mm apart (Figures 6.44 A, B, G) in positions that relate to the $\wedge$ Gothic arches (Figure 6.44 D, E). The tips of the arches point to the tops of these ridges, some of which stain densely (Figure 6.44 C). The width of the ridges varies with position in the elliptical circumference of tusks with wider ridges along the flatter edges and the narrowest ridges along the inside curve of the more acute side of the ellipse (Figure 6.44 F).

The ridges in elephants are wider than those in mammoths (Figure 6.44 G). The average width in elephants measured on tusk profiles like Figure 6.45 E is 4.22 mm, significantly wider than the 2.10 mm measured on separated sheets of mammoth dentine like those in Figure 6.44 B. In a crude experiment,

stretching the ridge profiles of a mammoth to match the size of those in an elephant also increased the Schreger angles to about the values found in elephants. Conversely, shrinking an elephant profile made the Schreger angles match those of a mammoth (Figure 6.44 H–K).

(Opposite page)
Figure 6.44. The /\/\ tips of Schreger pattern arrays point to the peaks of ridges at the cementum-dentine interface. A, B. Incompletely preserved mammoth tusks often split at the cementum-dentine interface to expose the ridged surface. Scales = 1 cm. Natural surfaces. C. Profiles at the tusk periphery show the forming stages of new outermost Schreger columns as new ridges arise. Dentine at the peak of each ridge stains as if it were the outermost Schreger column. The ridge elevates it above the columns on each side, causing the staggered rows. Elephant transverse profile. Mercury sulfide stain. Scale = 1 mm. D. Mammoth and E. Elephant transverse profiles show that the $\wedge$ peaks begin below each ridge. The number and position of $\wedge$s corresponds to the number and position of ridges. Scales = 1 cm. F. The Schreger angle diminishes from the periphery to the core and from the flatter to the more convex side of the ellipse. Plots of angle X distance follow smooth curves. Scale = 1 cm. G. Dentine is ridged at its interface with the cementum with wider ridges in elephants than in mammoths. The average width in these elephant samples is 4.22 mm, significantly wider than that of mammoths at 2.10 mm. Measurements on profiles of elephant tusks (E) and on surfaces of mammoth tusks separated at the dentine-cementum interface (B) did not take into account the variations in position around the circumference. H. Ridges occur in both the cementum and the dentine at the time of their formation. Transverse profile at the base of an elephant tusk. They are lost at the surface as the cementum increases in thickness. I–L. Stretching the profile of ridges in a mammoth to match those of an elephant increases the Schreger angles to about the values expected for an elephant. Conversely, shrinking the profile of an elephant to match that of a mammoth decreases the Schreger angles to values approximating those of a mammoth.

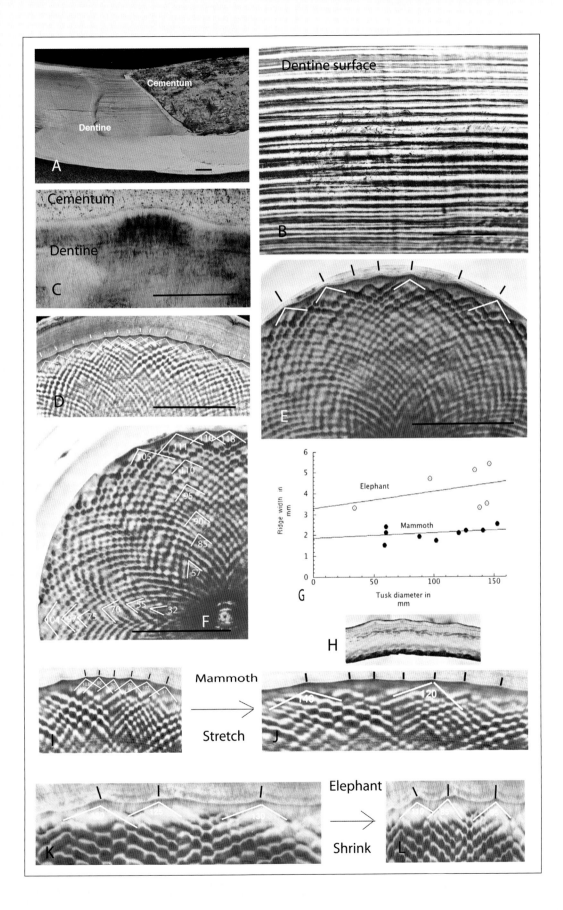

Dentine surface

Cementum

Dentine

Cementum

Dentine

A

B

C

D

E

F

G

H

Mammoth

Stretch

I

J

Elephant

Shrink

K

L

117

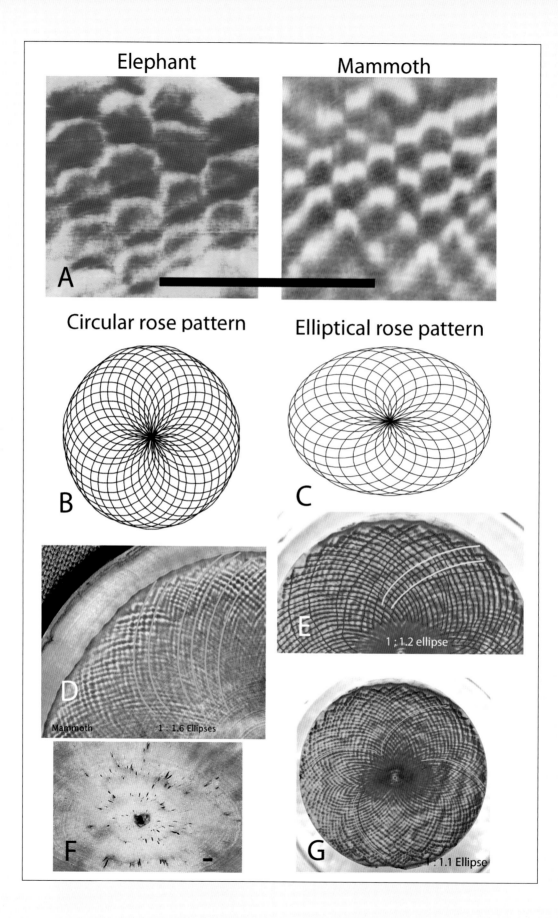

Elephant

Mammoth

Circular rose pattern

Elliptical rose pattern

A

B

C

D

Mammoth   1 : 1.6 Ellipses

E

1 : 1.2 ellipse

F

G

1 : 1.1 Ellipse

Figure 6.46. The phase shift of dental tubules in elephant ivory results from their staggered starting position on the ridged cementum, which also causes the feather pattern in transverse and tangential profiles. A. Radial out of phase tubule waves. B. Oblique radial view of the cementum/dentine interface. The tubules are formed out of phase by beginning at the ridged edge of the cementum. The depth of the ridges then determines the phase differences between waves. C, D. The waves reverse the extent of their phase difference in the circumference, matching the waves in the cementum. In transverse and circumferential profiles the filaments appear as short lengths cut from the waves. Since neighboring filaments are out of phase radially, the pattern of short and long lengths form diagonals to the radius that are reversed when the phase shift reverses. E. The amplitude of the waves declines from the periphery to the core as tubules are lost, resulting in narrower VVVs.

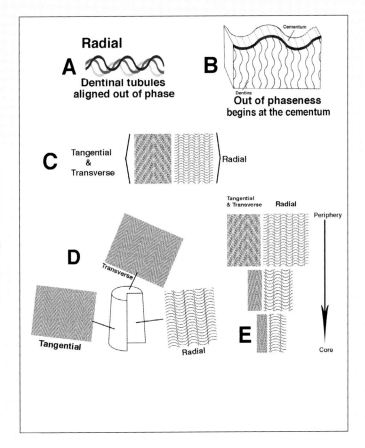

(Opposite page)
Figure 6.45. Changes in column dimensions lead to Elliptical Rose Schreger patterns. A. Transverse profiles of the outer regions of tusks show elephants have columns nearly twice as wide as those of mammoths (about 1.2 mm to 0.6 mm in these preparations). The radial dimensions are not very different (1.2 mm and 1.0 mm), giving width/radial length ratios of about 1 for elephants and 0.7 for mammoths, the kind of differences leading to the angle differences portrayed in Figure 6.22. Methylene blue stain. Scale bar = 5 mm. B. The rose pattern created by rotating a circle around a point one radial length from the center. C. The rose pattern created by rotating an ellipse around a point one short radial length from the center. D. Mammoths have patterns like those created by ellipses with radial ratios of about 1:1.6. Parts of an ellipse with a 1:1.6 ratio in green are a good fit to the Schreger pattern. E, G. Elephants have patterns slightly more elliptical than a circle that is easily distinguishable from a mammoth ellipse. In E, the yellow lines outlining parts of the path of a 1:1.2 ellipse follow the Schreger pattern overlaid in red. In G, the red lines outlining parts of the path of a 1:1.1 ellipse follow the Schreger pattern overlaid in green. The measurements are too crude to separate ratios of 1:1.1 from 1:1.2. F. Cylindrical spaces containing nerves are perceived as lines radiating diagonally from the eye of a tusk. In small samples these might be mistaken for the blood vessels in bone. Transverse profile of an elephant tusk stained with methylene blue and black marker pen. Scale = 100 mm.

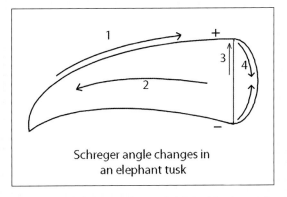

Figure 6.47. Schreger angles vary with position in a tusk. Arrows show the direction of increases in angle in the positions marked. 1. Angles and ridge size just below the cementum increase as the tusk grows in diameter. 2. Angles decline in the length of the tusk as the columns starting at the periphery grow narrower as they become the core. 3. In transverse profile angles made from columns formed at the periphery are larger than those formed later towards the core. 4. Angles and ridge size increase from the narrow to the broad sides of the ellipse. + and - indicate the additional change in angle between the concave and convex sides of a curved tusk.

Differences between elephant and mammoth ivory

Feature	Elephants	Mammoths
Distance between ridges at the dentine-cementum interface	About 4mm	About 2mm
Column width	Up to 1.3mm	Up to 0.8mm
Column radial dimension at periphery	About 1.2mm	About 1.0mm
Ratio of column width to radial dimension	About 0.9	About 0.7
Mean Schreger angles {Espinoza, 2000 #45; Espinoza, 1990 #36}	*Loxodonta* 124.2±13.4^0 *Elephas*	*Mammuthus* 73.2±14.7^0 *Mammut*
Schreger angles from comparable regions in similar sized tusks.	More than mammoths	Less than elephants
Dimensions of ellipse describing Schreger pattern = change in ratio of circumferential to radial dimension of columns	about 1:1.1	About 1:1.6
Colour	White to cream	Cream to deep brown
Density	1.78	1.7 or less

Table 6.5. Differences between elephant and mammoth ivory. Statistically different sets of data are hard to apply since measurements vary so much with position in the tusk that is often not known (Figure 6.48). However, some values can be used to identify a group whatever the origin of the sample. The most promising are column dimensions and the changes in those dimensions that determine the ratio of the Schreger ellipses.

Ridges begin at the forming base of the tusk where the combined width of dentine and cement is only about one mm wide. The cementum in this position is therefore also ridged. This gave rise to the hope that a simple inspection of the surface of the cementum might distinguish elephants from mammoths. However, the cementum covers over the sharp ridges as the tusk grows, making them hard to resolve when their growth is complete after leaving the socket. The wear on exposed surfaces then polishes the ridges away, often through to the dentine at the tip. African elephants have two sizes of ridge, a fine one about 1 mm wide that may have a diagonal cross-hatch patterning tending to survive abrasion except at the tip, and a coarser one of 4–5 mm that is lost when no longer protected by the gum. Mammoths have a much thicker cementum than elephants.

Column dimensions and the Schreger pattern. The dimensions of the columns influences the pattern in two ways. The ratio of length to width determines the angle (Figure 6.38) and the change in dimensions in the progression from the periphery to the core determines the change in angle causing the curved elliptical pattern.

The influence of dimensions on angles. The description above leads to the idea that the difference between Schreger angles in elephants and mammoths is due to differences in the dimensions of their columns, their basic units of construction. Figures 6.45 A, B show the considerable difference between elephant and mammoth columns in typical transverse profiles close to the periphery. Typical elephant columns near the surface are about 1.3 mm wide compared to 7 mm for mammoths, the same ratio as the ridge widths. These dimensions are illustrative rather than definitive since they vary with position in the same way as the angles that they determine. Precise species determination would require measurements to be taken in all positions in the tusk, as with angles. However, column measurements can be made on much smaller samples than are needed to measure the angles. If a column is wider than 1 mm, it is almost certainly from an elephant and if more than 0.8 mm, it is most probably elephant. The converse is not necessarily true, since elephant columns become as narrow as mammoths in their progress through the core (Figure 6.43, 45).

The influence of changing dimensions on curves. In order to fit on a curved surface like that in a cylindrical tusk, the columns must become smaller (or fewer) in their circumferential dimension in the inward progression from column to column in the segment. This would cause the straight diagonals in Figures 6.38, 39 to become the curves observed as the family of rose patterns that are created when circles or ellipses rotate about a center (Figure 6.45 B, C). The rose patterns, like the column dimensions, are characteristic of the species, but they depend on more than the width to depth ratio of the column. The curves depend on the change in the ratio of width to depth. The curves do not match the Schreger lines perfectly as there are occasional zigzags due to losses of complete columns. Elephant patterns are only slightly elliptical with ratios near 1:1 (Figure 6.45 B, E, G). Mammoth patterns have ratios of about 1:1.6 (Figures 6.44 D, 45 D). The curves represent a summation of the angles. Matching elliptical templates with the curves exposed in transverse tusk profiles for species determination is a much quicker task than measuring all the different angles at various depths within the tusk.

The functional advantage of the elliptical arrangement of the columns is easy to visualize. Imagine a simple radial arrangement as in Figure 6.2 C. To fill the space, units at the periphery have to be eliminated as the secreting surface retreats to the core. This would leave radial fault lines susceptible to cracking from lateral stress. Twisting such a radial structure into a rose pattern (Figure 6.45 B, C) both enlarges the surface at risk and changes it from a straight plane to a curved one.

The origin of the VVV staggered Schreger pattern. The cause of the out of phase alignments of wavy dentinal tubules is simply explained by their origins at the ridged surface of cementum as in Figure 6.46. If they started from a plane surface they would be in phase. Starting from a waved surface determines the extent to which they are out of phase. This in turn determines the VVV pattern.

Conclusions on the use of tusk measurements in Proboscidian taxonomy

There is a hierarchy of structures beginning with the frequency of ridges and the positioning of the columns, their staggering, and differences in size leading to changes in their proportions. The linkage of these features suggests they are causally related through their development. A transverse profile from the periphery to the center is a temporal record of the changes in development that took place from the tusk tip to the forming face at the base. These quantitative differences in the columns that reflect changes over time are summarized by the ellipse patterns in which they culminate. The ellipse patterns and the structures that generate them are therefore good candidates for use in taxonomic discrimination. Unfortunately the position where measurements are taken also influences the outcome (Table 6.4). The four quarters of an elliptical transverse profile are symmetrical, differing only in being mirror images. Superimposed on this are the consequences of tusk curvature that elongates the ellipse, causing the more convex surfaces to have obliquely cut columns, changing their Schreger angles. The curvature combined with the change in diameter also causes the more convex ends to differ, introducing a further asymmetry. The influences of tusk shape and development on Schreger angles is summarized in Figure 6.47. Most tusks also have a slight helical twist, which removes symmetry altogether and creates right and left handed tusks. In its detailed pattern, a tusk approaches uniqueness. Only single measurements with known provenance can discriminate between tusk patterns. For this reason the measurements given are from small samples and illustrative rather than large and statistically significant but definitively futile. Fortunately, some of the dimensions in Table 6.5 can separate elephants from mammoths. For example, if a column is greater than 1 mm wide it is not from a mammoth, whatever part of a tusk the sample has come from. The most comprehensive and possibly the most useful measurements are the size and proportions of peripheral column profiles and the proportions of the ellipses. Some of the features discriminating between elephant and mammoth tusks are summarized in Table 6.3.

Development of the waved pattern

*It may be that my Lord will lead
me to a closer way of truth than this.*

Prayer of a Pious Mussulman

In the waved model presented for elephant ivory and banded hippo ivory, waved dentinal tubules are aligned with one another in laminae in the radial/axial plane that are out of phase by regular increments in adjacent laminae. This presents problems for their growth. To maintain the angles while adding new tubule material at the cell surface of a growth zone (Figure 6.2 B), adjacent cells would have to move relative to one another axially—not impossible in engineering, but unusual in biological development.

Growth in tubules that create wavy or patterns. It is easy to visualize growth in a simple tusk like that of an orca (Figure 6.5). Cells subtend tubules with similar orientations. As the dentine increases in thickness, the tubules can elongate in unison in the same direction. But to create an out of phase waved pattern requires circumferentially adjacent cells to have differently orientated tubules. To accommodate an increase in dentine thickness their cells must move in directions determined by the orientations of their tubules. Relative cell positions must therefore move to accommodate differing tubule orientations. Cell shuffling is unlikely. Epithelial cells have many desmosomes tending to keep them stuck together. Changes in relative position usually result from changes in an epithelium as a whole. The most likely solution lies in contractions of the cell's cytoskeletons to cause a cyclical wave-like axial motion, tip to base and back, concurrent with dentine deposition (Figure 6.48).

6. 9. Discussion—laminar architectures

This description of ivory structure is an exercise in the interpretation of radial plywood-like structures assembled from dentinal tubules arrayed in laminar sheets. The toughness of ivory depends on its resistance to forming cracks and their confinement once they have begun (Nalla et al., 2003). Much of the structure described may be an adaptation to prevent the propagation of cracks by spreading the load and avoiding homogeneity. The results are summarized in Figure 6.4. Elephants and hippopotamus arrange their dentinal tubules within laminae to form waved arrays, normal to the forming face in elephants or angled to it in hippopotamus. Pigs have evolved skeins of curly dentinal tubules. The narwhal has crossed helices, cementum against radial laminae of dentine. Presumably the arrangement of opposing spirals of hard tissue, pitting the cementum against the dentine, creates increased mechanical resistance to bending. The double spiral also gives more weight to the proposal of Currey (Brear et al., 1993), following D'Arcy Thompson (126) that the helical structure may be a mechanism for creating a straight tusk. The other systems leave the dentinal tubules within laminae having a constant radial orientation but orient them at various angles to the axis. A common variable feature is the presence of a granular matrix. Since plywood-like structures occur in the cementum (Nalla et al., 2003), and waved arrays are merely a complex plywood, it is perhaps surprising that simple plywoods were not found in the ivories studied.

The architecture of ivory is easily understood by considering the complexity introduced in successive steps of organization in the progression from linear radial dentinal tubules to three-dimensional waves. It is important to realize that it is very hard to fit tubules into a three-dimensional space without either a great deal of filler space or layering as in laminae. The waved laminae of proboscideans have the closest packing, while some pigs, such as wart

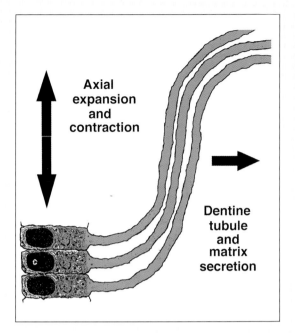

Figure 6.48. Cells secreting dentine must move in directions determined by the orientations of their tubules when their dentine increases in thickness. If the only movement is radial or radial diagonal, then tubules would have a straight trajectory as dentine is laid down around hem. The waved pattern of tubules observed requires a synchronous oscillatory axial movement. Epithelial cells have many desmosomes tending to keep them stuck together that would ensure changes in the epithelium as a whole, changes in relation to the secretory surface. The most likely cause of the waved tubules may be from contractions of the cell's cytoskeletons causing a wave-like axial/lateral motion.

hogs with their curled tubules, have the loosest fit. There are two variables, lateral alignment to make laminae and orientation of dentinal tubules within laminae. The first step is the radial arrangement of dentinal tubules found in most teeth and the featureless ivory of hippopotamus incisors. The second step involves the axial/lateral alignment of radial dentinal tubules into radial laminae. The dentinal tubules may be radial/transverse or radial and angled to the axis. The third step, occurring in banded ivories, involves changing the orientation of the dentinal tubules in each lamina from one lamina to the next. Variations in the changing orientation allow the formation of the modified waves making up the Schreger columns in proboscideans.

Ivory, by definition, is the dentine of large teeth, but teeth became large in response to many different evolutionary pressures. The

most striking feature of ivory is how each group has responded differently to meet their respective mechanical challenges and the limitations of developmental processes. Teeth are structured primarily to resist axial compression. The relatively unspecialized structure in whales and the forwardly projecting incisors of hippopotamus continue to meet this need. Elephants and hippopotamus have evolved curved tusks as levers that must resist bending, and it is here that waved architecture causes most modifications from simple tooth structure. Functionally, the orientation of laminae and dentinal tubules may give strength appropriate for a tusk, i.e., resistance to lateral stress from bending, rather than just resistance to axial compression as in teeth. Dentine in tusks is maximally stressed from bending closest to the surface. This allows them to be cylinders (at least in part) without loss of strength. The same argument can be applied to the dentinal tubules themselves. They lose little resistance to bending by being cylinders rather than rods.

This study is incomplete in that it does not show the relation between calcified collagen fibers, the object of much study (e.g., Su and Cui, 1999; Nalla et al., 2003), and dentinal tubules. However, it does provide a structural basis for future correlations between microscopic and molecular levels. The staining of dentinal tubules with the touch of a fine marker pen on a polished surface is a revealing tool to identify the kind of ivory used to make antiques.

Conclusions

In covering this wide field I am very conscious of interpretations presented with only the data that I have had the time and opportunity to gather. In this discussion on ivory structure there are bound to be errors and gaps in understanding. I have been fortunate to correspond with Dr. A. Virag, who kindly shared with me the paper that he is about to publish (131).

Chapter 7
Keratin,

The External Skeleton of Vertebrates

7.1. Introduction

Two molecules, collagen and keratin, define the evolution of vertebrates. Collagen, while not unique to vertebrates, has evolved as their speciality, particularly when calcified in bones and teeth. It is their preferred material for growing and modifying gross structures. Keratin is even more characteristic of vertebrates as their dead external protective covering.

Although horn is more versatile than bone in the things that can be made from it, horn artifacts are much less common. The reason is that bone is more durable, surviving undamaged unless eaten by carnivores with very acid stomachs like dogs or Bataleur eagles, or exposed to wet acid soil. Few animals have mastered the art of digesting keratin. Owls swallow their prey whole, complete with hair, feathers, and fur that they cannot digest. With gastronomic sensibility they elect not to send this baggage through their system but eruct it in pellets. If all organisms had this limitation on the digestion of keratin, far more horn and hair artifacts would survive, but several insect groups have discovered how to do it. Horn as well as hair can be a food source for clothes moths, tortricid moth larvae. Only the larvae feed on keratin, but they have mouth-parts just as tough as the main destroyers of horn, larder beetles of the genus *Dermestes*, Dermestidae. Insects can be much better than we are in separating horn from plastic: they have to be, their lives depend on it. Insects of many kinds dine on dead bodies. They are specialists, maggots go first, taking the soft parts. The last bits to go are horns and hooves, made from very nutritious but hard, chemically resistant keratin.

A group of beetles in the family Dermestidae, have the mouth parts and guts to do the job. Most of them belong to fifty-three species of the genus *Dermestes*, three of which became worldwide pests known as larder beetles, eating bacon, cheese, woolen carpets, and anything else in the days when we had larders. The adult beetles are 7–9 mm long with blackish wing covers and whitish scales (Figure 7.1 A). Most of the feeding is done by the larvae, active six legged creatures covered with tufts of hairs. The most famous is *D. vulpinus*, used by museums to clean dried flesh from skeletons. There are also many species of *Attagenus* and *Anthrenus*, some of which are pests. In a natural environment dermestids are important recyclers. I have seen them transform piles of Gnu horns to dust in weeks.

For the antiquarian, dermestids are invaluable in another way. Beetle pests were much commoner in households of the pasts and often took bites out of precious horn objects as well as what they could find in the kitchen. But they didn't eat plastic. If there are gnawing marks, it is a certain indicator that

(Opposite page)
Fig. 7.1. Keratin eaters. A. Larva and two species of Dermestes or larder beetle that are the most common cause of damage to keratin. Their bite marks are an invaluable clue that an object that looks like keratin is keratin and not a plastic imitator. This is particularly useful for the identification of tortoiseshell that has many good plastic imitators. B. A tortoiseshell comb has several Dermestes bite marks enlarged in C and D. E. Bite marks on a horn walking stick. Horn is easier to identify, but these bite marks are instantly conclusive.

Keratin Eaters

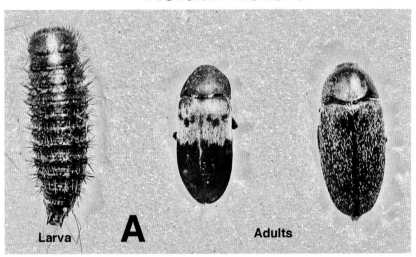

A

Larva

Adults

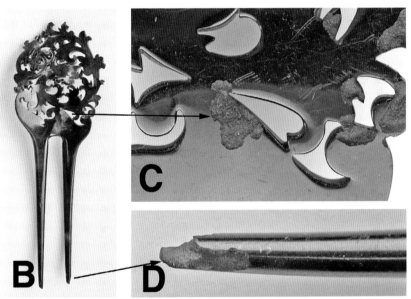

B

C

D

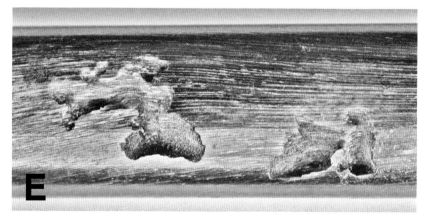

E

7.1

the object is made from keratin, and also that it is probably old (beetles are rare in houses these days). The marks are easy to spot with a hand lens or even by eye. They are pits about 3 mm wide showing the bite marks left by the beetle mandibles that scraped them out (Figure 7.1 B–D). They can be very destructive; more often the beetle has only had time to take a few bites before moving on. Small bite scrapes are surprisingly common. Seven out of the 12 small horn cups older than 50 years that I have in my collection have such bite marks.

7.2 Keratin Derivatives

Basic structure

Textbooks and papers from nineteenth century histologists bury their observations in terminology. It seems that everyone wanted to describe a new layer by naming it after himself, adding useless description rather than functional explanation for structure. Nowhere is this more apparent than in studies on epidermal derivatives, where dense nomenclature buried useful observation. In principle, different kinds of structure can be simply derived from the way that the keratin forming epithelium is folded and the kind and rate of deposition of the keratin. All keratin structures begin with dividing cells in a basal epithelium that form layers of linked cells that fill progressively with keratin filaments as they flatten towards the outside before being sloughed off. Human skin takes about forty-eight days from dividing cells at the base of the epidermis to shedding of dead cells at the surface (56),(99).

(Oppsite page)
Fig. 7.2. All keratin structures result from the division of epidermal cells that fill with precursor granules and filaments before dying. Skin forms like this. Nuclei and organelles disappear as the cells flatten and fill with filaments before being sloughed off on the outside. Differences in structure result from the kind of folding of the epidermis and the type of keratin filling the cells. Soft hydrated keratins are found in skin and hard dehydrated keratins form other protective structures. Scales, plaques of hard keratin overlying bones in reptiles and birds, form the simplest kind of surface protection. Hairs, characteristic of mammals, are cylinders of keratin forming by growth from the bottom of a tubular infold. Feathers, the characteristic structures of birds and dinosaurs, are more complicated. Dermal structures such as blood vessels form part of the core of the shaft that bears barbs held together by side branches of barbules. Horns, characteristic of the Bovidae, are cylinders of hard keratin around a core of bone projecting from the skull. Rhinoceros horns have a simpler structure. They are cylindrical outgrowths of keratin embedded in a keratin matrix, each cylinder forming above a papillae. Baleen forms the filter system that allows whales to feed on krill and small fish. Sea water passes between sheaves of keratin enclosing hair-like fibers that break free at the edges to form the filter. Nails (and claws, hooves, talons) are like scales growing at the tips of all vertebrate digits. Keratin is secreted on one side of the nail plate as it matures and slides over the nail bed.

Keratin derivatives

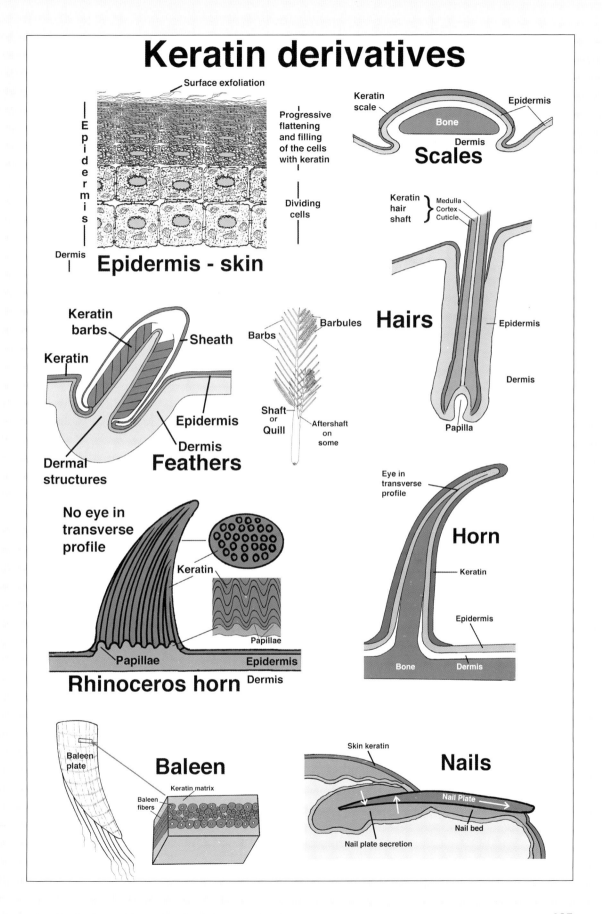

Epidermis - skin

Surface exfoliation

Epidermis

Progressive flattening and filling of the cells with keratin

Dividing cells

Dermis

Scales

Keratin scale

Bone

Epidermis

Dermis

Hairs

Keratin hair shaft — Medulla, Cortex, Cuticle

Epidermis

Dermis

Papilla

Feathers

Keratin barbs

Sheath

Keratin

Epidermis

Dermis

Dermal structures

Barbs

Barbules

Shaft or Quill

Aftershaft on some

Rhinoceros horn

No eye in transverse profile

Keratin

Papillae

Papillae

Epidermis

Dermis

Horn

Eye in transverse profile

Keratin

Epidermis

Bone

Dermis

Baleen

Baleen plate

Keratin matrix

Baleen fibers

Nails

Skin keratin

Nail Plate

Nail bed

Nail plate secretion

7.3. Skin, Vellum, and Leather

I shoot the Hippopotamus
With bullets made of platinum,
Because if I used leaden ones
His hide is sure to flatten 'em.
The Hippopotamus.

The Bad Child's Book of Beasts
Hilaire Belloc

Structure and properties

Skin is two layered, epidermis and dermis above a fatty connective tissue layer. The dermis is often the thickest layer of the skin below the cystine rich keratin of the epidermis (Figure 7.3.1). It contains many structures—blood vessels, nerves, sebaceous glands, hairs, sweat glands—but collagen and elastic fibers are the main structural components. It is their properties that determine those of the sheets and containers that are made from skin. Collagen fibers are strong and inelastic, properties that made skins and tendons (with bone) some of the first multipurpose natural animal materials (see Table 2.3).

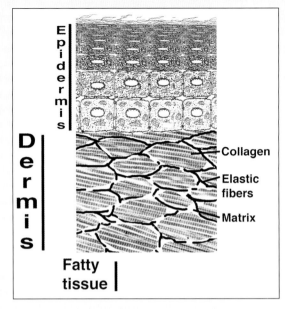

Figure 7.3.1. Skin consist of two layers above fatty tissue with keratin the main structural element in the epidermis and collagen in the dermis. The dermis contains many structures—blood vessels, nerves, sebaceous glands, hairs, sweat glands—but collagen and elastic fibers are the main structural components. The dermis, below the cystine-rich keratin of the epidermis, is often the thickest layer of the skin. Its properties have made it suitable for sheets, coverings, and containers.

Tensile strengths of some natural materials

Material	Tensile strength, p.s.i.
Cartilage	430
Fresh skin	1500
Tanned leather	6,000
Fresh tendon	12,000
Fresh bone	16,000
Human hair	28,000
Silk	50,000
Nylon thread	150,000

From {Gordon. J.E., 1978 #196}

We can demonstrate that the tensile strength of collagen exceeds that of glass very easily. If a careless laboratory worker (or kitchen hand) leaves a gelatin (= collagen) solution to dry out in the bottom of a glass vessel, it sticks to the surface and dries to the consistency of a jelly bean. A layer of glass then breaks away as it shrinks further since the adhesion between collagen molecules and between collagen and the glass is stronger than between glass and glass. It is no surprise that Stone Age man knew what he was doing when he dressed in skins. So did the armorers of nations throughout the world before the advent of metal and guns when they dressed their fighting men in heavy skin or leather. Tendons are the collagen extensions of muscles at their origins and insertions and not part of the skin, but their properties and uses are similar to skin strips used to make string.

In the spirit of an age when nothing was wasted it was customary for farmers to create tough, long lasting whips from bull penises (Figure 7.33.3 G) by twisting them and pulling them out two or three feet. If this seems a good length, consider the early whalers who, in the same spirit, valued the six-foot penises of sperm whales enough to flay them and to stretch their skin out into a sheet large enough to make an Inverness Cape.

Scarification. Scarification, the art of forming patterns of deep scars by rubbing particles into wounds to keep them open, was performed for many purposes, magical, medical, religious, rights of passage, adornment, clan and tribal identity. It is commonest in Africa and Australia suggesting that it preceded tattooing, which is rare in those continents but widespread throughout the rest of the world.

Tattooing. Scarification probably led to tattooing, the introduction of stable particles such as charcoal to spaces between cells in the dermis, leading to a more or less permanent fine patterning in the skin. Tattooing is made possible by the permanence of the dermis, where particles find a permanent home. The particles may be diluted as the dermis

increases in area or thickness, but unlike the epidermis that grows only to be shed, the dermis remains in place. Tattooing began in the modern western world when sailors voyaging in the Pacific returned with tattoos after living happily and intimately with local inhabitants, later spreading widely aboard whaling ships. While on the *Endeavour* during Captain Cook's first voyage of discovery in the Pacific, Joseph Banks records how in Tahiti it was a traditional "right of passage" to have solid black buttocks as well as decorative patterns tattooed over much of the body. He, and most of the crew, came back with tattoos in 1771. Lieutenant Bligh was on that expedition and later captained the ill-fated *Bounty*, on which all but one of the mutineers were tattooed (1). The "native" type tattoos of that period have evolved to become "high art" in western youth (Figures 7.3.2 D, E).

Vellum, parchment, papyrus, and leather

Little I ask: my wants are few …
… of red Morocco's gilded gleam
And vellum rich as country cream.

Contentment
Oliver Wendell Holmes,
1809-1894

Vellum is skin from almost any mammal, commonly calves or sheep, but even from pigs, horses, and camels, prepared to take writing or printing ink. The word comes from the Latin *vellus*, the skin of any animal, through the Old French *vélin*, meaning calf skin, the same root that gives us veal, calf meat. The use of vellum dates from the second century BC in Asia Minor, but it was slow to spread in competition with papyrus, from which we get the word paper although paper is not made from papyrus. Papyrus, used by both Romans and Egyptians, was made as early as 3,000 BC from a river sedge, *Cyperus papyrus*, localized to the Nile. However, as the Roman Empire spread through Europe away from the source of *Cyperus papyrus,* it became more

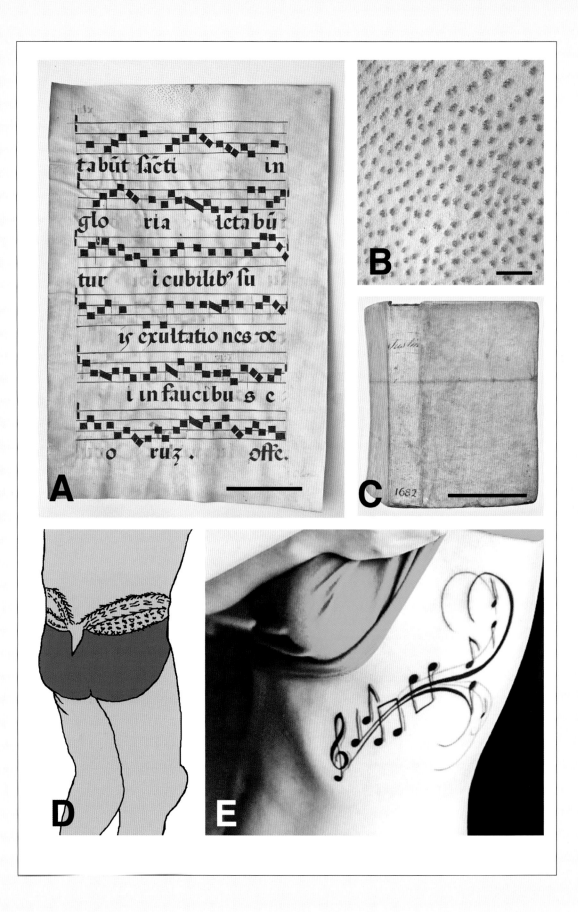

convenient to use the skins that were found everywhere. Vellum replaced papyrus until it in turn was superseded by true paper. True paper prepared from plant cellulose fibers by the eunuch T'sai Lun in the Court of the Chinese Emperor Ho-Ti in 600 BC began to be used in Europe in the twelfth century AD. It spread with the Arabs to Egypt and Spain and from there to the rest of Europe, where it came into general use as an essential part of the revolution from the introduction of the printing press in the fifteenth century. Between the times of papyrus and paper, illustrations and the written word were stored on vellum (Figure 7.3.2).

Terminology is imprecise. Vellum usually indicates quality, but it may mean made from the unsplit skin, parchment being used for split skins, but parchment may also mean paper made to look like vellum. The best quality vellum comes from young or even stillborn fetuses. Skins are soaked in water, hair removed, bleached in lime, stretched, dried, and the surface finished by being abraded with fine pumice and whitened with chalk and talc. The skins were often split, making them thinner and more translucent, the inner surface being made into vellum and the outer hair surface into leather. Vellum is still used for important documents because of its durability. Its strength also made it suitable for drumheads and lamp shades (but not made from the tattooed skin of Buchenwald inmates, probably a myth exposed as a post war exercise in allied propaganda).

Containers

The heads of medieval English criminals were hard-boiled after execution before being impaled on spikes for exhibition. This blackened them, denaturing their proteins, making them more resistant to the weather, and prolonging the show. Although the executioners did not know this, they were continuing a skill dating back to early prehistory. The skins of whole animals were made into bags and filled with entrails to be boiled into soup over the fire, much as more recent Boy Scouts have been taught how to boil water in paper bags. Relics of these techniques survive around the world in the use of air-filled whole skins as floats. In coastal nineteenth century Scotland, floats for fishing nets were made from the skins of dogs. The head, legs, and other body orifices were sealed and the skin tarred and inflated. Dog skins, like other large furry mammals, lack sweat glands, producing a skin without small holes.

Smaller containers were made by stretching skins over forms. The Kikuyu box in Figure 7.3.3 D, E was simply made by stretching skin with the hair side outermost over a round wooden stick and holding it over a fire to singe off the hair and dry the skin. The surface was scraped clean and cut from the pole to give a clean edge. Drying was completed by filling the box with hot ashes. A second stick with a slightly different diameter was used to make the lid.

The natural shapes of udders and scrotums were used to make bottles to store perfumes and scented oils in India up to the middle of the twentieth century (Figure 7.3.3 C, F). Hair and epidermis were scraped off a goat scrotum tied to give the neck of a bottle around the end of a bamboo tube. It was then blown up and dried over a fire. These bottles remained in use until replaced

(Opposite page)
Figure 7.3.2. The durability of skin. A. Vellum changes little in color with time. The *Missal* written on vellum of stretched calves skin in 1606 is as unblemished and colorful as if it had just been made. B. An enlargement from A, with hair follicles, shows that it is made from unsplit skin. The piece is too thick to be the outer surface of split skin. C. Vellum withstands wear. The *History of Justin* was bound in 1682 and has been used by many hands, but its cover shows little sign of wear. It is thin vellum lacking hair follicles and is made from the split inner surface. D, E. Tattoos last the lifetime of the individual because particles inserted into the dermis remain there, unlike the keratin that is continually shed. D. A Tahitian tattoo recorded by Joseph Banks in his journey with Captain Cook on the *Endeavour* (1768–1771). The buttocks are entirely black and much of the body has patterns. Such tattooing was a rite of passage for Tahitian men. E. In contrast, a modern (2011) tattoo may be an exercise in artistic expression. Scales, A, C = 5 cm, B = 1 mm.

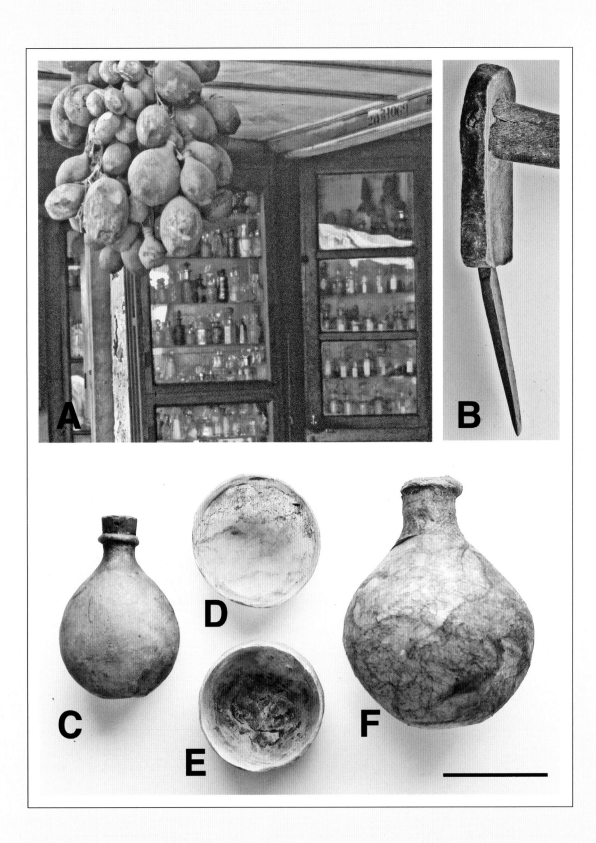

by cheap plastic towards the end of the twentieth century. Bunches of skin bottles, like exaggerated pawnbroker signs, were the outdoor symbols of perfume vendors for many years (Figure 7.3.3 A). The sheep caecum, a blindly ending tube just larger than its human homologue, the appendix, lent itself to the creation of soft, pliable condoms for use by strict Jews forbidden to use synthetic materials for the purpose.

More delicate and larger containers were made from the endodermal equivalents of the surface skin such as the urinary bladder. Balloons made from pigs' bladders were part of a jester's equipment, and continue to be used in authentic reproductions of Morris dancers.

The makers of stringed instruments knew the properties of strips of skin (rawhide) when they used cow gut to string lutes. (Shakespeare knew this and much more about the properties and uses of hides and guts, which is one of the best pieces of evidence that the commoner from Stratford on Avon familiar with practical matters wrote the plays and not some rich aristocrat).

Thick skins for heavy wear. Skins are ideal for use as hinges because the only friction used in bending is internal in the fine structure, functioning without the friction in metal bearings. Thick skins of elephants, hippos, and buffalo are also suited for mounting tools such as adzes and chisels (Figure 7.3.3 B). More frequently these functions were born by skin made into leather.

Leather. Protein denaturation by heating over a fire may have been the origin of leather, since wood tar contains tanning agents such as polyphenols and quinones. Protein treatment for leather making is complicated in detail and too big a topic to be elaborated on here, but the principle is simple. Proteins contain many hydrophilic reactive groups such as $-NH2$ or $-OH$ that make them soluble in water. Tanning agents cross-link such groups in adjacent skin proteins, mainly collagen in the dermis, creating giant, hard, insoluble hydrophobic polymer sheets. These are then worked physically to soften them into leather. Many tanning agents, such as quinones or metal ions like chromium, can cross link proteins. Other agents were used primarily to remove particular components of skin as a preliminary to tanning. In the Middle Ages, dog poop was gathered from the streets as a valuable commodity used to prepare skins. The world famous tannery in Fez that produces "Morocco Leather" still uses pigeon poop. Different kinds of leather depend on the skin components that survive such treatments as much as on the tanning process.

Shagreen.

Shagreen is a special kind of leather made from the skins of sharks and rays, members of the ancient group of cartilaginous fishes classified as elasmobranchs, characterized by their rough, protective, sandpaper-like skin, with its embedded enamel denticles. Rays were especially favored as they provided large flat areas of skin. In the process of leather making, the denticles were removed to create interesting slightly raised oval patterns. Shagreen was originally made in ancient China and later in Japan from the skins of the cow tail stingray, *Pastinachus (Hypolophus) sephen*, common in shallow waters of the Indo-Pacific. The wet skin was draped over a wooden form and allowed to dry, shrinking to its new shape before being polished, as in the Chinese spectacle case in Figure 7.3.4 C and the Japanese knife and ivory chopstick case in Figure 7.3 D. These old shagreens

(Opposite page)
Figure 7.3.3. The uses of skin. A. Skin bottles used as signs to advertise a perfume shop in India in the 1960s. B. Elephant, hippo, or buffalo skin used as a seat for a steel adze. Kenya, nineteenth to twentieth century. D–F. Skin was used after little treatment for containers of all kinds. C, F. Perfume bottles, India, nineteenth century. Probably made from goat scrotums. D, E. Pill box, top and bottom, Kikuyu, Africa, early twentieth century. Made from stretched surface skin. Scales C–F = 5 cm. Both external (epidermal plus dermal) and internal (e.g. bladder) surface skins may be used.

Reptilian skin of the marine turtle *Eretmochelys imbricata*

> *The turtle lives 'twixt plated decks*
> *Which practically conceal its sex.*
> *I think it clever of the turtle*
> *In such a fix to be so fertile.*
>
> The Turtle
> by Ogden Nash

Introduction

Reptile's and bird's feet have a covering of stiff keratin scales separated by regions of soft skin to create a body armor that is both protective and flexible (Figure 7.2). Dermal bones, local plaques of calcified collagen, support the scales. In the Chelonia, tortoises' and turtles' dermal bones fuse with one another and the ribs below them to form a rigid, protective, boxlike shell around the thorax and abdomen, creating a body of ten segments, the shortest of any vertebrate (except frogs). The shell bones are covered by

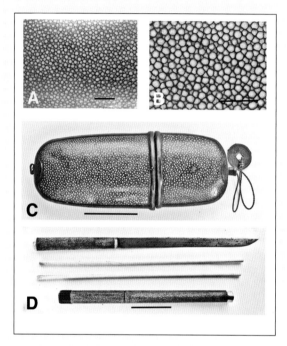

Figure 7.3.4. Shagreen, skin of the cow tail stingray, *Pastinachus (Hypolophus) sephen*, tanned and dyed green with denticles removed. Other elasmobranchs or skates and sharks are also used. A, B. Surface view of the skin. C. A typical use for shagreen to cover a nineteenth century Chinese spectacle case.

The hawksbill turtle, *Eretmochelys imbricata*

Hawksbills are the smallest of the sea turtles, but even so they may grow up to a meter [three feet] in length and weigh 80 kilograms [176 pounds]. The largest recorded weight is 127 kilograms [300 pounds]. Several characteristics distinguish them from other sea turtles. Their elongated, tapered head ends in a sharply pronounced and hooked beak-like mouth, with a sharp tomium, the cutting edge of the beak. Their heads have two pairs of prefrontal scutes; their arms have two claws on each flipper; as protection from abrasive corals in their environment they have very thick scutes on their carapaces and plastrons; and the scutes on the rear margin of

were usually colored green by treating them with copper arsenate made from copper sulfate and arsenious oxide (Figure 7.3.4 A, B). Occasionally they were light brown, perhaps faded from the green. Recently shagreen made from the cow tail stingray has become an expensive fashion item using modern dyes to create exotic colors. Other leathers have sometimes been patterned to create faux shagreens.

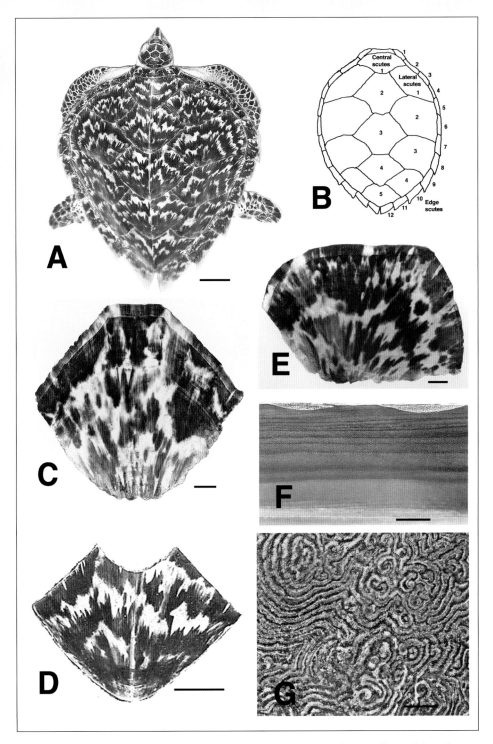

Figure 7.4.1. Tortoiseshell structure. A–B. Dorsal view of the hawksbill turtle, *Eretmochelys imbricata*, and outlines of the scutes. C. Central scute 3, separated from the underlying bone. E. Lateral scute 2. The bands on anterior edges show the extent of new growth. D. Outline of the exposed central scute 3 from A, with the overlap covered by the more anterior and lateral scutes missing. Compare C and D to see the overlap. F. Tortoiseshell is deposited in layers showing up as bands in transverse profile. Darker regions retain the remnants of cells with melanin granules. G. The layers are not uniformly flat but deposited in a complex pattern characteristic of tortoiseshell. View from the forming face. Scales: A = 5 cm, C, D, E, G = 1 cm, F = 1 mm.

the carapace point outwards, giving a serrated look. Males are similar in size to females but have longer claws, thicker tails, and somewhat brighter coloring than females. Hawksbills are also distinguished in their ecology, being the only turtles feeding primarily on sponges and coelenterates. Their average life span in the wild is thirty to fifty years.

Distribution

Hawksbills have a worldwide distribution mostly in tropical waters, with two subspecies, *E. imbricata imbricata* from the Atlantic and *E. imbricata bissa* from the Indo-Pacific. They migrate across open ocean waters to nest throughout their range, but spend most time feeding in shallow lagoons, mangrove swamps, and coral reefs. They avoid deep waters, preferring coastlines where sponges are abundant and sandy nesting sites are within reach (34, 79).

In the Atlantic, *E. i. imbricata* populations range from Long Island Sound and Massachusetts to Florida, the Gulf of Mexico, and the Caribbean to the Brazilian coast, and on the other side of the Atlantic from the Cape of Good Hope to the frigid waters of the English Channel.

E. i. bissa is tropical and subtropical. The Indo-Pacific populations extend from the Red Sea and Persian Gulf along the east coast of Africa to the southern Asian coasts, Indonesia, and northern Australia. The Pacific range extends from Korea, Japan, and northern New Zealand, most of the Pacific islands to the west coast of the Americas from Chile to the Baja peninsula.

Present status

Since 1996 all hawksbills trade has been banned by CITES because they are critically endangered, although it is hard to know exactly how endangered because of their worldwide distribution and migratory habit.

Human fishing practices threaten hawksbill populations with extinction. The most wasteful killing is of young hawksbill turtles for stuffed souvenirs, an unnecessary luxury trade that has had a major impact on turtle populations. Commercial trade in tortoiseshell (= *bekko* in Japanese, the term for the hawksbill carapace) has declined worldwide since CITES came into force in 1975 and since 1983 when commercial trade in turtles was prohibited under most circumstances for the seventy-eight countries that were then part of CITES. Unfortunately, France and Japan took "reservations" that allowed them to continue to trade. Between 1962 and 1981, Japan imported about 30,000kg [66,000 pounds] of worked *bekko* a year, the equivalent of almost 800,000 hawksbills, mostly from Panama, Cuba, and Indonesia, then major exporters of tortoiseshell. In addition, between 1950 and 1992, Japan imported about the same weight of raw *bekko* shells a year adding up to the loss of more than 1.3 million large hawksbills.

In 1989, CITES concluded that global hawksbill populations were depleted or declining in fifty-six of sixty-five countries where data were available. In 1991, pressured by a U.S. embargo of fishery products and support from the 172 member countries of CITES, Japan agreed to end its tortoiseshell imports but with government support the Japanese industry has remained intact by using up its stockpiles of *bekko*. This led to a shortage of raw shell that has pushed up the price to $1,000 per kilo, a sure way to encourage the illicit harvesting that is now rampant, including imports to Japan from South East Asia. Global volume of trade has been reduced, but a lack of reliable data on population levels in the numerous hawksbill populations leaves the illicit tortoiseshell trade an unquantified but pervasive threat to hawksbill recovery.

It is now illegal to import or export any turtle products since the entire family Cheloniidae has been listed by CITES. In spite of this, tourists from around the world continue to buy tortoiseshell articles in local markets in Vietnam, the Caribbean, Dominican Republic, Central America, Colombia, and Venezuela, although they are often seized by customs on return to their home countries. Whatever the exact numbers of turtles killed, world trade has caused and continues to cause long-lasting effects on hawksbill populations.

Scute shape and growth

The bone shell covered by scutes consists of a dorsal carapace and a ventral plastron. Bone plates below the scutes interlock and grow around their edges in a pattern similar to that of the scutes (Figure 7.4.2 D, E). The carapace has a single dorsal row of five keratin scutes flanked on each side by four large scutes separated from the ventral plastron by twelve small scutes that curve around the edge (Figure 7.4.1 A–E). The plastron consists of a paired row of large scutes.

In the giant tortoise *Chelonoidis nigra* from the Galapagos (Figure 7.4.2 A) and other tortoises, scute growth is around all the edges, unlike that in most turtles. Growth in the hawksbill is forward at the front and back, causing the forward edge to position itself under the scute in front of it and the rear edge to overlap the scute behind it (Figure 7.4.2 B). Growth in the area occurs largely at the front of each scute, leading to the elongated pattern of dark blotches radiating from the narrower posterior edge (Figure 7.4.2 A–E). Although the shapes of the keratin plates look at first glance to match the shapes and patterns of the bones, their edges do not coincide but lie between those of the bone plates, suggesting that dermal and epidermal growth are independent (Figure 7.4.2 D, E).

The Japanese developed a technique for gently heating the dorsal carapace so that the keratin scutes came away without damage to the epidermis that secreted them. The turtle was then released to grow another shell. Scutes on the plastron are more sensitive, their removal causing death.

Diet

Their near relatives are carnivorous but hawksbills are omnivorous with an unusual main diet of sponges (a turtle is estimated to eat more than 500 Kg [1100 lbs.] a year) and floating jellyfish, including the dangerous Portuguese man o'war (*Physalia physalis*) armed with stinging nematocysts. The hawksbill's scutes protect their bodies from the stings, but leave their eyes vulnerable, which they therefore close when they feed. Perhaps this is why so many die while trying to eat floating plastic bags.

The diet containing poisonous nematocysts can make their flesh toxic. In spite of this, hawksbills are eaten as a delicacy in many parts of the world. Hawksbill turtle soup is still served in the Caribbean. As far back as the fifth century BC, hawksbills were eaten as delicacies in China, where various tortoiseshell concoctions—*T'u-p'l, Kuei-pan, Kuei-chia*—had medicinal uses (5) to "open up meridians and activate the lo passageways." If that doesn't work, try *Ti-lung* (earthworms). Turtles and tortoises gathered from the countryside could still be found stacked high in late twentieth century Chinese markets. In contrast to the hawksbill, the commonly eaten green turtle, *Chelonia midas*, is herbivorous, feeding mainly on sea grasses. It gets its name from its green fat and cartilage called *calipee*. In times past turtle soup was served at the annual banquet of the Lord Mayor of London. Perhaps the possibility of being poisoned from soup made with the wrong kind of turtle may give new meaning to the activities of the waiters who would serve the soup with the question, "Would you care for a little of My Lord Mayor's green fat."

Scute structure and color

The color and structural properties of their scutes have made hawksbills famous as the source of tortoiseshell (Table 7.4). Tortoiseshell scutes have an attractive pale yellow to amber background patterned with light to dark brown almost black radiating streaks; they soften with heat when hydrated, allowing them to be shaped and molded, are hard and fine textured allowing their surface to take a fine polish, have a low thermal conductivity giving them a feeling of warmth against the skin. Their scutes are also thicker than those of other turtles as an adaptation to cope with wear from abrasive corals encountered when they forage reefs for their preferred food of sponges.

Tortoiseshell is deposited in layers that show up as bands in transverse profile (Figure 7.4.1 F). The layers are not deposited uniformly parallel to one another but in a complex pattern diagnostic for tortoiseshell (Figure 7.4.1 G). The pattern is three-dimensional, most easily seen on the untouched forming face as a series of whorls somewhat like Liesegang rings (though unrelated to them in their formation). The whorls correspond to slight differences in the timing of deposition of new keratin layers, leading to differences in elevation as if a sandy seashore had been swirled into curves rather than into ripples from waves parallel to the shore. The pattern may also show up in planes overcut (i.e., polished with too much pressure so that layers with slightly different composition or orientation are preferentially removed) parallel to the forming face, sometimes but not always allowing it to be seen in artifacts. The clarifying hot water treatment used to prepare tortoiseshell for making artifacts diminishes the diagnostic pattern by squeezing out surviving cell spaces and layers.

The color in light yellow regions is due to the keratin. Such regions are translucent but never completely transparent, always slightly cloudy by eye due to the survival of parts of the cells that contain the keratin. Cells are more obvious in darker regions due to the melanin granules clustered around their nuclei. The various shades of light brown to black depend on these cells and the kinds and concentrations of their melanin (Figure 7.4.1 F).

Working tortoiseshell

Tortoiseshell can be worked to shape very quickly on a 220 grit lap or drum followed by 600 grit followed by polishing on wet leather or felt charged with alumina, cerium oxide, or iron oxide. It is very heat sensitive. Removing one small burn spot may require the regrinding of a whole surface. Try to clean and polish by hand without using power tools. If you must use power tools to clean and polish, use a low speed and a 5 cm or wider diameter wet buff. Reduce the pressure that causes heating by holding the workpiece in the hand rather than supporting it on the bench.

7. 4. Hooves, Claws, and Beaks

Definitions

Skin keratin can be locally specialized into hard sheets at the tips of the digits of most mammals, birds, and reptiles, and some amphibia, and sometimes around the mouth (Figure 7.2) (7). They are claws when curved and pointed, nails when flat with a curved edge instead of a point as in humans and some other primates. Hooves are nails large and strong enough to bear the weight of the animal, as in horses and cattle. Ungulates are any mammals with hooves. With the advent of DNA sequencing, their relationships with other groups have changed but they still form a natural group with two branches, the odd-toed horses, tapirs, rhinoceros' (Perissodactyla) and the even-toed cattle, deer, pigs, camels, and more distantly related hippos (Artiodactyla or more properly Cetartiodactyla). Beaks are hard keratin around the mouth in birds and reptiles.

Hooves

In principle hooves of both even- (Figure 7.5.2 A, B, C) and odd-toed ungulates (Figure 7.5.2 J, K) consist of five functional components and the connections between them. (1) A central rod of articulating digital bones can be moved by (2) tendons attached to the end bone that connects at the tip to the inside of (3), a peripheral diagonally cut cylinder of hard keratin with pad of soft elastic hydrated keratin at the bottom. Cushions (4) lie between the horn and the bones, and (1 & 2) are embedded in skin and connective tissue (5). The simplicity of this structure is often obscured by terminology and detail (15).

History. Until the advent of internal combustion engines, cities, towns, and farmlands almost throughout the world supported large populations of horses, the main means of transportation. Estimates for the domestic population of horses in the U.S. were 8 million in 1867, 21.5 million in 1915;

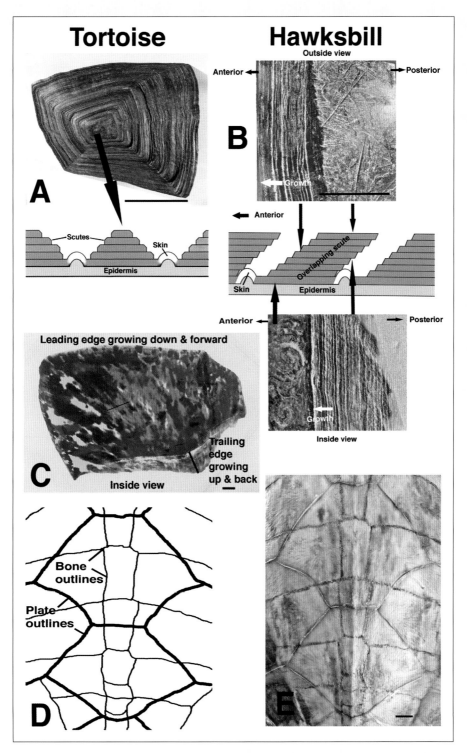

Figure 7.4.2. Tortoiseshell growth. A. A scute from a tortoise like this *Chelonoidis nigra*, from the Galapagos, grows around all the edges, unlike that of turtles such as the hawksbill, *Eretmochelys imbricata*, B, which grows at the front and back, causing the scutes to overlap. C. A scute from the plastron (ventral surface) showing the leading edge close to the epidermis and the trailing edge overlapping the more posterior scute. D, E. The scute outlines on the bones of the carapace are positioned between the growing bone edges, showing the independence of dermal bone growth and epidermal scute growth. Scales: A = 5 cm, B, C, E = 1 cm

the U.K. had 3.3 million in late Victorian times. After death, their skins were a mainstay of tanneries and their bones were a valuable substitute for ivory and essential for glue making, but although hooves were readily available in massive quantities they were only used for occasional decorative items such as snuff boxes and never became important commodities for things other than glue, animal feed, and fertilizer. Cattle contributed horns to the economy as well as meat, skin, and bones, but not hooves. The importance of horses and cattle has led to detailed knowledge of hoof structure, but the cause of their hooves not becoming an industrial commodity is not addressed. The reasons may lie in their structure and awkwardly shaped small sizes. Perhaps by the time it was realized that hooves could be pressed and molded, cheaper synthetic plastic substitutes had become available. Claws and beaks were even more limited in their industrial uses. Illustrations of structure are included here to encourage artisans to think of using this beautiful material in their creations and to enable antiquarians to identify hooves on the rare occasions that they may be encountered.

Structure. Hoof keratin is a fiber in matrix composite (12) (125). The key to understanding its structure lies in a change in the orientation of components from that in skin (Figure 7.5.1). Skin functions as a protective covering forming and shedding layers parallel to the forming face. Hooves meet stress in the length of the hoof at right angles to the skin. They accomplish this by rearranging the epidermis around papillae projecting as tubules at right angles to the surface. Microscopy shows a progressive filling of the tubule space by keratin layers in much the same way as epidermal layers of keratin are shed to make skin keratin, but with an orientation normal to the surface rather than parallel to it. Unlike the relatively smooth surface of the skin from which they are derived, all hoof keratin has tubules forming keratin cylinders separated either by a randomly arranged hard keratin matrix or

by soft hydrated laminae in pad keratin. Hard keratin forms in parallel layers around tubules that are fine and straight (Figure 7.5.2 G, H). In the central hydrated pad, the tubules are wider and distorted, sometimes helical, as might be expected from the softness of their keratin (Figure 7.5.2 D, E, F). Tangential profiles (Figure 7.5.2 D) have a pattern similar to that indicating helicoidal architecture for chitin in insect cuticle (75). This suggests that the laminae may be in plywood-like layers with a progressive regular change in orientation of their keratin components. The cylinders are probably a developmental mechanism for obtaining keratin sheets normal to the main stress but in the pad they could also be responsible for maintaining the hydration necessary for softness.

Growth. The basic structure of hoof keratin is that of cylindrical sheets parallel to the filament surface from which they have parted, separated by keratin in a reticular pattern uniformly resistant to stress (11, 12, 67, 125). Wear around the edge of the cylinder of hard keratin is compensated by growth in length from the base and diagonal growth of lamellae from the inside (Figure 7.5.2 A, B, I). The pad is exposed to wear over its whole surface with growth over that surface (Figure 7.5.1 and 7.5.2 A). The growth patterns confirm the derivation of the hard keratin from an enlarged nail (Figure 7.5.2 A, B, J), and the pad as a second round of adaptation from skin. Both use tubules to change the keratin orientation by 90° from that in skin.

Claws and hooves in other mammals. Elephants have very large toenails, although they are only distantly related to ungulates. African elephants have four nails on their front feet and three on the hind, separating them from Indian elephants with five nails on the front and four on the hind, sometimes allowing the country of origin to be determined when the feet are made into waste baskets.

Bird Beaks. The loss of teeth with the evolution of beaks has had profound consequences. Horn is tough, but much softer than tooth enamel. As a consequence, birds

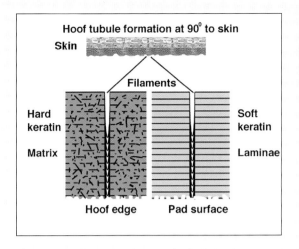

Hoof tubule formation at 90⁰ to skin

Skin

Filaments

Hard keratin

Matrix

Soft keratin

Laminae

Hoof edge

Pad surface

Figure 7.5.1. The change from soft skin requires rigidity and toughness for the hoof shell and soft elasticity for the pad. Cylinders of epidermis from the forming face turn through 900 to create a fiber in matrix structure.

Figure 7.5.2. Ungulate hooves. All hoof keratin forms around cylindrical extensions (filaments) from papillae on the epidermis. A. Artiodactyl (even-toed) hooves consist of a partial cylinder of hard keratin lined on the inside by lamellae and making contact with the ground by a hydrated soft elastic pad. Saggital profile of one of the terminal pairs of an Artiodactyl hoof to show the main components and directions of keratin growth. Wear around the edge of the hard keratin is compensated by growth in length from the base (arrows). Wear on the pad takes place from the inside normal to the surface. B. Transverse profile of C, an elk hoof. D–F. Soft hydrated cow pad keratin. D. Distorted or twisted rather than straight filament profiles appear in tangential profiles as expected if the soft elastic keratin is deformed by a helicoidal plywood-like arrangement of keratin laminae around the filaments. E, F. Twisted or helical filaments traverse laminae in transverse profiles. G, H. Hard keratin. The filaments are straight in longitudinal G. and transverse profiles. I, J. Perissodactyl (odd-toed) hooves have a structure similar to Artiodactyls but differing in detail. I. Saggital profile of a Perissodactyl hoof. J. Horse hoof.

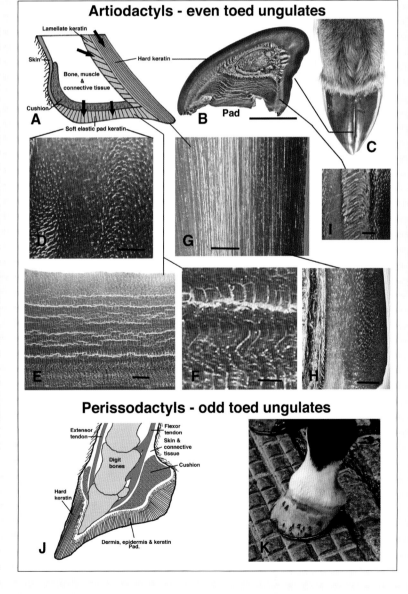

Artiodactyls - even toed ungulates

Lamellate keratin

Skin

Hard keratin

Bone, muscle & connective tissue

Cushion

A

Soft elastic pad keratin

B Pad

C

D

G

I

E

F

H

Perissodactyls - odd toed ungulates

Extensor tendon

Flexor tendon

Skin & connective tissue

Digit bones

Cushion

Hard keratin

Dermis, epidermis & keratin Pad.

J

K

swallow hard stone grit to grind up vegetation that they swallow whole. The only beaks that have commercial significance come from the Helmeted Hornbill, *Rhinoplax vigil.*

The Helmeted Hornbill from the Malay peninsula, Sumatra, and Borneo is one of fifty-five species in the family Bucerotidae. It is now "near threatened." All the hornbills have an enlarged upper bill or casque, most of which are shells of beak keratin around a bone cavity. Unlike other hornbills, the casque of the Helmeted Hornbill is solid. Together with the skull and bill they weigh up to 300 g, ten percent of the bird's weight. This keratin casque known as hornbill "ivory" or *angang gading* to the Javanese is fine grained and takes a good polish like very superior ivory but deeper yellow with a superficial bright scarlet layer. Its qualities have made it one of the most expensive natural materials used for carving in South East Asia, especially Java and Japan.

Hornbill was introduced into China from Borneo in 1371, and has been carved there ever since. In the eighteenth century hornbill snuff bottles were especially prized. By the nineteenth century, the Ho-a-ching shop in Canton had developed techniques to make jewelry for the foreign market. The people of Java and Sumatra were also pioneers in their use of *angang gading*, where the Dutch supported the industry for the European trade.

Claws are a common ingredient in folk jewelry, notably those of grouse coupled with citrine and smoky quartz by the Scots.

Conclusions. The failure of hooves, claws, and beaks to become a commercial commodity in spite of their abundance has many causes, mainly the pieces are too small, awkwardly shaped, and lack uniform properties. Their structure has much to teach us about the mechanics of natural materials. Unless a fad develops for creating models of the mythical Norse ship *Naglfar,* that was made entirely from toenails and fingernails, they are likely to remain of biological but not commercial interest.

7.6. Horns

The preyful princess pierc'd and prick'd a pretty pleasing pricket. Some say a sore: but not a sore, till now made sore with shooting.

Shakespeare
Loves Labours Lost IV II 58
(Pricket = two year old buck,
sore = four year old buck).

"When the males are provided with weapons which in the female are absent, there can hardly be any doubt that these serve for fighting with other males:"

Kudu, from Darwin, *The Descent of Man*
Sexual selection, the Law of Battle

*Why, with horns that jar and with fiery eyes,
Should the male stags fight for the shuddering does.*

The Gazelles
T.S. Moore

Biologists may criticize those who conflate horns and antlers, and yet the two are structurally more similar than they care to admit. They both occur in even-toed ruminant ungulates (Table 7.6.1). Deer form the family Cervidae that grow antlers, annually shedding bone outgrowths temporarily covered with skin. The others have horns, permanent bone outgrowths covered by layers of hard keratin. One family, the Antilocapridae, have horns that in some ways resemble antlers. Their horns are branched and their surface is shed. They also have a horn structure quite different from all other ungulate horns with longitudinal, hollow, hair-like filaments somewhat like the hard keratin of hooves (Figure 7.6.7). The surface display of keratin in most horns makes us forget that, like antlers, their strength lies primarily in their bone core, the keratin often being only a very thin protective layer (Figure 7.6.3 A, B). Horns are protective devices for bone outgrowths from

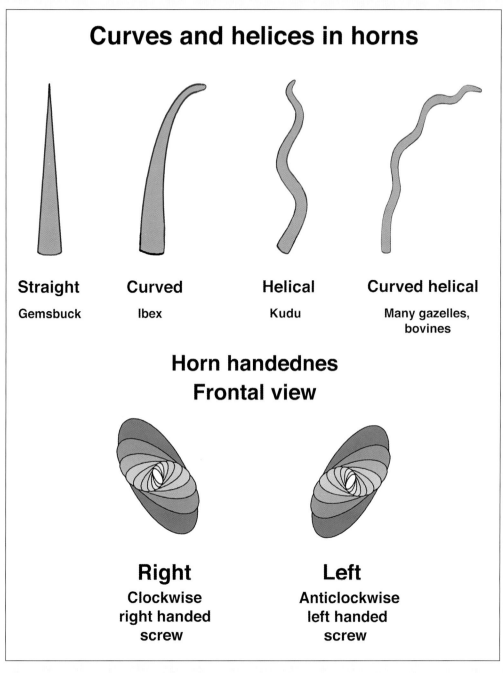

Curves and helices in horns

Straight	Curved	Helical	Curved helical
Gemsbuck	Ibex	Kudu	Many gazelles, bovines

Horn handednes
Frontal view

Right
Clockwise
right handed
screw

Left
Anticlockwise
left handed
screw

Figure 7.6.1. Curves and helices. The daunting variety of horn shapes may be simplified as cones distorted with two variables, curves and helices. The simplest horns are straight (growth is uniform around the base). Straight horns may also be helical, as in markhor goats and Racka sheep. In more complicated horns, the curves lie in one plane with greater growth on one side of the base. A constant growth gives the horn a long, flat C shape (ibex). A varying angle can give a hook (chamois). In helical horns, the angle changes from plane to plane by a constant amount like a corkscrew (an elevated growth rate moves around the base), or varying amount like a short screw. The most complex shapes occur when a helix is imposed on a curved horn screw (an elevated growth rate moves around the base, which has a biased elevated rate on one side). In practice, most horns are a complex mixture, even in the examples given. Right and left bilateral embryonic gradients are reflected in the handedness of horns. Right horns twist clockwise and left horns twist in an anticlockwise direction.

the skull. Unlike antlers, with a yearly life span, their long life has enabled them to evolve and function in several ways through the life of the animal, not just as tackle for offensive males in the brief breeding season. The Bovidae, comprising 135 species of cattle, goats, and antelopes, form the largest family, including abundant species like cattle and buffalo whose horns have been economically important in the past. Horns from rarer species have evoked a new wave of contemporary interest by very skilled artisan knife makers.

Classification. Horn or antler bearing animals are all even-toed ungulates (having paired hooves, Figure 7.5.2), with chambered stomachs for fermenting cellulose in their diet, making them ruminants. There are a forbiddingly large number of them. The classification of those most commonly met with is outlined in Table 7.6.1.

Cattle origins. Domestic cattle have multiple origins with several rounds of domestication from two strains of humpless taurine *Bos taurus* and a humped zebu strain (51). About 10,000 BP, one humpless taurine strain domesticated in northeast Africa, spread through east Africa, to the south. In about 8,000 BP, the second taurine strain was domesticated in the fertile crescent region of what is now Turkey. Some 2,000 years later, a humped zebu strain was domesticated in the civilization of the Indus Valley of what is now Pakistan, and spread via sea routes to the horn of Africa. These strains are now mixed worldwide in a multibillion dollar beef and milk industry. Two adaptive features characterize the horns: size and wall thickness (Figure 7.6.3 C). Warm climate cattle such as zebu are adapted to lose heat from large, thin-walled horns that have a thin vascular bone lining. Temperate and cold climate taurine cattle horns are smaller, adapted for defense and sexual selection, mostly with thick horn and a bone core. There are now about 800 breeds of domestic cattle.

The American bison, *Bison bison,* often called buffalo but only distantly related to true buffalo, the Asian water buffalo, *Bubalus bubalus,* and the African buffalo, *Syncerus caffer*, is a relative newcomer to North America, migrating over the Bering Straight some 10,000 years ago and replacing the steppe bison, *Bison priscus*. There are two subspecies: Plains bison, *Bison bison bison* are smaller, not as heavy, more faintly colored, and have a more rounded back than wood bison, *Bison b. athabascae*. In the early nineteenth century, American settlers slaughtered the Plains bison, killing off some fifty million animals mainly for their skins, but some for sport (record Plains bison horns measured as much as 55 cms [1.8 ft.] along their outside edge). Guns and horses increased the rate of the slaughter, tipping the balance towards extinction after thousands of years of the much milder Amerindian kills. This was the time when the English cutlery market expanded to meet the needs of the new middle class created by the Industrial Revolution. Bison horn was used for handles, replacing the more expensive and scarce ivory, but most was wasted as they were killed primarily for their hides or sport and the carcass allowed to rot. By the 1850s the bison was almost extinct, the population reduced to some 300 animals. As the bison were exterminated, their horn was replaced by the even less expensive bone and plastic. Conservation has brought bison back from extinction to about 500,000, but this includes many with genes from domestic cattle and only about 15,000 range free in natural wildlife habitats. The microscopic structure of bison horn is similar to that of cattle described as follows, but they differ in coarser features (Table 7.6.2). Cattle horns are more elongate, whereas bison tend to be in a tighter continuous curve (Figure 7.6.4 A–E).

Helices in Natural Materials

Material		
Ivory		
Elephant, mammoth and mastodon tusks		Slight
	Left	Clockwise
	Right	Anticlockwise
Mythical Unicorn		Anticlockwise
Narwhal cementum		
	Left	Anticlockwise
	Right	
Dentine microlaminae		
	Left	Clockwise
	Right	?
Pigs		Slight
	Upper Left	Anticlockwise
	Right	Clockwise
	Lower Left	Anticlockwise
	Right	Clockwise
Hippopotamus Dentinal tubule helicoid orientation		Anticlockwise
Elephant Dentinal tubule helicoid orientation		Anticlockwise
Horns		
All Ungulates		Slight to strong
	Left	Anticlockwise
	Right	Clockwise
Pronghorn Antelope		Slightly
	Left	Clockwise
	Right	Anticlockwise

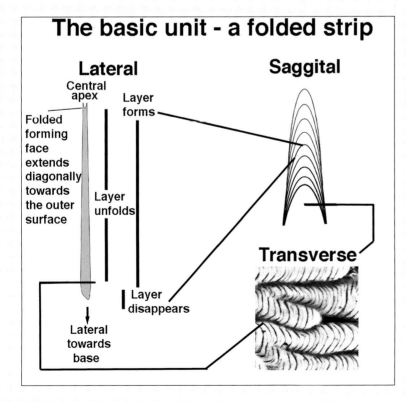

The basic unit - a folded strip

Lateral

Central apex

Folded forming face extends diagonally towards the outer surface

Layer unfolds

Lateral towards base

Saggital

Layer forms

Layer disappears

Transverse

Figure 7.6.2. The basic repeating unit in bovine horn structure is a folded strip. A bovine horn in a simplified saggital view shows stacked conical layers of keratin, but these layers are not flat and not continuous. They are composed of axial repeating units lying lengthways and side-by-side in the circumference. Each unit is folded more sharply anteriorly and flattens out towards the base, causing the edges between units to appear as lines in tangential profiles.

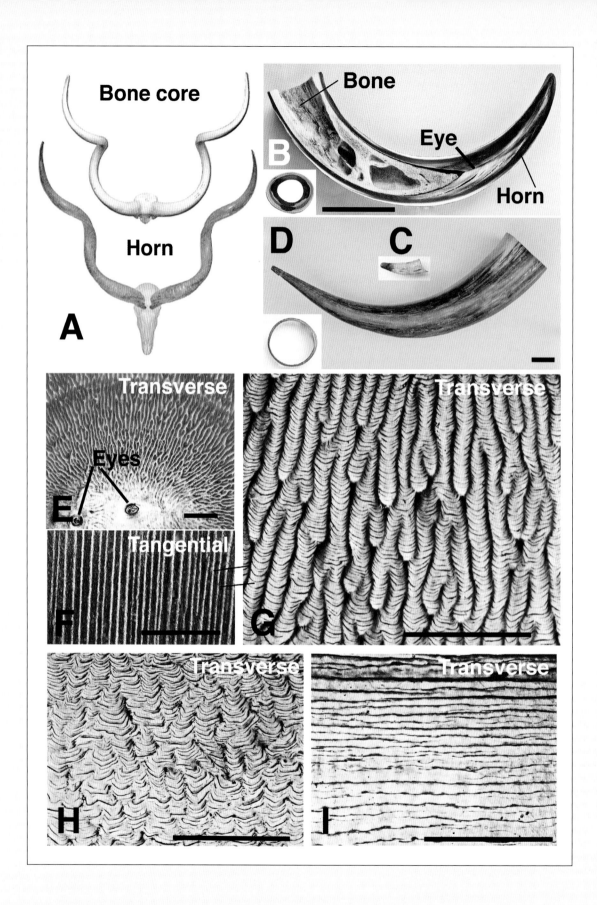

Figure 7.6.3. Bovine horns. A–D. Horns consist of a keratin layer over a bone core. A. These Kudu (*Strepsiceros strepsiceros*) horns show the thin layer of keratin coats the bone core. B. The strains of most temperate cattle descended from *Bos taurus* in the fertile crescent tend to be small with relatively thick keratin and robust bone cores (inset), adapted for defense and herd dominance, and relatively smooth outer surfaces. C. Typical horn on the same scale as D. Some are almost solid keratin. D. Tropical descendents from the Indus Valley gave rise to zebu cattle strains having large horns with thin bone and keratin walls adapted to encourage heat loss (inset). Horns vary in their angle of curvature and change the angle along the length. Bovine horn structure. E–I. E. Transverse profile of cow horn near the tip showing the stacks of folded strips radiating from a dominant central eye. The eye is the remnant of the forming face above the bone core. There are frequently two or three eyes near the tip but one becomes dominant and the others disappear. F. The folded strips appear as longitudinal ribs on the forming face or in any tangential view. G. Higher resolution shows the curved folding of the strips stacked in columns that flatten (H) towards the base, becoming almost complete layers (I) at the base of the horn. Scales: B, D. 5 cm. E, F, G. 1 mm.

The European bison or wisent, *Bison bonasus*. Unlike American bison that position their horns for charging, wisent horns point forward through the plane of the face, allowing the bulls to fight like domestic cattle (77). Their structure reflects this. Both form almost continuous curves with wisent's horns pointing forward from the side and American bison's horns pointing upwards and forwards.

Goat and sheep origins. Goats (*Capra hircus*) were domesticated from wild *Capra aegagrus*, also known as the bezoar, by Neolithic farmers in the Near East beginning about 10,000–11,000 years ago. All domestic goats today are descended from a few animals, but from different places. Early domestication centers were probably in the Central Iranian Plateau and Eastern Anatolia, including Northern and Central Zagros, a finding consistent with archaeological data identifying Eastern Anatolia as the likely origin of almost all domestic goats (94). Today there are more than 300 breeds living in climates from high altitude mountains to deserts.

Sheep were domesticated from the Asiatic mouflon, *Ovis orientalis*, in Mesopotamia at least as early as goats, probably in two separate waves for European and Asian breeds. Some breeds are probably very old, as the earliest Sumerian texts record 200 different words for kinds of sheep by about the third millennium BP. Their domestication was favored by their non-aggressive behavior and quick reproduction.

It is interesting that although goats and sheep were both among the earliest animals to be domesticated by peoples with much the same lifestyles—herding for milk and meat—their mythologies are so different. Goats pulled Thor's chariot but they are more often associated with Satan and the lustful Greek god Pan. Sheep and lambs are at the other end of the scale in the Abrahamic tradition of sacrifice and gentle beneficence. Goats deserve more esteem. Even sheep respect them. A single goat was often introduced into a sheep herd to kill venomous snakes, a role recognized in the markhor goat (*Capra*

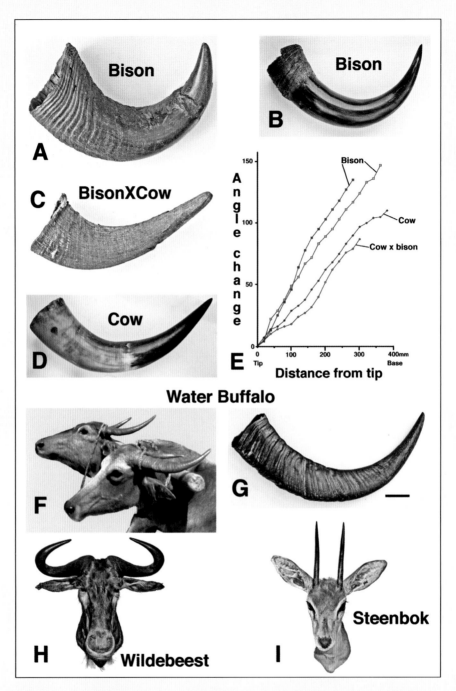

Figure 7.6.4. Bison horns. A. Bison (*Bison bison*, American buffalo) horns are thick, with a rough surface marked by growth rings and, unlike cattle, their curve continues with the same angle. B. Polished horn. C. Two-year-old male horn from a commercial bison herd bred for meat showing in the changing angle of curvature along its length that it has cattle genes. D. Cow horn for comparison with bison (A, B) and hybrid (C). E. Horns can be compared by measuring the angle of the curve along the outside edge from the tip (origin) to the base (still growing). The slope gives the angle of the curve. The departure from a straight line is a measure of the change in angle along the length. Bison horns lie in a narrow range of straight (= constant angle change) and steep slopes (= tight curves). Cattle are variable, as would be expected after a millennium of selection for domestic characteristics. Horns from bison herds grown for their meat are cattle-like. F, G. Water buffalo, *Bubalus bubalus*. H, I. Examples of the great variety of shapes in other Bovid sub families. H. Alcelaphinae, Blue or common wildebeest, *Connochaetes taurinus*. I. Neotragini, Steenbok, *Raphicerus campestris*.

falconeri), the name deriving from the Persian mar, for snake, and khor, eat.

Horns most used in commerce. Horns from all the families in Table 7.6.1 have probably been used whenever they became available but they leave no mark. Beetles and moths have destroyed them. Only in countries where there is a written record or where artifacts were of such value that they were carefully preserved do we know that they existed. More recently horns from the family Bovidae subfamily Bovinae, such as cattle (*Bos taurus*: numerous from early times but between 1950 and 1990 the Western World's desire for beef doubled the cattle population to five to six billion, a cow for every human), American bison (*Bison bison*), and to a lesser extent water buffalo (*Bubalus bubalus*), yaks (*Bos mutus*), and African buffalo (*Syncerus caffer*) became commercial commodities. Horn products have lost their importance in competition with plastics. In the subfamily Caprinae, domestic sheep (*Ovis aries*), domestic goats (*Capra aegagrus hircus*), descendents of the wild goat (*Capra aegagrus*), as well as the mountain goat (*Oreamnos americanus*), muskox (*Ovibos moschatus*), and bighorn sheep (*Ovis canadensis*) are well known, some from trophies, others from artifacts made from their horns.

Horn Shapes—curves and helices. Any museum display of horns shows a daunting variety of shapes that are at first difficult to understand (Figure 7.6.1). Growth in the simplest horns is uniform around the base, giving rise to a straight conical structure. The structure of more complicated horns may be simplified as conical growth distorted to create curves and helices by one or both of two variables. Growth in some horns is greater on one side of the base, causing a two-dimensional curve to form. The shape of the curve varies with the growth rate, but it is a flat C in one plane. In helical horns, an elevated growth rate moves around the base, changing the angle in three dimensions from plane to plane by a constant (corkscrew) or changing amount. The most complex shapes occur when an elevated growth rate moves around a base that also has a biased elevated rate on one side. A helix is then imposed on a curved horn. In practice, most horns are a complex mixture, even in the examples given to represent straight, curved, and helical horns in Figure 7.6.1. Embryos have right and left gradients from the center that are reflected in most structures (e.g., hands, ears), including horns. Right horns twist clockwise and left horns twist in an anticlockwise direction.

Bovine horns may occur in cows, but are larger in bulls. They tend to have relatively smooth surfaces and circular or oval cross sections with curves mainly in one plane and a small tendency to become helices. We may correlate the shapes with their multifunctional uses, protection, herd behavior, moving vegetation, with only a limited degree of male fighting. Caprine horns, in contrast, have a much bigger role in sexual selection, usually being much larger in males and sometimes absent in females. They often have flattened, triangular, or irregular rectangular cross sections with raised surfaces and strong curvatures very often also in helices. The raised surfaces correspond to annual growth cycles, but are most enlarged on forwardly directed knobs of male horns that prevent slipping in clashes with their opponents in sexual combat.

Bovine horn structure. In principle, cattle horns are stacks of elongated conical shells formed by the detachment of sheets of cells filled with keratin from the forming face on the inside (Figures 7.6.2, 3). However, the details of this simple arrangement make the structure much more complicated. Horns have two problems to solve: they must be tougher than simple stacks of sheets prone to cracking between the sheets, and their development must allow deposition from the periphery to the core and from the tip to the base that is simple and possible.

Cattle horns consist of a keratin layer over a bone core (Figure 7.6.3 A–D). The inner face tends to be smooth, except in very large, thick-walled horns that develop longitudinal ridges, like bison, towards the base. Temperate cattle descended from temperate *Bos taurus* can be almost solid horn for part of their length. From the much larger horns of zebu cattle have thin walls. In both kinds of horn, the bone core projects to the tip as an eye in transverse profile, the relic of a compressed forming face. There are frequently two or three eyes near the tip, but one becomes dominant as it continues in the bone core. The structure changes from tightly folded sheets in the tip surrounding the eye to flattened sheets around the bone core nearer the base. In profiles parallel to the surface straight longitudinal lines in the length of the horn might be misinterpreted as longitudinal filaments like those in hooves, pronghorns, baleen, or rhino horns, but they are the cut edges of folded layers (Figure 7.6.3, 2G). This draws attention to the basic unit in bovid horns—the folded strip (Figure 7.6.2).

Horn is a multilayered structure with 10–20 layers per mm stacked up on one another approximately in a succession of cones with increasing diameter corresponding to growth layers (Figure 7.6.3 J). The cones are not flat and uniform but divided into longitudinal strips, each strip being narrower towards the tip and wider towards the base to accommodate the horn's increasing diameter. The strips stack up on one another in columns. Towards the horn tip each strip is folded into a curve, making it narrower in the circumference. The edge of each curve meets up with that of the next strip. Longitudinal profiles of these edges give the appearance of longitudinal filaments mentioned above.

As a horn grows, it increases its cross-sectional area from tip to base, space that must be filled by the growth of the layers (Figure 7.6.3 D, E, F). Several different mechanisms contribute to this growth. 1. The strips are wider towards the base. 2. The curves at the tip flatten out towards the base, increasing the circumference. This is demonstrated in the strips that flatten from CCC shapes to III shapes in transverse profiles as they progress from tip to base (Figure 7.6.3 E, H, I). 3. Stacks

of layers form radial columns that appear, disappear, or branch (Figure 7.6.4 E). The obvious solution to decrease the number of layers from periphery to core during growth would seem to be for the fusion of column branches from the outside to the inside, decreasing the cross section by a succession of Y branches. However, the branches are oriented in the reverse of this. They actually branch towards the inside. Columns reduce space occupied on the inside by not being deposited (Figure 7.6.3 D, E). Functionally, the deposition of folded rather than flat keratin sheets would reduce the possibility of propagating cracks.

Bison horns. The microscopic structure of bison horn is similar to that of cattle described above, but more difficult to resolve because of its opacity and dark color. They differ in coarser features (Table 7.6.2), tending to be thicker and heavier with a longitudinally ridged rather than a smooth inner face. Cattle horns are more elongate, whereas bison tend to be in a tighter continuous curve (Figure 7.6.4 A–E). Horns can be compared for differences in curvature by measuring changes in the angle of the curve along the outside edge from the tip (a record of the angle of the new horn) to the base (the angle at the still growing surface). The slope gives the angle of the curve, a steep curve signifies a tight angle. The departure from a straight line is a measure of the change in angle along the length. A straight line signifies a constant change in angle. A curve indicates change in angle as the horn curve flattens or tightens. Bison horns lie in a narrow range of straight lines with steep slopes in agreement with their appearance as tight curves having a constant change in angle. Natural selection of bison has kept those with horns having a particular functional shape. Cattle horns, on the other hand, after millennia of domestic selection for diverse features, have many kinds of slopes and curves. Horns from commercial bison herds bred for meat have many cattle features: thin walls, surface little marked by growth rings, and the absence of longitudinal folds on their inner surface and their shape (Figure 7.6.4 E). Contemporary "bison" horns on the market come from "bison" meat packers. The horns are heated in ovens to sterilize them and blacken their keratin before sale to craftsmen making powder horns. Their shape, thin walls and absence of longitudinal folds on their inner surface suggests that the genes for their horns are more from cattle than bison.

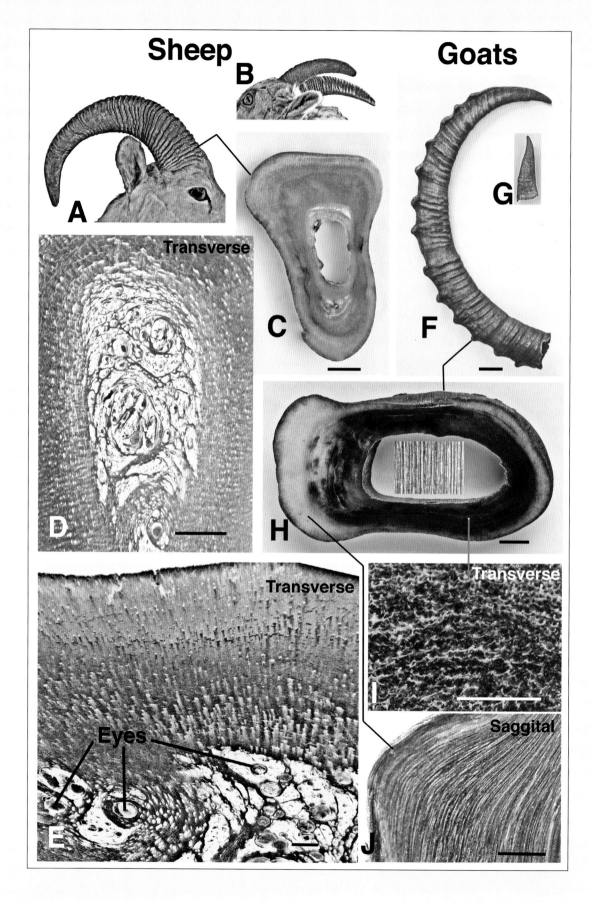

Sheep

B

A

Transverse

C

D

Transverse

Eyes

E

Goats

G

F

H

Transverse

I

Saggital

J

Caprine horns, sheep, and goats.

Although sheep horns tend to be helical and goats curved, horn shape does not separate them. For example, the Racka race of sheep (*Ovis orientalis*) have straight helices very similar to those of markhor goats (*Capra falconeri*). Nor does size separate them. Both sheep and goat horns vary in size from small to very large. Ram's horns are large compared with those of their ewes (Figure 7.6.5 A, B) and even within the *Capra* genus, horns such as those of the ibex are very large compared with domestic varieties (Figure 7.6.5 F, G).

Caprine horns have a similar structure to those of bovines in that their keratin is also in folded strips, but they differ in many ways. 1. Their transverse shape is irregular compared with the circular or oval profiles of bovines. Large sheep horns tend to be triangular in cross section, accommodating the helical shape. Large goat horns such as the ibex tend to be more rectangular in cross section (Figure 7.6.5 C, H). 2. The forming face where the folded strips arise is therefore also irregular and the resulting keratin sheets are often folded in complex ways. 3. The single dominant "eye" of bovines (Figure 7.6.3 E) that carries on in the bone core is multiple in Caprines, perhaps hundreds in the musk ox. Each eye is surrounded by keratin cylinders creating a structure like "birds eye maple" (Figure 7.6.6 D, F, G). We may correlate this with the different mechanical properties required for the massive head butting of buck Caprines compared with the milder defensive activities of bull cattle. 4. Sheep have yellowish brown horn and goats tend to be dark brown to black, the dense color being mainly localized in discrete cell fragments rather than dispersed in the keratin (Figure 7.6.5 C, H). 5. Spaces around the eyes fill with air. After polishing, these spaces become more visible as a central white core filled with polishing compound (Figures 7.6.5 D, E; 7.6.6 D, E, F). This has several possible consequences—lower density, shock absorption, heat insulation. 6. The curved edges of the folded strips outline spaces that contain soft, light colored material that may also be infiltrated by polishing compound, but only at the exposed surface. The spaces line up like longitudinal fibers with a crescent shaped outline in cross section (Figure 7.6.5 D, E).

(Opposite page)
Figure 7.6.5. A–E. Sheep. F–J. Goats. Both sheep and goat horns vary in size from small to very large. A. Ram. B. Ewe. F. Ibex, *Capra* sp. G. Domestic ram goat, *Capra hircus*. C. Large sheep horns tend to be triangular in cross section, accommodating the helical shape. Bighorn sheep, *Ovis Canadensis* ram. H. Large goat horns such as this ibex, *Capra* sp., tend to be more rectangular in cross section. Sheep have yellowish brown horn (C) and goats tend to be dark brown to black. Insert of tangential profile of ibex, showing general similarity of all ungulate horns. (H, I, J). The general structure of caprine horns resembles that of bovines in that the basic repeating unit is a folded strip (I, J), but they differ in having multiple "eyes" and air spaces around the eyes (D, E). The large air spaces become filled by polishing powder during tissue preparation. There are also spaces between the curved folded strips forming longitudinal rods with crescent-shaped cross sections. These small spaces may fill with polishing powder at the surface, but they contain their own characteristic pale material through their length. Scales: E. 1 mm; J. 5 mm; C, D, H. 1 cm; F. 5 cm; I. 100 m.

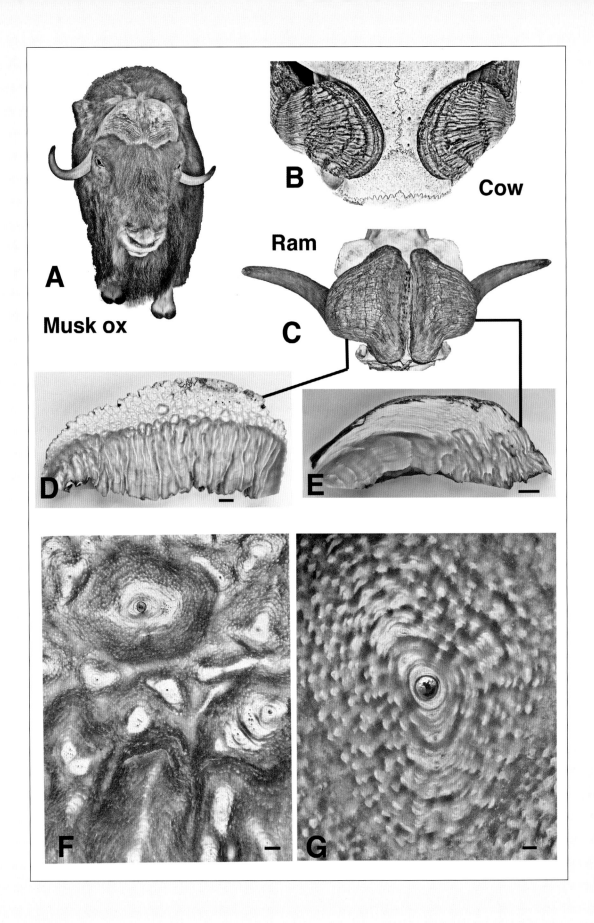

A
Musk ox

B
Cow

Ram
C

D

E

F

G

These Caprine features are most easily seen in horns of the musk ox, *Ovibos moschatus*. (Figure 7.6.6 A). The forepart of the skull of bull musk ox are covered by the bases of their horns in a protective sheath or bos (C), that cows with their smaller horns lack (B). The bos has many eyes with two orientations. Those formed most recently are at about 90° to the bone (D, F, G). Those formed earlier, forming the outside barrier, are parallel to the surface, pointing laterally from the center (E). The structure of the cow horn (B) shows how this has come about. The cow horn is like a smaller version of the outer layer of the bull, consisting of laterally directed eyes. In bulls, this layer is thrust away from the surface by the formation of a thick layer of eyes pointing directly away from the skull surface. The combination of multiple eyes, their orientations and that of their component folded strips, together with the extensive air-filled regions, must surely have functional consequences for toughness, lightness, and heat insulation.

(Opposite page)

Figure 7.6.6. Musk ox, *Ovibos moschatus*. Bull musk ox (A) have the base of their horns covering the forepart of the skull in a protective bos (C). Cow horns (B) are smaller and the bases do not extend to cover the skull. D, E. Transverse and saggital profiles of the male horn base show the characteristic multiple eye structure with many white cores containing small air spaces. The eyes arise from the horn base and turn laterally through 900. F. Transverse profile of individual eyes. The multiple core structure consists of eyes surrounded by keratin sheets and air spaces. G. Profile of a single "eye" showing the cylinder composed of folded strips similar to those making whole cattle horns (Figures 7.6.2, 3). Scales: D, E. 1 cm; F. 1 mm; G. 100 mm.

Horn structure of *Antilocapra americana* (Pronghorn).

The pronghorn antelope has branched horns that it sheds, unlike all ruminants other than deer (Figure 7.6.7). The horns have a broad base, a single fork with one short branch. Record horns measure as much as 44 cms along the outside edge (A, B). Bone extends for about half the length of the horn up to the fork, giving an impression of strength with a distinct laminar bone layer on the outside surrounding an even, spongy core without air pockets (C). It lacks the pedicel found in deer. Only horn keratin is shed from this permanent bone core (D). Above the fork, the horn is composed of longitudinal hair-like keratin filaments embedded in a matrix (E, F). The filaments are longitudinal but at a slight angle to the axis allowing them to grow by increasing in length and by adding more filaments around the base of the horn. The lumen of the keratin horn extending beyond the bone core has a characteristic white component resembling that in goat horns (D, G).

Conclusions on horn structure. Except for *Antilocapra*, the basic structures of all the horns examined are variants of the basic folded strip unit most clearly displayed in cow horns. The gross structure may also be simplified and more easily understood as the result of differing rate of growth at one side or progressively around the base of a horn to create curves or helices. Selection on these two features in male rivalry, individual and herd protection, heat exchange and conservation, has resulted in the great variety of horn shapes, often convergent in otherwise not closely related subfamilies, but all a tribute to the properties of keratin.

Mythology—the Cuckolds Horns

The cuckoo then on every tree
Mocks married men, for thus sings he:
Cuckoo.
Cuckoo, cuckoo, O word of fear,
Unpleasing to a married ear.

Shakespeare
Loves Labours Lost (1594–5)

By Shakespeare's time, the root word cuck (an alternative to the slang word for excrement and a transfer from the slang word for penis by the transposition of u for o) was well established as a descriptor for marital infidelity and with it the cuckolds horns. Samuel Harsnet blames the Catholic Church for frightening poorly educated parishioners into paying dues to protect them from devils with horns. In "A declaration of Egregious Impostures" he says "… the devil comes from a smoky black house, he, or a lewd prior … with ugly horns on his head, fire in his mouth, a cows tail in his breech … claws like a bear … and a voice like a lion … was enough to make their hair stand upright." But horns did not always have this negative association. In the Old Testament (2 Samuel 22:3 and Psalms 18:2: "God … is my shield and the horn of my salvation.") and in texts of classical writers, the horn was a symbol of power and dominion. Alexander the Great was depicted with horns and the Norse heroes and gods had horns on their helmets. It was in this spirit that Michael Angelo's (1475–1564) statue depicted Moses with a rather diminutive pair of horns (perhaps partly as a result of an early mistranslation of Exodus 34:29–30, "The skin of his face shone" as "The skin of his face sent forth horns"). From the fifth century BC, the Horn of Amalthea was associated with good things, an abundance of food. Zeus accidentally broke the horn of Amalthea, the goat that raised him. In remorse, he gave her a magical horn that would fill with whatever she wished for, originally depicted as a Cornucopia or Horn of Plenty filled with fruits and flowers that also became a symbol for a woman's fertility, a change that preceded the cuckolds horns. Dionysus began as a relatively innocent god of wine, but later became adorned with the horns that befitted his more randy lifestyle. Pan began life with the haunches, hind legs, and horns of a goat, but was an innocent god of nature, only later becoming more strongly connected with fertility, morphing into the devil, "Auld Hornie," or "Auld Cloutie," the devil with cloven hooves. In King Arthur's court, the horn was a symbol of virtue but also a test to detect cuckolds. Morgan Le Fay sent Arthur a "Horn of Fidelity," a drinking horn that had the magical property that "no lady could drink of it who was not to her husband true." Only 4 of the 100 court ladies passed the test. (This may compare unfavorably with contemporary North America, where one out of ten children believed to be fathered by heads of families have been shown by genetic testing not to be his).

There has been a change in the meaning of horns from commendation to cuckoldom and Satanic ritual, but over a much longer period than between the lives of Shakespeare and Michael Angelo. Many different trends may have led to the change. The strongest probably began in the early Christian era when Christianity had to compete with local horned gods. Over centuries the Catholic Church managed to conflate horns with Satan. Another, much later, may have been a technique used for the identification of capons. In an earlier time, capons were made by castrating cockerels that were then released back to feed freely in the yard. When the time came to cull them from the flock, this is claimed to present a problem of identification. Which birds were just plump cockerels and which had been castrated? The solution was to cut off their spurs and implant them into their combs at the time of castration. The spurs grew into small horns in their new location, in spite of low testosterone (a modern experiment is needed to confirm this), making it easy to recognize in a head count (why not just amputate the comb on one side) which birds in the flock had been caponized. The image coupling horns with castration may have contributed to the identification of horns with the cuckold.

Beaks. The beaks of the Helmeted Hornbill (*Rhinoplax vigil*) are the source of hornbill "ivory," which was introduced into China from Borneo in 1371 and has been carved there ever since. Hornbill snuff bottles were prized in the eighteenth century. In nineteenth century Canton, the Ho-a-ching establishment made hornbill ivory jewelry for export. Hornbill ivory (*angang gading*) was also carved by the people of Java and Sumatra, an industry subsequently supported by the Dutch for the European trade.

Figure 7.6.7. A. The pronghorn antelope, *Antilocapra americana*, is the only ruminant other than deer with branched horns. B. Side view of the horn. The horns have a broad base and a single short branch. C. Transverse profile above the base where the horn is composed only of keratin having a characteristic white component in the core. D. Below the branch, the broad base has a bone core. E. Transverse profile of the horn. The keratin is composed of longitudinal hair-like filaments embedded in a matrix. F. The keratin consists of longitudinally arranged hair-like filaments in matrix. Tangential profile. G. Transverse profile of the horn core with filaments surrounded by matrix and the white component resembling that in Caprines. Scales: C, F, G. 1 mm. D. 1 cm. E. 100 mm.

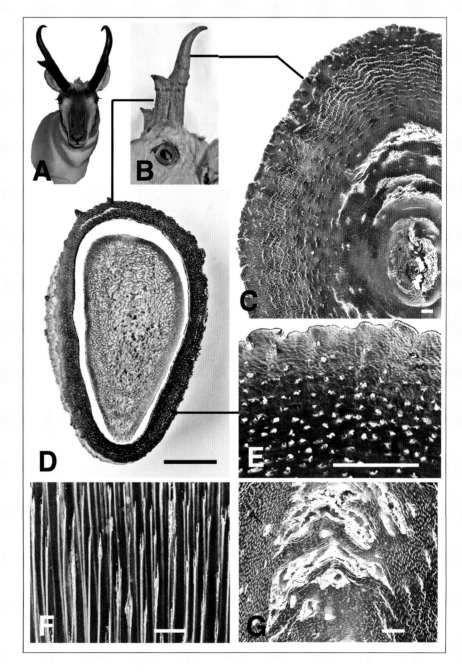

7.7. Hair, Wool, and Quills

Behold thou art fair, my love; ... thy hair is as a flock of goats ...

Song of Solomon, 4. v. I

Hair. Hair and feathers characterize the two main lines of evolution from our reptilian ancestors, hair in mammals, feathers in birds and dinosaurs. The basic structure of a hair is that of a rod of elongated cortical cells filled with keratin filaments protected by a cylinder of flat cuticle cells containing hard keratin. The keratin filaments of the rod determine the mechanical properties and the cuticle cells determine the surface properties (Figure 7.7.1).

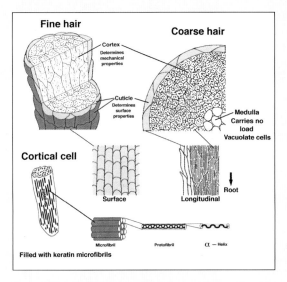

Figure 7.7.1. Hair structure. The shape and size of cuticle cells create species specific patterns. Cuticle cells are separated from the underlying cortex by a basal lamina. The mechanical properties of hair come from the semi-rigid cylinder of cuticle cells and from keratin microfibrils filling the elongated cortical cells. Sometimes, especially in coarse hair, there is a central medulla of vacuolated cells containing keratin precursors such as eleidin.

That this basic structure is little altered in the few derivatives (porcupine quills, pangolin scales) is a tribute to its efficiency as a protective heat-conserving coat. The finest hairs are little more than 10 m in diameter. It would require only one or two red blood cells to stretch from one side to the other. When woven into cloth, such fine hairs are among the most valuable of all natural materials. Five Tibetan antelope have to be slaughtered (illegally) to create the wool for one shahtoosh shawl that may sell for $15,000 (Table 7.7.1). A noticeable difference from feathers is the absence of physical colors. Nearly all coloration of hairs is due to pigment in the keratin of the cortex.

The heat conserving properties of wool and fine hair continue to make them important in commerce. When horses were common for conveyance, horse hair was a cheap commodity, useful for its strength and elasticity to stuff furniture. Now it is a specialist item for bow strings made from Chinese white horse tails and a multibillion dollar wig industry.

Kinds of hair. There are two kinds of hair. Down or undercoat hairs next to the skin are responsible for insulation. Guard hairs give color and protect the down hairs. Down hairs are abundant, fine, light-colored, and wool-like, trapping air in an insulating coat (Table 7.7.1). Guard hairs (Kemp fibers) are sparse, coarse, long, colored and straight, oriented to extend over the down and allow rain and snow to drip off. Guard hairs differentiate in various body locations as vibrissae, eyelashes, eyebrows, genital coverings, beards, etc., but remain similar structurally. Both down and guard hairs arise from clusters of follicles and have basically the same structure (Figure 7.7.1). Some human scalps have both down and guard hairs. Variations in hair structure occur due to differences in the cuticle, the cortex, and air spaces within the cortex (fusi), melanin granules in the cortex, and the extent of the medulla, whether it is continuous or in separated columns.

Species or variety	Origin, status and distribution.	Common name of hair	Hair diameter
Chiru, Tibetan antelope. *Pantholops hodgsonii.*	Above 5,000 meters in Tibet (China) with a small population in India. Endangered. Import and export from 151 CITES countries illegal.	Shahtoosh, from the Persian shahtush, king of fine wools.	10-12μm
Angora rabbit. *Oryctolagus cuniculus.*	Originally from Ankara (=angora), Turkey, now world wide with several sub breeds.	Angora.	10-20μm Long wool.
Musk ox. *Ovibos moschatus.*	Northern tundra of Canada, Alaska and Greenland.	Qiviut, Musk or arctic ox.	11-15μm
Changthangi or Pashmina goat. *Capra hircus var*	Himalayas in Nepal, Pakistan, north India. Now farmed in Mongolia, increasing desertification. Processed in Kashmir.	Pashmina, Fine cashmere often blended with silk	12-16μm
Numerous Cashmere goat varieties. *Capra hircus laniger.*	Mongolia, China. Numerous new varieties being reared throughout the region and Australia.	Cashmere	12-21μm
Shamina or Changra pashmina. *Capra hircus var.*	High Himalayas of Nepal.	Shamina, finer pashmina trademarked Changra Pashmina	14μm or less
Llama. *Lama pacos.*	Originally in Peru, Bolivia and Chile, now also in Australia, USA, Canada and Europe.	Alpaca.	14-28μm
Merino sheep. *Ovis aries var.*	Originally from Asia Minor, now worldwide wherever climate is suitable.	Merino.	8-24μm
Persian lamb. *Ovis aries, var platyura.*	Central to West Asia, spread worldwide wherever climate is suitable.	Karakul. Persian lamb.	29+μm
Sheep, many varieties grown for wool & meat. *Ovis aries var.*	Worldwide, estimated population over a billion in 2008.	Wool	8-60 μm
Angora goat. *Capra hircus var.*	Originally from Angora in Asia Minor, now widely distributed.	Mohair	Kids 22-27μm, adults 40+μm
Human. *Homo sapiens.*			50-90μm
Elephants, African and Indian.			~1.5x2mm, Tail bristles.
American porcupine. *Erethizon dorsatum.*	Throughout USA and Southern Canada.		2mm quills.
African porcupine. *Hystrix africaeaustralis.*	Africa South of the equator.		7mm, large quills.

Table 7.7.1. Hair, wool, and quill diameters. Arranged in order of diameter. Five slaughtered Tibetan antelope are needed to create wool for one shahtoosh shawl woven in China that sells for about $15,000. Original data and (14).

Cuticle. The cuticle is a hard, protective cylinder responsible for a hair's surface properties, its role as a protective barrier, and some of its mechanical strength. A layer of flat keratin-filled cells form overlapping scales to create the stiff cylinder that gives hairs their shape. Scales have characteristic sizes and shapes that allow species and sometimes individual identification invaluable in forensics (97). Edges are important in determining interactions with other hairs. The forward edge of each scale may project slightly above the surface so that hairs may tangle rather than slide smoothly over one another, especially in wool. The secretion of lipids (lanolin in sheep) over the cuticle creates a hydrophobic barrier that protects the cortex and makes the whole fleece water resistant. Twenty percent of a newly sheared sheep fleece may be lanolin. Removal of the barrier with detergents allows water and dyes to penetrate between the cuticle cells through the basal lamina to the cortex.

Cortex. The cortex consists of elongated cells filled with keratin microfibrils (Figure 7.7.1). The main differences in various keratins arise from their sulfur content. If there are many cysteine disulfide cross-links, then there is very little flexibility as in horns, claws, hooves, or nails. In wool, hair, and skin keratins there are fewer disulfide cross-links that allow some stretching with a return to normal after the relaxation of tension. Hair color depends on melanin granules in the cortex. Fusi begin as fluid spaces but dry out into air spaces creating degrees of lighter colored or whiter hair.

Medulla. As in other cylindrical structures (Chapter 3, Figure 3.1), lateral stress cancels out in the center so that structures giving mechanical support can be absent without affecting the strength of the cylinder. Some hairs take advantage of this and fill the center with a medulla of vacuolated cells rather than keratin filaments (Figure 7.7.1). The extent of the medulla varies consistently with the species. It may be a continuous rod or broken up into characteristic segments. In many fine hairs the medulla may be absent, but in others it forms a continuous rod of cells or intermittent segments with characteristic shapes and patterns (59). These vacuolate cells contain eleidin. Eleidin is a colorless translucent precursor to keratin present in the skin, notably in the lips, where its translucency allows the color of blood to define human facial patterns. We may suppose that enough keratin precursors can be available during the initial formation of fine hairs, but for larger structures, taking longer to form, a local supply of precursors is needed.

Development. Hair development begins with the generation of fine unpigmented hairs (lanugo) over most of the surface of the fetus in the twelfth week in humans (66). Lanugo is usually shed before birth when the follicles change their function to the formation of down hairs and guard hairs and their distribution and growth cycles to the adult pattern. After birth most hair follows a growth cycle characteristic for its particular location. Human body hair, for example, grows for three to five years, followed by a seven to fourteen day transition to three to four months rest before shedding and return to growth from a revived papilla. Growth in length occurs by multiplication of cells in the papilla at the base of the follicle (Figure 7.2).

The sparse body hair in all humans has posed a problem since Darwin drew attention to it. He supposed that women with less hair were more desirable, sexual selection for less hair being more powerful in evolution than the advantage of more hair for protection.

Wool

To wear the arctic fox, you have to kill it.
Wear the underwool of the arctic ox—pulled off it like a sweater,
Your coat is warm; your conscience better.

The Arctic Ox
Marianne Moore, 1986

Sheep's wool has the general structure of undercoat hair with surface scales, a cortex, and in some varieties a medulla, ranging in diameter from the coarsest at 60 mm in diameter to 8 mm in the finest Merinos (Table 7.7.1). It differs from most hair (Table 7.7.2) in growing continuously with rates varying from 4–8 cms pa in Merinos to 25–46 cms pa in Black Faced Sheep. Growth is in tufts of up to twelve fibers giving an average density in Merino sheep of 5–8,000 per cm^2.

Material	Hair	Wool
Growth	Cycles. Human cycle of 3-5years growth followed by 3-4months rest before shedding and regrowth from papilla. On the head may grow throughout life.	Continuous.
Width	Usually thicker but commercial species very fine.	Variable but selected for thinness.
Scales	Smooth.	Edges project.
Felting	With difficulty.	Easily felted.
Medulla	Absent in fine hairs, present in coarse ones.	Absent in wools selected for fineness.
Shape in cross section	Usually nearly circular	Flattened or oval
Crimps or waves	Usually straight or slightly wavey, occasionally curley.	Curly, high frequency waves.

Table 7.7.2. Differences between hair and wool. The flattened shape of wool in cross section encourages the formation of waves in three dimensions.

Felting is the process of matting fibers together permanently without weaving them; indeed, it came about before weaving. Any fibers can be felted to some extent but the properties of wool—scales and waving—make it the easiest fiber to felt. The edges of the scales tangle more easily with one another than those in hair. Wool tends to be oval rather than circular in cross section, a flattening of the fiber that encourages the formation of waves. Whereas hair is often straight, wool is waved at a frequency of 2 per cm in coarse wool to 10 per cm in the finest Merino. In a long, complicated process these properties make it possible to squeeze hot wet wool together and harden it into felt that continues to compete successfully with plastic imitations.

Not all hair from sheep is wool. Kemp fibers (kemps) are straight outer coat hairs distributed through the wool that are shed periodically.

Quills

Two rodent families, the old world Hystricidae (eleven species) and the new world Erethizontidae (17) (142) (88), have evolved into porcupines independently, their hairs becoming quills but of rather different kinds (Figure 7.7.2 E–G). Well known representatives are the African porcupine (*Hystrix africaeaustralis*), with long, hard, heavily built quills (~7 mm x ~20 mm) and the North America porcupine (*Erethizon dorsatum*) with short, thin, and soft but sharp quills (~2 mm x ~10 mm). The African porcupine quill has a very strong, rigid structure created by a thick cuticle with radial extensions of the cortex into a vacuolate medulla. In contrast, except for the hard tips, the American porcupine has soft quills, easily bent, having only a thin, soft layer of cuticle and cortex around a vacuolated medulla.

Elephant Tail Bristles

Having pull'd out of an elephants-tayl a black Hair, and cut transversely from it a thin scale, I exposed it to my Microscope, which represented in the thick of that Hair about an hundred little specks somewhat whitish, and in each speck a black point, and in some few of those black points, a little hole; and this hair consisted withal of united Globules, which yet I thought I should have found bigger in this thick hair of so bulky a Beast, than indeed they were.

Anthony van Leeuwenhoek
Philosophical Transactions of
the Royal Society (1674)
Quoted in (144)

(Opposite page)
Figure 7.7.2. Hair and quill structure. Most mammals have an undercoat of fine white hairs next to the skin protected by longer, colored, robust guard hairs with structures like that in Figure 7.7.1. A. Undercoat and guard hairs of woolly mammoth. B. Dog (Sheltie) guard and undercoat hairs. C, D. Longitudinal and transverse profiles of elephant tail bristles. Unlike typical hairs, they have a fibrous structure symmetrical about each side of a flattened axis. Each bristle is formed from several hundred keratin fibers in matrix. The outer fibers are cylinders, often hollow, the inner fibers narrow and rod-like. E, F. African porcupine quill, transverse profile and surface view. The thick cuticle and radial extensions of the cortex into a vacuolate medulla create a very strong, rigid structure. G. American porcupine, undercoat, guard hairs, intermediates between guard hairs and quills, quills, transverse profile of quill. Except for the hard tips, the quills are easily bent, having only a thin, soft layer of cuticle and cortex around a vacuolated medulla. H. Pig bristles, formerly a valuable commercial item, are rigid hairs. I. A concave circular plane with a sharp circumference was used to remove bristles from dead pigs and crop them from live ones. Scales: D = 0.1 mm, all others = 1 cm.

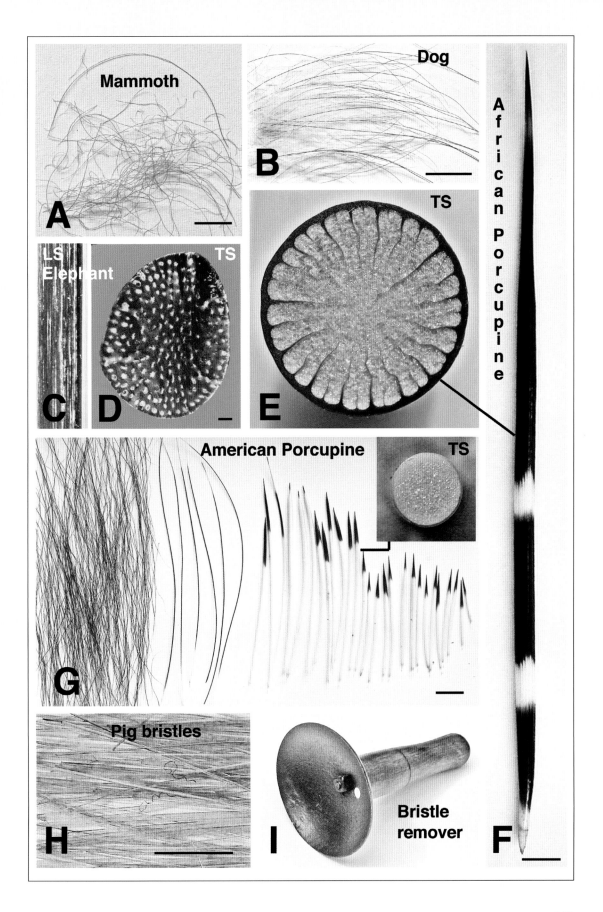

Mammoth

Dog

LS
Elephant

TS

TS

A
f
r
i
c
a
n

P
o
r
c
u
p
i
n
e

American Porcupine

TS

Pig bristles

Bristle
remover

163

Elephant tail bristles emerge in strips on each side of the tail allowing it to function like a fly swatter. The flattened black bristles are about 1.5–2 mm in diameter, much larger than typical hairs, with a fibrous structure symmetrical about each side of the flattened axis (Table 7.7.1, Figure 7.7.2 D). Each bristle is formed from several hundred keratin fibers in a matrix. The outer fibers are often exposed on the surface, the cuticle cells having worn away with use. The outer fibers are hollow cylinders, the inner ones narrow and rod-like. They could have arisen by the fusion of several papillae or more probably by the division of a large papilla similar to that in the genetic malformation *Pili multigemini* together with a simplification of structure.

Conclusion. Mechanical constraints have caused hair to evolve in two different directions from fine, flexible hairs composed of a cylindrical cuticle around a rod of cortical cells containing longitudinally arranged keratin microfibrils (Figure 7.7.1). One has evolved resistance to bending, the cortex becoming a hard, rigid cylinder with the center filled with vacuolate medullary cells (e.g., porcupine quills). The other has evolved a structure with lateral flexibility that allows repeated bending due to a cortex of longitudinally arranged keratin microfibrils without a medulla (e.g., elephant tail bristles).

7.8. Whale Baleen

The ocean's whales are big as ships.
Their giant mouths they fill
And filter out the fish and krill.
I wonder what they do for chips.

Anon.

Introduction. Baleen meant whale in the sixteenth century, the word coming from the middle English *baleyne,* which in turn came from the old French word *baleine* and the Greek *phalaena*. The term was then transferred to the commodity, as baleen, inaccurately termed "whalebone," became a valuable byproduct of the whaling industry.

Order Cetacea
    Suborder Mysticeti Baleen Whales
        Family Balaenidae, Right Whales
  Genus *Balaena*
    B. mysticetus, Bowhead
  Genus *Eubalaena*
    E. glacialis, North Atlantic or Biscay Right Whale,
    E. japonica, North Pacific Right Whale,
    E. australis, Southern Right Whale.
        Family Balaenopteridae, Rorquals
          Subfamily Balaenopterinae,
  Genus *Balaenoptera*
    B. Physalis, Fin
    B. borealis, Sei
    B. brydei, Bryde's
    B. edeni, Eden's
    B. musculus, Blue
    B. acutorostrata, Minke
    B. bonaerensis, Antarctic Minke
        Subfamily Megapterinae
  Genus *Megaptera,*
    M. novaeangliae, Humpback
        Family Eschrichtiidae
  Genus *Eschrichtius*
    E. robustus, Grey Whale
        Family Neobalaenidae
  Genus *Caperea*
    C. marginata, Pygmy Right Whale

Table 7.8.1. Order Cetacea. The right whales, Balaenidae, were the main source of commercial baleen in the nineteenth and beginning of the twentieth century, first the North Atlantic right whale, then the bowhead. Although the rorquals were later killed in enormous numbers for their oil, their plates were smaller and their mechanical properties less suitable. The baleen market was also changing with fashion and competition with synthetic plastics. Rorqual baleen could not compete and was presumably discarded. Bryde's whale is pronounced "Broodus" after the discoverer.

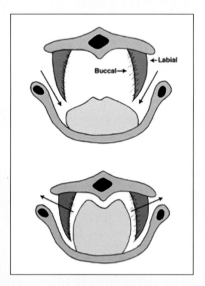

Figure 7.8.1. Sea water and krill are sucked in below baleen plates (Figure 7.8.2 A–B) hanging from the upper jaw of right whales when the mouth opens. Krill are filtered from the sea water passing out through the plates as the mouth closes.

Whale Baleen Plates					
Kinds of whale and baleen shape	No of plate-pairs	Colour	Filament Diameter in mm. Filament density = no per mm²	Length x width cms	Width to length Ratio
Right whales, Balaenidae.					
Bowhead, *Balaena mysticetus*	325 - 360	Dark gray to black	0.045 – 0.37. Very fine to fine. 74.4 sd 4.6	430x30 450x36	14 12.5
North Atlantic or Biscay Right whale, *Eubalaena glacialis*	225 - 250	Black	0.12- 0.17 Very fine	232x26	9.0
Rorquals, Balaenopteridae.					
Fin, *Balaenoptera physalus*	262 - 473	Asymmetrical; the right front 1/3 is creamy yellow, alternating on the left with blue gray.	0.3-0.9 Medium -Coarse	76x30 99x29 24- 30x11- 13	2.5 3.5 2.2- 2.3
Sei, *B. borealis*	320 - 380	Black, light brown to white fringe.	0.15- 0.25 Very fine - fine	86x24	3.5
Bryde's, *B. brydei*	250 - 350	Some front plates white, others black	0.4-0.7 Medium - medium Coarse.	73x20	3.6
Blue, *B. musculus*	320- 400	Dark brown to black. Black filaments.	Bimodal, 0.2 – 0.3, 0.4- 1.4 Fine and Coarse 4.5	94x36 85x27 100x53	2.6 3.1 1.9
Minke, *B. acutorostrata*	300	Yellow-brown, some black, gray banding	0.4 – 0.8 Medium. 5.6	46x14 13- 14x5	3.2 3.0
Humpback, *Megaptera novaeangliae*	270- 400	Dark gray to black	Bimodal, 0.1 – 0.2, 0.6- 0.8 Very fine & Medium Coarse 3.3	72x26 44- 49x21- 23 76x20 58x18	2.8 2.1 2.1 3.8 3.2
Other Baleen Whales, Eschrichtiidae					
Gray, *Eschrichtius robustus*	130- 180	Off white. Gray with yellow filaments.	0.9-1.1 Coarse	57x13 82x18 62x18	4.4 4.6 3.4

Table 7.8.2. Whale baleen plates. Growth occurs in width as well as length, so that their shape tends to remain about the same. In spite of the many variables (length from the tips of the filaments or from the place where they are embedded in matrix, age, length, and width along the curves or straight, position of plate from front to back, base angled to the length, degree of exposure of filaments), these measurements show that length to breadth ratios are markers for families and species. Right whales, Balaenidae, have ratios of 9 -14, rorquals, Balaenopteridae, range from 1.9 to 3.6 and the Gray whale, Eschrictiidae, is 3.4 -4.6. Words and measurements do not adequately describe the texture of the filaments that are fine hairs at the tip but wear away to broader bristles at the base, see Figure 7.8.2. Terms of coarse, fine, etc., often used to describe baleen filaments are misleading without numbers. Diameters of exposed filaments vary from 0.08–1.4 mm, and are grouped here more precisely as: very fine = below 0.2 mm, Fine = 0.2–0.4, Medium = 0.4–0.6, Medium coarse = 0.6–0.8, Coarse = above 0.8. Filament density, where available, is the number seen in transverse profiles like those in Figure 7.8.2. Some are bimodal with the fine filaments often overlooked. Where they have been measured, filament densities in right whales are thirteen to twenty times those of rorquals. Data are from original observations and several sources, including (96) (123) (120). The whale outlines are modified from those created by Chris Huh for Wikipedia and used here under the terms of the GNU Free Documentation License.

Baleen, or "whalebone," characterizes the suborder Mysticeti (Table 7.8.1) of the whale order Cetacea, the toothed whales and dolphins forming the other two suborders (see under whale ivory) (90). Instead of teeth, whalebone whales have several hundred plates of keratin extending as a fringe into the mouth on each side of the upper jaw as in the right whale above (Figure 7.8.1). Each plate has two keratin components: a core of hard filaments and a matrix of soft layers easily cracked and separable from one another (Figure 7.2). On the inner, buccal, surface the matrix wears away to expose the filaments as a meshwork, making the buccal surface of the plates on each side into filters (Figure 7.8.1).

The shape of their plates reflect feeding habits in the three main families of the Mysticeti (96), differing in their width to length ratios (Table 7.8.2). The mouths of right whales, Balaenidae, are bow-shaped to allow their plates to hang vertically. They provide the main baleen of commerce, with long plates (width to length ratios of 9–14) and very fine black filaments not much thicker than horsehair (Figure 7.8.2 A, B). They cruise through the sea with their mouths open to catch krill and very small fish. The rorquals, Balaenopteridae, have much shorter plates (width to length ratios of 1.9–3.6) and for the most part coarse filaments (Sei have fine filaments). They cooperate in concentrating prey that they then gulp into mouths made expandable by pleated throat grooves before squeezing out the water. Rorquals include the largest (blue whale) and the commercially most important whales, but their baleen had little use. The third family includes the gray whales, Escherichtiidae, (width to length ratios of 3.4–4.6) which specialize in stirring up prey from the bottom. The pygmy right whale, *Caperaea marginata*, in the Neobalaenidae is rare and not well described. An interesting fact is that baleen filter feeding is several hundred times more efficient in the ratio of muscle energy used to food energy acquired than is the predatory feeding of toothed whales.

History. Whaling began in the Bay of Biscay in the twelfth century from Spanish and what are now Portuguese ports. They targeted *Eubalaena glacialis*, which became known later as "right whales," because they swam slowly, were easily harpooned by hand from small open boats, and were retrievable after death, floating rather than sinking because of their large oil reserves. By the early nineteenth century, American and other European countries joined in the exploitation, leaving it close to extinction by the mid-1800s. Although protected since 1935, the Biscayan or North Atlantic right whale population is now the most endangered baleen whale with only about 300 left. There is also an arctic race of about 9,000, and two other species, about 1,000 *Eubalaena japonica*, the north Pacific right whale and 7,500 *Eubalaena australis*, the southern right whale in the Antarctic (Table 7.8.1). They have survived more from changes in fashion and industrial needs than from protection.

Bowhead whales, *Balaena mysticetus* of the Arctic, called "Greenland right whales" by Yankee whalers, occupied the same kind of economic niche for the Inuit and Aleuts as *E. glacialis* did for the early Europeans. Bowhead populations are estimated to have been more than 50,000 in early historic times. Blubber (*muktuk*) and muscles were energy rich

(Opposite page)
Figure 7.8.2. The structure of baleen plates. Matrix on each side of the central band of filaments often has cracks (C) in preparation for the shedding that allows exposed filaments to make the filter. A, B, C. Right whales only have fine filaments. Approximate values were calculated from the number counted per area. Bowheads have a wide central band of small densely packed filaments (C), 74.4 sd 4.6 per mm2, with an average diameter of 45 - 370mm and little central matrix. Rorquals have a bimodal distribution of filament sizes. D – M. Rorqual filaments (F, I, L) are only 3 – 6per mm2 and have a bimodal distribution of sizes (0.4 – 1.4 and 0.1 – 0.3mm). Outer rows of wide filaments enclose a central band of fine filaments resembling the much broader band in Right whales. Minke (I) has one or two irregular rows of wide filaments labially but only central fine filaments between the broad ones lingually (123). The structure varies front to back in whole plates and with axial and transverse position on each plate (123). A, B, C, Bowhead. D, E, F, Blue whale. G, H, I, Minke. J, K, L, M, Humpback. C, F, I, L are profiles to show the typical structure near the base of a plate. Scales, A, D, G, J, =10cm. B, E, H, K, =1cm. C, F, I, L, M, =1mm. J, from (123) by kind permission of L. Szewciw.

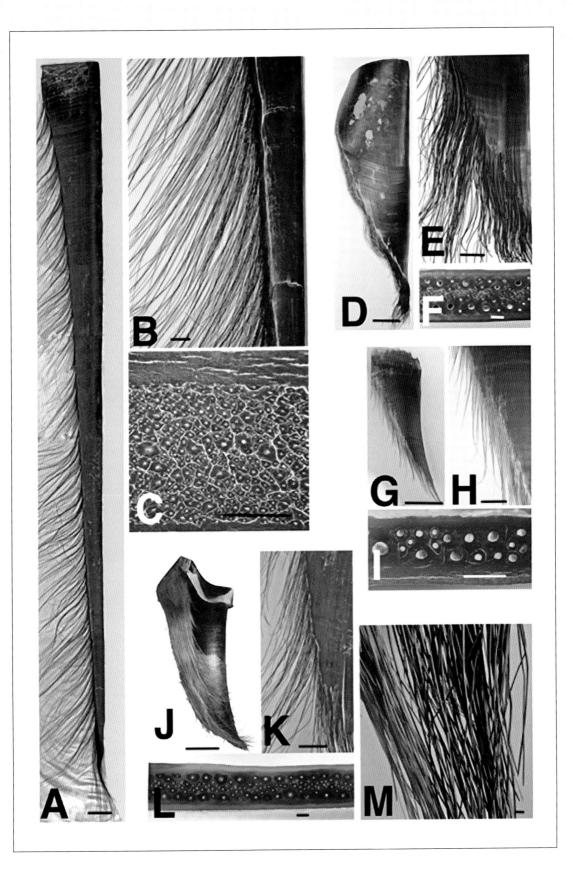

foods and baleen and bones were valuable for tool making and art works. The relatively mild predation by Biscayan and Arctic native hunters came to an end in the mid-nineteenth century when exploitation escalated with the introduction of steamships and explosive harpoon guns introduced in 1865 (17). Whale oil for lamps became a valuable industrial commodity and baleen was the preeminent plastic material used to make everything for which we now use synthetic plastics—skirt and corset stays, handles, baskets, buggy whips, fishing poles, brushes, brooms, and ladle handles. By the mid-nineteenth century, bowheads had been hunted almost to extinction. With protection, their population is now estimated to be about 8,500. They are now threatened by the toxic accumulation of environmental organochlorine (138).

It has been claimed that oil rather than baleen was the major contributor to right whale decline as it has been for blue whales. Only a thousand blue whales survive in the southern oceans from an initial population of a quarter of a million, with no recovery since protection in 1967. However, at the peak of whaling in 1853, more than 2,500 metric tons of baleen, worth $1,950,000, landed in USA (103). European whalers may have taken just as much. Contemporary photographs show outdoor storage areas as big as playing fields covered in teepee-like stacks of baleen plates. Minke are the only whales showing any substantial recovery in numbers since the International Whaling Commission introduced a moratorium on commercial whaling in 1982 that was largely ignored by Japan, which continued whaling for "research" using Britain's last whaling ships bought in 1962. Genetic analysis shows that Japanese markets sell meat and "bacon" from many whales in addition to minke (8).

In the last few decades, baleen has resurfaced as a material for modern craftsmen.

Baleen plate shapes. Baleen plates in early development are nearly rectangular, but the tongue wears the matrix away on the buccal face in a diagonal curve to form the approximately trapezoidal shapes characteristic for each species (Figure 7.8.2). The tip matrix has been exposed longest and wears to a point on the buccal face, curving to the unworn base that extends the full width of the plate. Differences in levels and types of calcium salts along the labial-lingual axis may also help produce the triangular shape of the plate (124). Filaments characteristic of the species are exposed along the length of the diagonal. This combination of initial shape and kind of filament exposed by tongue wear results in the species specific shapes (Table 7.8.2). Right whales are very long and relatively narrow with single plates weighing up to 2 kg. Rorquals are shorter and relatively broad. Large humpback plates may weigh 300 gms, minke 120 gms.

The length of the filaments forming the filter reflects the length of the plate from which they have separated. Bowhead plates have 30–40 cm long draping fringes. Rorquals have spikes up to about 10 cm long in minke, 15 cm in humpback and blue whales.

Baleen structure and properties. At its simplest, a plate consists of surface layers of matrix keratin within which filaments are embedded, sometimes close packed together (right whales) at other times with additional matrix between them (rorquals), (50, 41, 40, 103) and hardening by calcium reinforcement (50), (124, 123, 122). The rorqual structure is described in a detail that may never be repeated in Tycho Tullberg's classic paper *"Bau und Entwicklung der Barten bei Balaenoptera sibbaldii"* ("The structure and development of blue whale baleen"), which was published in 1883 in *Nova Acta Regiae Societatis Scientiarum Upsaliensis*, reviewed in (40). This structural principle for obtaining particular mechanical properties by embedding cylindrical structures in a matrix that we use currently to make composite glass or carbon filaments in resin was "discovered" by whales in their evolution some forty million years ago.

The structure shows why artisans preferred right whale baleen. Densely packed fine filaments (74.4 sd 4.6 per mm², average diameter of 130 mm) form a central band with little matrix (Figure 7.8.2 C). Some rorquals (blue and humpback) have a few central filaments larger than those of bowheads in a sandwich between rows of broad filaments. Others (minke) have two irregular rows of broad filaments labially and central fine filaments localized between the broad ones only on the lingual side (Figure 7.8.2 F, I, L). If baleen filaments are homologous to hair then the coarse filaments may be homologous to coarse guard hairs and the fine filaments to fine underhairs. However, these fine filaments are not recorded in the exposed surface filter suggesting that they may be a stage in development, growing to become broad filaments before emerging.

Baleen filaments are hollow and fluid-filled, sometimes with cells and debris, probably from both ends. This may not be just an accident of development, but a mechanism to maintain hydration influencing rigidity/plasticity, elasticity, and hardness. Baleen can become less rigid, even plastic, in fine hydrated filaments. Dehydration can set it in the shape assumed while plastic, rehydration restoring it to its original shape. This property was known to the Inuit of the Canadian Arctic who devised an ingenious wolf and fox killer dependent on baleen properties. A strip of baleen pointed at both ends was softened in hot water and folded into a small packet before being allowed to dry and set. The nub was hidden in bait for the wolf to gulp down into its warm, wet stomach where it returned to its pointy weapon shape, knifing through the gut wall. Hardness is related to dehydration. Air drying makes a-keratins harder, stiffer, and less extensible, properties preserved via shrinkage and chemical cross-linking of the surrounding protein matrix (123).

Commercial baleen was boiled for twelve hours, resulting in hydration and softening with collapse and consolidation of the cracks in the matrix. The treatment made it soft and plastic for molding: hardness and elasticity returned on drying (see Chapter 9 on artifacts and antiques). There were two main uses. Sheets were sawn into strips that were twisted to create rods with the equal radial mechanical properties needed for handles. Longer filaments in filters were uncovered by teasing them from the sheets before weaving into coverings for grips.

Baleen colors. Colors vary from off-white to yellow, brown, and black, influenced by fading, by developmental changes during growth and by the initial genetic properties of forming cells at the base which follow those of nearby skin color. Filaments are often darker than matrix, but may be bleached after they emerge from the plate to form the filter so that dark plates are often fringed with straw-colored filaments. Sei plates, for example, are almost black but the fringe of exposed filaments is pale brown to white. Transverse bands across the plate show that colors may change during development, sometimes in an annual cycle, but greater differences occur in longitudinal stripes where the plates arise from basal tissues that are stable in the color of keratin they form. Fin whales are especially interesting in this regard because they are asymmetrical. Somehow this may aid in the capture of shoals of fish that they frighten into tight schools before turning on their right side to engulf them. Their lower jaw is white or creamy yellow on the right side and mottled black on the left side. Their baleen follows this asymmetrical skin pattern. Bands of creamy-yellow alternate with blue-gray on the left side of the mouth. The right side is blue-gray with the forward third creamy-yellow (4). Gray whales are also handed. They feed by rolling mostly on their right side, which causes uneven wearing of the baleen.

Conclusion. The properties and availability of baleen (and horn) allowed them to play an essential roll as plastics at the beginning of the Industrial Revolution just when they were needed. They provided light materials for rods or handles that could be rigid or elastic. The art of fine metal plate engraving had been invented so that hot metal templates could be used to impress lasting patterns on keratin sheets. Functional objects of little value were made for the emerging middle classes rather than carefully conserved art objects for the rich. This set the stage for the same techniques to be used on synthetic plastics towards the end of the nineteenth century. Keratin had one major disadvantage—it was vulnerable to insect attack and the great tonnages of keratin used in the industry have all but disappeared. As a consequence, we may have overlooked the industrial importance of baleen as a plastic and in the development of techniques passed on to the synthetic plastic revolution of the late nineteenth and twentieth centuries.

The literature contains many descriptive measurements that are contradictory for various reasons. Readers are urged to make their own observations.

7.9. Rhinoceros horn

The Rhinoceros. You have a horn
where other brutes have none
*   Rhinoceros you are an ugly*
beast.

Hilaire Belloc, 1870–1953

[Rhinoceros] Hee is taken by
the same means that the Unicorn
is taken, for it is said by Albertus,
Isidorus and Alunnes, that above all
creatures they love Virgins, and that
unto them will come be they never so
wilde, and fall asleepe before them,
so being asleepe they are easily taken
and carried away.

Historiae Animalium de Quadrupedibus viviparis
(1551)
Conrad Gessner (1516–1565)

Introduction

Not all early descriptions of rhinoceros are so gentle. Julius Solinus wrote in his *Polyhistoria* "*...the Unicorne, a monster that belloweth horrible, bodyed like a horse, footed like an elephant, tayled like a Swyne, and*

headed like a Stagge. His horn sticketh out of the midds of hys forehead, of a wonderful brightness about four foot long, so sharp, that whatsoever he pusheth at, he striketh it through easily. He is never caught alive, kylled he may be, but taken he cannot bee." Translated by Arthur Golding, 1587 (69).

There are five species of rhinoceros, two in Africa—black rhino, white or square lipped, and three in India and South East Asia—Indian, Sumatran, and Javan (Table 7.9.1). They have gathered a considerable literature on their biology and influence on culture (115). There is also a voluminous and reliable literature on the Internet coming from zoos and organizations devoted to rhino protection.

The close similarity of the three species of Asian rhinoceros attracted Darwin's attention in 1842 in his first notes on the origin of species. He wrote that he preferred to believe in one law governing the transmutation of species than in separate acts of creation, just as the planets revolve in their orbits from one law of gravity rather than through separate volitions of the creator (108).

Rhinos are odd-toed ungulates, belonging with horses in the order Perissodactyla, family, Rhinocerotidae. White rhinos and the Indian rhino are the largest, weighing 1,800 to 3,600 Kg [3900 to 7900 lbs] and 3.6 m to 4.2 m [11.8 to 13.7 ft] long (record 4,500 Kg [9900 lbs] for a white rhino). They are colored grey like all the other rhinos, the name being a mistranslation of the Bohr/Dutch word "*wijd*" meaning wide and referring to the broad square upper lip that distinguished it from the pointed prehensile lip of the black rhino. The black rhino is smaller, up to 3.6 m [11.8 ft] long but more lightly built, weighing up to 1,400 Kg [3000 lbs]. The Javan and Sumatran rhinos are smaller still, weighing up to 1,000 Kg [2200 lbs]. They are all distinguished by their horns (Figure 7.9.1).

Present status and threats to survival. In the early 1800s there were probably several hundred thousand black rhinos and almost as many whites, somewhat fewer Indian, but still many thousands. Eighty-five percent of the world's population was killed between 1970 and 1987. Some threats are shared with other

Name	White	Black	Indian	Sumatran	Javan
Species	*Ceratotherium simum*	*Diceros bicornis*	*Rhinoceros unicornis*	*Dicerorhinus sumatrensis*	*Rhinoceros sondaicus*
Number of horns	2	2 Rarely more, up to 5 recorded	1	2	1 Often absent in the female
Record front horn length in cms.	159	136	55	82	27
Record rear horn length in cms.	45	57		19	
Estimated number surviving in 2004	11,100	3,600	2,400	300	60

Table 7.9.1. Rhino horn records—number, size, and length. Record lengths dating from early in the nineteenth century (135). Measurements are made on the outside curve.

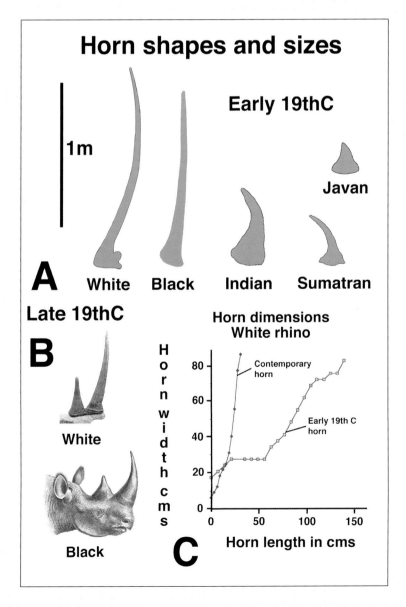

Figure 7.9.1. Size and shape change in nineteenth century horns. A. African rhino horns collected early in the nineteenth century were more than a meter long while good Indian ones were over half a meter. Approximately to scale. B. By the end of the century horns were less than a third of that length. For record sizes, see Table 7.9.1 C. A graphical comparison of the shape of representative horns shows how the growth trajectory changed from early to late in the nineteenth century.

wildlife—habitat destruction, but the more serious threats are specific for rhinoceros because of the value of their horns.

Asian rhinos were the first to suffer. For 2,000 years the conical shape of rhino horns made them suitable for Chinese craftsmen to carve elaborate cups of great beauty (21, 22, 57). The demand was small and only for the rich, but it was spread over a long period. Coupled with its use in medicine, this probably caused the extinction of the Chinese race of rhinos about 1,000 years ago. It may also have affected the populations of Sumatran and Javan rhinos that are now so low, but without the mass production of horn artifacts effects on populations were probably small.

The first big wave of destruction of African rhinos came with early nineteenth century big game hunting and horns collected as an industrial commodity. Nineteenth century hunters attacked them as if they were an unlimited resource, reducing hundreds of thousands to near extinction in an attitude to wildlife that we now find abhorrent. They were shot for raw material for the new market in walking sticks, umbrellas, and riding crops that was springing up with the demands of the new middle class made rich by the Industrial Revolution. Rhino horn had the advantage over cattle horn in being solid and in much longer lengths (Table 7.9.1). Horn craftsmen stocked up with half-meter lengths of Indian and meter lengths of African rhino horn. Ward records "sportsmen" shooting half a dozen rhino in a single evening as they came to drink at a pool. One called Andersson killed sixty in a few months (135).

Chinese medicine gave rise to the next wave of rhino destruction. Rhino horn, under the name of *His-chiao* or *Shui-niu chiao*, has had a place in Chinese medicine for almost as long as the Chinese love of horn cups (5). Indeed, it was intimately connected with the belief that rhino horn cups could detect and even neutralize poisons, a belief that spread to Europe in the Middle Ages. Rhino horn was/ is believed to clear fevers, "cool" the blood, "detoxify" and control convulsive spasms, given in doses of 2–8 fen (= 0.6–2.5 gm). There

is no evidence for horn having any beneficial effect, but belief trumps rationality, perhaps through the placebo effect. This placed little stress on rhino populations until the 1970s when the rise of affluence in Southeast Asia escalated the demand for horn as medicine to $50,000 a kilo = $50 a gram, which would make an 8 fen dose cost $125 (95). Nor is this the highest price being paid to smugglers. In Africa, where conservation had allowed the last free rhinos to rebound, poaching became big and dangerous business. Poachers are often better armed than wildlife officers and prepared to shoot rather than be captured, with tragic results to rhinos and humans.

Dagger handles crafted in Yemen and Oman created a threat to rhinos at about the same time as the expansion of horn as a medicine and for some of the same reasons—the spread of economic wealth. Rhino destruction increased as the Arab world became rich from oil and began to experience unprecedented economic development. Yemenis became wealthy during the oil boom at the beginning of the 1970s and daggers with rhino horn handles became affordable status symbols. Although the Yemen government had banned horn imports and domestic trade in horn dagger, craftsmen continued in their trade. An average of 75 Kg of rhino horn each year, enough for about ninety daggers and equal to about twenty-five rhinoceros, were smuggled into Yemen to make the handles for the traditional dagger, the *jambiya* or *jamboyya*, in the two years from 1994–1996. This had dropped to about 30 Kg by the turn of the century.

The *jambiya* dagger (also spelled *djambia, janbia* and *jambia* from the Arabic, جنبية *janbīyah*) is the essential Arab dagger, found throughout the world wherever Arabs have been. It has a short curved blade adapted for slicing in one movement as it is pulled from its sheath. The concave handles are made of wood, bone, or horn. The workmanship and material from which the handle is made determines its value, the most valuable being the *saifani* made from rhino horn. With age, this may turn to a translucent yellow called *saifani* heart, greenish yellow called *asadi*, yellowish white called *zaraf,* or translucent white, *albasali*. These antique *janbias* may be exceedingly valuable, costing as much as several hundred thousand dollars. *Keris* or *Kris* daggers from Indonesia, Malaysia, Thailand, and Brunei have asymmetrical wavy blades adapted for thrusting. Most have straight wood, bone, ivory, or horn handles, but some curve at an angle to the blade, especially those made of rhino horn. The most effective method for reduction of the rhino horn knife handle trade was the introduction of handles made from Indian water buffalo horns. In 2003, the average price for a rhino horn *jambiya* was $466 compared to $15 for one made of buffalo horn (82).

By 2004, the International Rhino Foundation estimated the populations of Black rhinos to be 3,610, white 11,100, Indian 2,400, Javan 60, and Sumatran 300 (Table 7.9.1). They are now among the worlds most threatened groups.

Horn size and shape. Contemporary illustrations of horns or views of those on living rhino have little relation to those living 150–200 years ago (Figure 7.9.1 A, B). African rhino horns collected early in the nineteenth century were more than a meter long while good Indian ones were over half a meter (Table 7.9.1). The length of horns on early white rhino is illustrated by records showing that they kept their heads forward and down so that their horns became worn at the tip from being pushed along the ground, a feat no longer possible for today's rhinos. Wear progressively along the length from the tips to the base may explain why early nineteenth century horns are relatively narrow (Figure 7.9.1). This would be a natural consequence of the most interesting finding of Hieronymus discussed below that the core is harder than the periphery (54). By the end of the century, horns were less than a third the length because their length had encouraged their exploitation for making sticks. Short Javan and Sumatran horns suffered a different pressure due to their shape, making them suitable for making cups.

One reason for the decline in length may be rhino's longevity, since they live for up to fifty years and their slaughter cut short their life spans. The shape of the horn is a record of previous growth from the tip where growth began to the base where the last phase of growth has occurred minus that lost by continued wear along the length (Figure 7.9.1 A, B). Changes in ratios of diameter to length could be due to differential wear, the characteristic conical shape being caused by a harder core keratin protected by melanin and the incorporation of calcium phosphate salts (54). This could be confirmed if observations on the relative proportions of hard core to soft peripheral horn were to show more hard core in old narrow horns than recent wide ones. It could also be confirmed if contemporary baby rhinos have narrow basal growth regions. Published pictures of baby rhino horns are not easy to interpret, but they seem to show a broad elevated base from which the horn arises, much as in adults. From this, a narrow horn emerges with dimensions similar to the tip of adult horns. It may be that both structure and changes in growth rate affect the shape of the horn. The relation between diameter and length for representative horns from early and late in the nineteenth century have growth trajectories that are not interchangeable, differing from the start either from differential wear or differential deposition or both (Figure 7.9.1 C). If it is from different rates of deposition, then early nineteenth century horns show periods of increase in length with a small progressive increase in diameter. Contemporary horns increase in diameter more rapidly during their lifespan. Selection changing genetics as has happened in elephants to reduce tusk size could be responsible. More probably, it is related to a change in nutrition as their habitat decreased in both area and nutritive quality. Selection and nutrition were probably acting much earlier than the nineteenth century. By the mid-sixteenth century, Portuguese traders were returning with live elephants and rhinoceros. King Manuel 1 of Portugal (1469–1521) was known to saunter through the streets of Lisbon with a menagerie of elephants and a rhino (63).

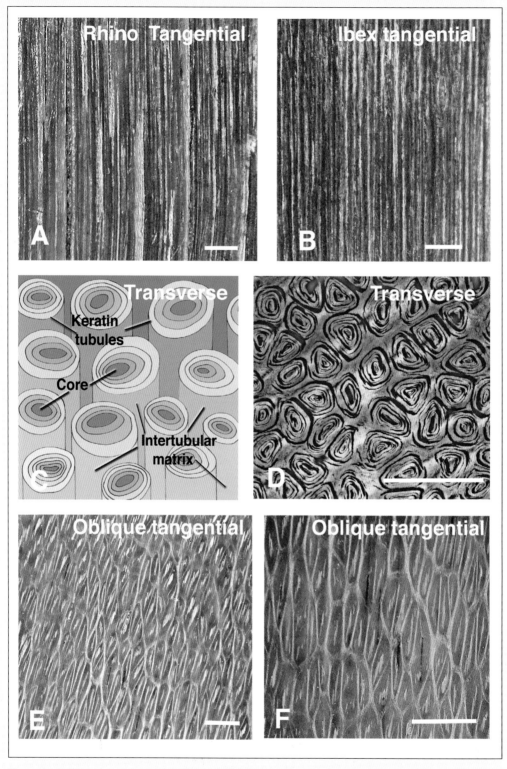

Figure 7.9.2. Rhino horn structure. A. Tangential profiles of rhino horn are difficult to distinguish from those of ungulates. B. Tangential profile of ibex horn for comparison with A. In both kinds of horn, the width and separation of the longitudinal components varies with the plane of intersection and does not help in their identification. C, D. Transverse profiles of rhino horns clearly separate them from those of ungulates. Rhino horn consists of longitudinally arranged keratin tubules separated by a matrix. The tubules are multilayered with characteristic cores of red to brown strands that may be capillaries or leaked blood. E, F. Tubules align in groups of 1–3. Matrices around the tubules form a reticular network in transverse or oblique profiles with wide matrices around groups and narrow matrices around individual tubules. Scale bars = 1 mm.

Structure. Rhino horn consists of longitudinally arranged keratin tubules (54), (80), (83), (116). They arise from papillae and grow quickly, as much as 9 cms a year on new horns after removal of the old ones (10). Surface views cut the tubule walls in various planes creating longitudinal lines with equally varied separations, as if the tubules had many different diameters. This makes it difficult to distinguish rhino from ungulate horn in either tangential surfaces or tangential cut profiles (Figures 7.9.2 A, rhino; B, ibex). However, the difference is obvious in transverse or oblique profiles that show rhino horn with tubules about 0.5 mm in diameter composed of concentric cylindrical keratin layers embedded in a matrix (Figures 7.9.2 C–F). The core of each tubule contains characteristic reddish threads that could be capillaries or leaked blood. In transverse or oblique profiles the matrix forms a reticular network with each tubule surrounded by a thin matrix but sharing a much thicker one with two or three other tubules.

7.10. Feathers

Mammals are dull creatures, perhaps reflecting their evolution crouched in a distant nocturnal past; their hairs are all the colors that melanin can produce, everything from brown to black. Birds, on the other hand, flew in the daytime and evolved brilliantly colored feathers in three different ways. They synthesize pigments of many kinds and deposit them in the keratin of their feathers as in the reds of the northern cardinal, *Cardinalis cardinalis* (Fig. 7.10.1.) They also absorb pigments from the food. Flamingos, *Phoenicopterus sp.*, in captivity can and do take up carotenoids that color their feathers, as happens in finches (54B), but in the wild the pink in their feathers comes from heme in hemoglobin in their diet. Flamingos are especially interesting in that their pink color

comes mainly from hemoglobin from several different sources, the common feature being their food of organisms that have independently evolved hemoglobin to enable them to survive the low oxygen levels in mud. There are six species from around the world feeding in muddy water where *Artemia salina* (Crustacea), and larvae of *Chironomus sp.* (Insecta, Diptera), have independently evolved hemoglobin to cope with the low oxygen. Thirdly, feather keratin can form stacks of thin, stiff, translucent sheets forming multiple interference layers as in the eye from a peacock *(Pavo cristatus)*. In this they rivaled the brilliant colors of insects obtained from stacks of chitin and tanned proteins.

Feathers are adapted for two main functions, as airfoils for flight and as downy plumes for insulation. All feathers are built on the same principle, a rachis with lateral barbules that interlock to form a smooth surfaced vane that is strong and light, or barbules that do not interlock but create an insulating down. An adaptation for their role as airfoils is the ease with which their barbules can separate and reattach. Instead of having to repair a rent in a permanent structure (like the skin of a bat) feather barbules can separate when stressed and reattach (Figure 7.2). Flight feathers are asymmetrical around a stiff rachis allowing them to fit together with their neighbors to create a seamless airfoil (Fig. 7.10.2). Contour feathers are symmetrical and interlock to make the whole body a smooth airfoil. To meet the second function of feathers—insulation—barbules at the base of the rachis transform into plumes and some may have a small after feather. Plumes form from barbules that do not interlock. Down feathers are made from nothing but plumes. Most feathers have some degree of plume development at their base, giving insulation to the whole body except for a strip below the wings allowing cooling during flight. Bristles and filoplumes are feathers simplified to a rachis with very reduced or simplified barbules or plumes (Fig. 7.10.2).

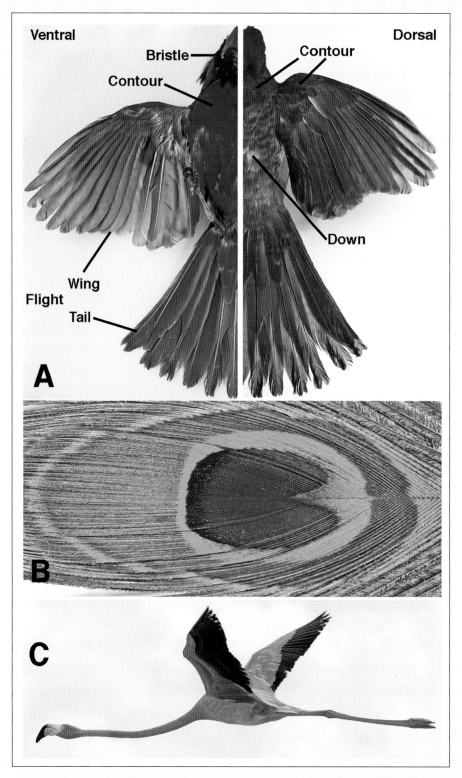

Figure 7.10.1. Feather colors. The color of feathers may be caused by pigments synthesized by the bird itself as in A, the northern cardinal (Cardinalis cardinalis); B, by interference colors as in this eye from a peacock (Pavo cristatus) feather; or C, by heme from hemoglobin in its food of Chironomus larvae coloring this Mexican flamingo (Phoenicopterus ruber) pink.

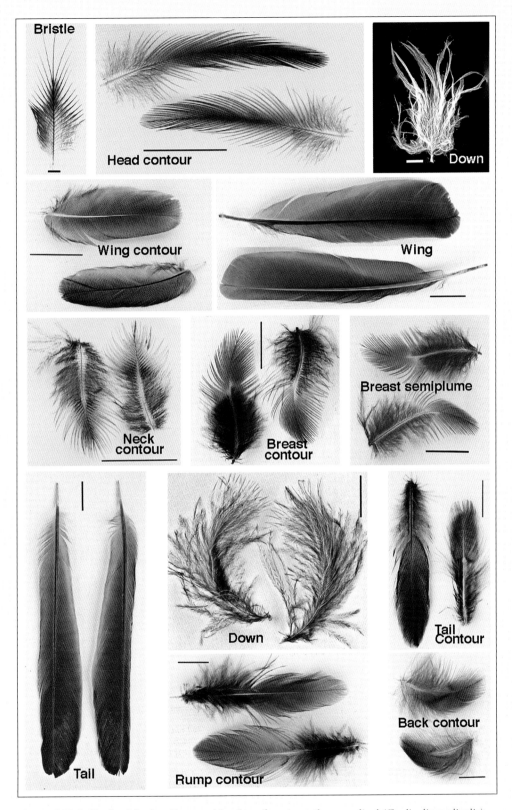

Figure 7.10.2. Kinds of feather illustrated by those from a northern cardinal (Cardinalis cardinalis). All feathers are built on the same principle, summarized in Figure 7.2.

Chapter 8

Other Materials

Black Things

Black materials have long been used to make small objects, especially during Queen Victoria's prolonged mourning after the Death of Prince Albert in 1861. The materials include: argillite–Haida slate; black agate and jasper; black ceramics–jasperware; **black coral**; black glass and obsidian (volcanic glass); black volcanic ash; **bog oak** (Ireland); **ebony**; **jet** and coal; minerals: psilomelane, manganite, quartz; papier-mache; pressed horn; vulcanite or ebonite–vulcanized rubber. There is only space here to describe four of these briefly—black coral, bog oak, ebony, and jet. Pressed horn is dealt with under horn antiques.

Black corals, order Antipatharia

Black coral is highly prized by jewelry craftsmen for its hardness, durability, and fine polish. There are about 230 species in 42 genera worldwide. The ones most valued have a shrub-like structure with the main trunk up to 2 cms in diameter (Figure 8.1 A1, 2, 3). All are from deep water and are being wrenched from the bottom by trawlers, later to be washed up onshore and wasted as raw material. Cuban craft markets, for example, are filled with black coral jewelry made in Taiwan, although the shores of Cuba facing the US are littered with black coral debris. Those with similar structures are difficult to tell apart, making it hard to identify species at risk.

Coral is secreted as a central core from cells restricted to a thin layer at the surface. Growth can be exceedingly slow. Some corals that live for more than 4,000 years add layers only 4–35 m wide per year, another feature that puts their survival at risk. The chemical composition of the skeletons of *Antipathes fiordensis* from New Zealand and *A. salix* from the Caribbean, have been studied (45). Both have 10–15% chitin associated with a tyrosine-rich fraction and 50% protein, and contain 2–5% halogens, iodine and bromine being dominant. Unlike arthropods with their chitin in layers changing orientation in a crossed helical structural organization (see the section on ivory structure), the chitin in black coral forms fibers that wind in anticlockwise spirals (60).

(Opposite page)
Figure 8.1. Other materials. A1. Black coral. Species of Antipatharia most favored for jewelry grow like small trees in very deep water. The tree is composed of very thin layers of chitin and tanned protein deposited by a layer of cells on the outside. A2, 3. Longitudinal and transverse profiles. B. Bog oak. Oak wood tanned by long exposure to tannins in Irish bogs was carved in the late 1800s into many small items like snuff boxes. C. Vegetable ivory—tagua nuts (Phytelephas macrocarpa, Family Arecaceae). 1. Whole nut. 2. Skin partly removed. 3. Nut with slice removed to expose the endosperm. 4. The surface in three magnified to show the cell structure. The endosperm is a uniform composite of polygonal cells with cellulose cell walls, making it ideal for taking the fine detail of impressions (5, 6), cutting into buttons, (7), or carving (8). It can also be dyed almost any color. D. Jet is Araucaria wood fossilized like coal but with a higher proportion of mineral oil and a harder, tougher, more uniform texture. Rough blocks are a dull grey (1) but take a glossy luster with polishing (2). They can be carved with fine detail (3). Chains are made by gluing together broken single links rather than by carving. E. Coquilla nut (Attalea, oil palm nuts, Family Arecaceae). Unlike tagua nuts that resemble ivory, the structure is wood-like since they come from the shells of the palm nuts. This is also their limitation. They can be turned into beautiful small containers but there is no 3-D mass to carve. The color varies from orange-brown 1, to dark brown 2). Scales, A1 = 5 cm, A2, 3, C4 = 1 mm, all others = 1 cm.

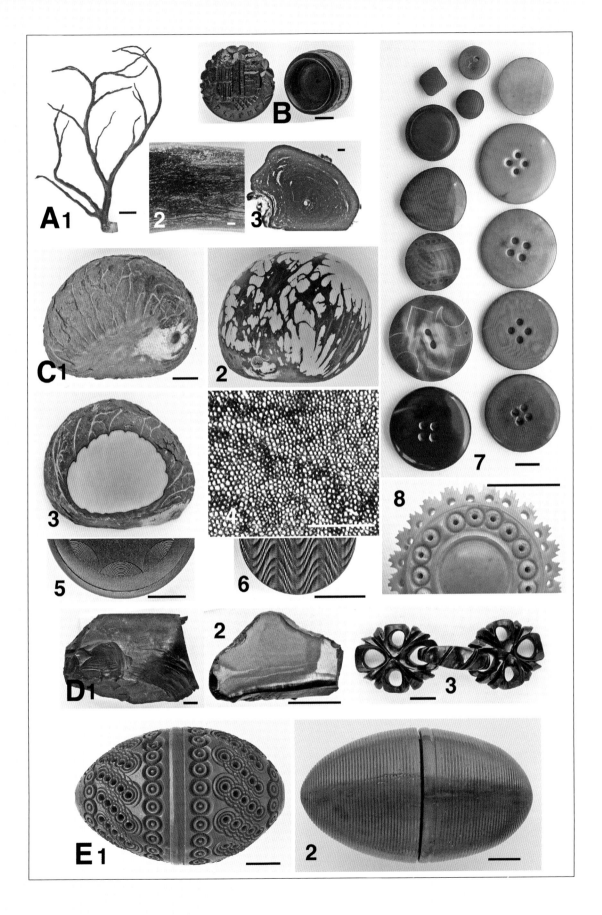

Jet. Hardness: 3–4 on Mohs' scale, density: 1.3, composition: carbon containing twelve percent mineral oil. Jet is *Araucaria* wood fossilized in marine deposits from the Jurassic 180 million years ago (93). It is almost featureless by eye, the wood structure usually only becoming visible by microscopy. Jet differs from coal in its toughness. Its most characteristic feature is the high black gloss achieved after polishing (Figure 8 D1, 2, 3). High quality jet occurs below a band of limestone in Whitby, North Yorkshire, England, where it has been mined since the bronze age or even earlier. Jet deposits of various qualities, including some as good as that from Whitby, are found throughout the world. Large pieces of high quality come from Utah.

Bog oak. Wood in quaternary bogs may react with tannins to become a hard, dark material ideal for carving (Figure 8 B). When first retrieved from a bog, the wood is soft enough to carve easily, becoming hard as it dries, preserving fine detail and a good polish. Almost all "bog oak" came from peat diggers in Ireland, where rather crude, small broaches, pots, and animals were carved locally in Victorian times. The blackness of the broaches made them popular in response to Queen Victoria's mourning of Prince Albert.

Ebony. The heartwood of many trees ceases to transport water and dies. This presents a problem, how to prevent rotting so that it may continue to function mechanically and keep the tree upright. The answer is to transform the heartwood chemically into something that prevents decay, most commonly by tanning with phenolics that crosslink to produce hard, dark, resistant wood. The best known of these heartwoods occur in nearly 500 species of the genus *Diospyros*, ebony or persimmon, in the family Ebenaceae (30, 104). Most occur in the tropics, notably in India, Ceylon, West Africa, and Indonesia. Their properties make them valuable woods for fine carvings, inlays, and special projects like the black pieces in chess. They are black, fine grained, take a high polish, and with a density greater than one, sinking in water.

Vegetable Ivory

Tagua nut ivory. Plants are fertilized in two parts, one part becomes the embryo with chromosomes from its male (pollen) and female (unfertilized seed) parents. The other part, the endosperm, receives three sets of chromosomes, two male and one female, and becomes a food reserve for the developing seed. The endosperm in palm nuts is large, simple, and structurally uniform, with cells having thick walls enclosing oils, proteins, or carbohydrates. The main constituent of the walls is cellulose, the structural polymer made by plants from b linked glucose units packed together in long chains that are chemically inert, unaffected by animal enzymes. These properties make some endosperm peculiarly suitable as a substitute for ivory. The endosperm from the tagua nut (*Phytelephas macrocarpa*, Family Arecaceae), the best known vegetable ivory, is even superior to real ivory in its structure. Its composition from polygonal cells that are almost the same in every direction give it uniform properties in three dimensions (Figure 8 C1–8). Tagua nuts are also known as Corozo and Dum nuts (the latter particularly when immature and used for food), but other palm nuts have been used. The main exports are from Ecuador, South America, where whole nuts are carved into heads and torsos for the tourist industry. In the past, the main use of vegetable ivory was in button making. In the nineteenth century, British buttons were "in;" from high society fashions to missionaries' clothing, the heathen buttons played their part. By the middle of the nineteenth century, the bone and horn that allowed Birmingham to supply buttons to the world were replaced by cheaper and more easily worked vegetable ivory, only to be replaced in its turn first by plastic and, in the 1950s and '60s, by zippers.

When first cut, the natural color of tagua vegetable ivory is an attractive cream, very like ivory. A hand lens shows the cellular structure, easily distinguishing it from bone or any kind of ivory. The cream color fades to a rather dull brown, not at all like old ivory. Few old buttons were stained, perhaps because the main expansion of the button industry preceded the development of the synthetic chemical industry that began in 1856 with Perkins Mauve. More recent buttons are often stained black, red, and pink.

Up to 100 species of *Attalea*, oil palms, Family Arecaceae, come from Mexico south to Brazil (Figure 8 E1, 2). The **Brazilian feather palm tree,** *A. funifera,* from the coast of Brazil, is the source of a reddish brown nut about 8 cms long popularly known as the coquilla nut. Although sometimes referred to as vegetable ivory, it is not made from the endosperm like the tagua nut but from the shell. Its structure is wood-like, similar to that of a coconut, making it popular with wood turners for making thimble and needle cases.

Boxwood. The treatment of wood is outside the scope of this book, but boxwood is a special case. It looks rather like bone or ivory and has many of the same properties taking superb detail in carvings. Like bone, it is often turned for handles, though not for cutlery, perhaps because it absorbs both greasy and aqueous stains too easily. It is easily recognized by the xylem vessels characteristic of wood and the absence of osteons characteristic of bone or the dentinal tubule patterns of ivory. Very old boxwood changes to brown rather than the mellower cream of ivory.

Plastics. Plastics are defined as materials that while liquid can be poured into shapes that they retain after becoming hard. Horn and tortoiseshell are soft enough to be deformed when hot, but they can only be made to take shallow, non-reentrant patterns—the characteristic patterns of pressed horn. If the patterns are more three-dimensional, they are either carved or made by filling moulds with plastic. Problems in identification arise when the moulds have been copied from original artifacts. The artifact Netsuke is coated with rubber latex, which is stripped off when set and used as a mold for the plastic. The plastic then copies in microscopic detail all the surface patterns of the original. For example, plastic copies of facetted jet beads may have the original scratch marks left

after polishing, napkin rings may have the slightly raised pattern of the crossed spirals of elephant ivory. The copies are not confined to expensive items like Netsuke and old carvings. Plastic toggles matching the color and surface patterns of horn tips may fool the unwary. Always look into the piece to verify that the pattern is also there below the surface. It is not sufficient to see the pattern from a brightly reflecting surface.

Celluloid. Cellulose acetate and nitrate were some of the earliest plastics, easily distinguished from natural materials by their flammability and solubility in alcohol (the surface becomes sticky with a small drop of alcohol). An early attempt to use them to replace ivory for billiard balls led to explosions when hit firmly (cellulose nitrate is "gun cotton").

Bakelite. Leo Baekeland was a Belgian chemist who had immigrated to the United States. Eastman Kodak paid him 3/4 million dollars for a photographic paper he had developed, enough to finance his laboratory to do the independent research on plastics, his consuming interest. He was looking for a plastic material that could replace shellac as an insulator in the rapidly expanding electrical industry. After five years, in 1907, he had a liquid that would harden into an amber colored solid with the exact form of the mold. This was the first completely synthetic plastic, a thermoset polymer made from phenol and formaldehyde. He called it Bakelite. Bakelite's properties are the result of reactions at any of three different positions on the benzene ring of the phenol component, allowing multiple cross linkages. It is an electrical insulator, tough, heat resistant, unaffected by light or water, solvents, salt, or acids, and it doesn't crack or discolor, burn or melt. It can also be given any color. Many of its properties were similar to ivory, making it an immediate success as a material for knife handles and billiard balls.

Chapter 9

Artifacts and Antiques

"… bring forth out of his treasure things new and old."

St. Matthew 13:52

9.1. Introduction

The previous chapters aimed to help collectors value their pieces by correctly identifying the natural materials from which they were made. Many museums have artifacts from the pre-plastic period, but every flea market contains similar undiscovered treasures, if only we learn to identify them. Displays in shopping malls or markets in the second half of the twentieth century, even in third world countries, are dominated by mass produced goods made of plastic. Similar goods were in use a hundred or more years ago, but they were made individually from natural materials such as bone, ivory, horn, antler, and wood. Craftsmen often made them in large numbers, but for a discriminating market. For example, in 1887, Sheffield cutlers produced 72,000 handles a week, and one of their suppliers of raw materials stocked 122 tons of ivory. Tableware was only one use for the precursors of plastics. There were also drinking vessels, culinary utensils, and tools for the kitchen, ladies boudoir accessories and jewelry, tools and handles for everything in science, medicine, war, and commerce. That these articles have survived is a testament to the toughness of natural materials and to their superb craftsmanship. That we might still want to possess such objects is a tribute to their beauty, achieving elegance through functional simplicity of design. They reward us with an atmosphere of quiet patience indifferent to time.

The first part of this chapter is a tribute to the skills of past craftsmen and the stories that their artifacts tell (9.2, 3, 4). The second part describes how to date artifacts (9.5), how to identify the materials used to make them (9.6), and what they may have been used for (9.7). The final section relates the properties of natural materials to their utility (9.8).

9.2. Intellectual Interest and Value

Were it not for imagination, Sir, a man would be as happy in the arms of a chambermaid as of a duchess.

Samuel Johnson, 9th May 1778
Boswell's Life of Johnson, Vol. iii, p. 341

The historian in every collector. Just as it is the pleasure and duty of a historian to make the past come alive with words and imagination, so it is the pleasure and duty of the collector to put his objects into a context that brings to life the period when they were created. The historian may only have myths and tales, architecture, and texts at best to create his story. His world overlaps with fiction and historical novels. The collector works with a more complete world of reality—objects that create but also confine his story. The facts presented are the major part of the story, the same for all, limiting the role for imagination in their interpretation.

Values. In his descriptions of antiques and the people who desire them, Thatcher Freund dwells on the unique and costly objects acquired by the rich and famous. Even the buyers of antiques in the $25,000 range are at his low end (39). Connoisseurship rules. Love is based on monetary value determined by a critic or dealer's personal sense of beauty. But love can depend on what an object tells us directly as much as by beauty determined by dealers. Objects bought for only a few dollars may be desired as much as more valuable objects but loved for a different reason. They are loved for what they tell us about the past, revealing more about their previous owners and ways of life than do expensive art objects or uniquely crafted furniture. Objects tell stories, but however expensive a chair, it may only tell us that its owner sat on it. Old needles may tell us what they did while seated. A set of cutlery valued at a few dollars may tell us more about the manners of those seated at the table than the table that sells for millions. Facts take the place of indefinable art. A love of small objects depends more on our knowledge and intellectual ingenuity than on the fashion of their perceived artistic value.

9.3. Windows on the Past Antiques That Tell Stories

The purpose of the preceding chapters has been to describe the **materials** used to make everyday objects, essential for an understanding of how, when, and for what purpose they were made. Now we must make those **artifacts** tell their stories. We do not need to rely on museums. We can step away from objects protected behind glass to touch, feel and smell our own small antiques that have a special interest as keys to past ways of life. Such windows need study before they disappear. Here are typical examples of the way **imagination, observation,** and **history** uncover the past in different ways.

"Old 'Ath 'ower" and a simple tube of horn

The horn in the illustration is nondescript at best, just an old piece of cow horn, perhaps just a waste scrap, thin, worn at the edges, clean inside but unpolished (Figure 9.1 A).

There is nothing about it that might tell us what it was for, if indeed, it was "for" anything. Could it have been used as a funnel? Hardly likely, there is little difference in diameter between the ends. Was it a scoop from an apothecaries dispensary or a measure from a food jar from the ancient equivalent of a corner store? When we put a thumb over the narrow end we can fill it as a scoop with any manner of things and just as easily empty it out into a twist of paper. Sugar is the most likely candidate, for the horn holds about 29 gms of soft brown sugar, depending on the packing, very close to 1 oz. avoirdupois (28.35 gms). It also holds almost exactly 31.1 grams of white pourable sugar, equal to one troy ounce. It holds forty percent more salt than sugar, and only forty percent as much tea, amounts that do not correlate with any units. Black powder for old muzzle loading guns was a possibility, but this would have been eight percent heavier, also losing any correlation with units of measurement. The measured weight of sugar is probably not a coincidence and is surely close enough to known units for a country store where both rroy and avoirdupois units were both used for bread and other food. It conjures up an image given to me by an elderly English astronomer colleague from his youth in North Yorkshire. His family would send him on errands to buy two penny worth of this and three penny worth of that from the small grocery shop in the village where he lived. It was run by "Old 'Ath Ower," who got his name from his usual response after cutting a small piece of cheese—"'ath ower" meaning a "halfpenny over what you asked for." I imagine this now distinguished astronomer as a small boy approaching a bare wooden counter with little for sale but the essentials, flour, butter, salt, sugar. "Please for a penny twist of sugar, Sir." "Old 'Ath Ower" twists a piece of rough paper around the horn to make a penny sac and fills it from the horn.

Jane Austen (1775–1817)

The little bit (two inches wide) of ivory on which I work with so fine a brush as produces so little effect after much labour.

Jane Austen, Letter, 16th December 1816

Jane Austin spent most of her life practicing to write. Success only came six years before her death when four of her novels were published, followed posthumously by two more. Her family had progressed from trade as wool manufacturers to respectability as landed gentry without land, a position that allowed Jane to observe and write about the social scene about her. Her family gave her support but there was little money. Education came from her father, rector of a small parish, a sinecure that allowed him to earn extra money by farming and tutoring. We live in a society that is flooded with cheap paper and it never occurs to us that in Jane's time writing paper was expensive. How could she afford the masses of paper needed for draft after draft?

The answer is that she didn't use paper for drafts. She wrote with a lead pencil like that in Figure 9.10 J on the tiny ivory leaves of the writing pads referred to in her letter. Six ivory leaves like those in Figure 9.1 C have an area of 153 cm², about a quarter of a sheet of foolscap (or twice that if she used both sides). We may imagine Jane spending her days writing and rewriting sentences in minute script on such ivory tablets before transcribing the finished result into ink on precious paper. The pads figured could even be hers, unless some collection or museum has pads with good provenance like those referred to in her letter. Writing pads like this usually had several blank ivory leaves protected by covers of tortoiseshell or ivory scrimshawed with decorative scenes as in Figure 9.1 B. Before photography or steel engraving, such descriptive scrimshaw was one of the cheapest kinds of illustration.

Careful observation may give crucial clues to artifact secrets where imagination is not enough, as in these examples.

A collection of combs

A strip of bone, horn, wood, metal, etc. with teeth, used for disentangling, cleaning, and arranging the hair, or for keeping it in place.

The Oxford Universal Dictionary

Combs used to remove knots from human and animal hair or to push down the threads in the weft of looms, are among the oldest archaeological artifacts. Many Roman and Anglo-Saxon combs, like the horn examples in Figure 9.1 D, but made from bone, ivory, or the outer surface of antlers, have survived. Most such old combs differ in an important detail from those made by the Iroquois in the fifteenth century (Figures 9.1 D2 and 3). They had no holes. The Iroquois combs had holes; holes that tell us something.

An important stage in social development came when people began to own things. For the first time in their history they had possessions—ornaments, clothes, weapons, toilet articles, **combs**. In the absence of a concept of personal possessions came a second set of problems: how to protect them, how to keep them for yourself. In the absence of a concept of theft, objects were

(Opposite page)

Figure 9.1. Artifacts that tell stories. A. A simple tube of horn with no distinguishing marks. See text 9.3.1 A for the story that it tells. B. The scrimshawed ivory covers to a typical writing pad from the early nineteenth century. The covers would have enclosed about six thin ivory leaves for writing notes like those in C. See text 9.3.1 B for the story that it may tell. C. A later nineteenth century tortoiseshell covered pad with six ivory leaves having a combined area of about half a sheet of foolscap paper. D 1–8. A collection of combs. 2. Comb of bone or antler with four teeth, "Neutral" Iroquois (1500–1600). 3. Effigy Comb of bone or antler with four teeth, Neutral Iroquois c. 1525 (*reproduced by kind permission of the London Museum of Archeology*). The other combs are horn but could just as easily have been made of antler or bone. Nit combs (8) were usually made of ivory or horn. Combs similar to 3 (a nineteenth century horse curry comb) have been made of bone for human use in various parts of the world for thousands of years. See the text 9.3.2 A for the clues that give information on a past way of life. 2 and 3. Scales = 1 cm.

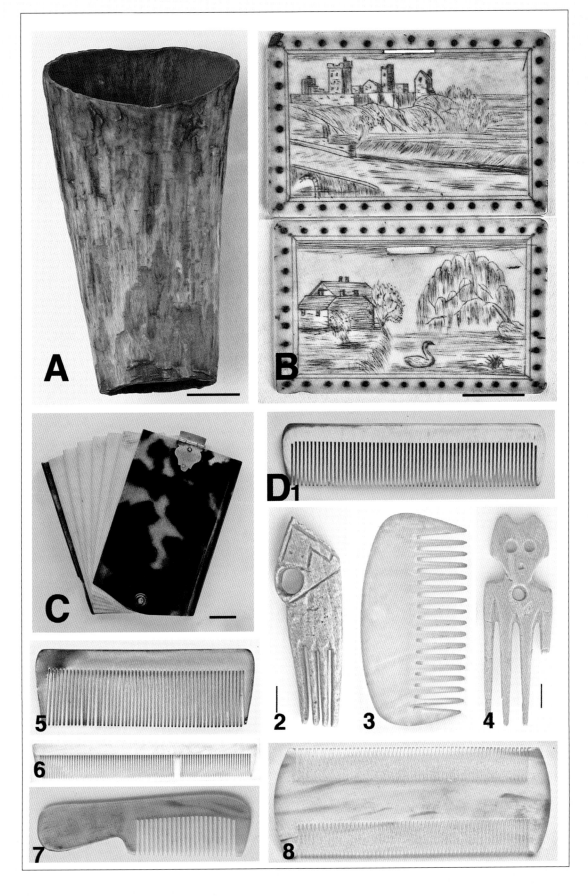

only possessions if they were in your space. The first stage was to keep them with you. The second step was to keep them in a larger space that was also yours. The Iroquois combs illustrate the first step. The combs had holes in them so that they could be hung on the body as functional tools doubling as readily available adornments. The Iroquois had communal great houses for shelter and sleeping, but no personal living quarters or space equivalent to a safety deposit box. Possessions were protected by carrying them. The other combs without holes illustrate the second step, being protected by storing in personal spaces such as dressing tables, hand-bags, pockets, and on barn shelves. The concept of theft developed from the integrity of these spaces.

Taking and using other peoples' objects in societies that did not and could not protect their possessions predated the concept of theft. Theft could only arise in societies that kept things in guarded spaces. Failure to realize this had tragic consequences. Captain Cook's hard line on theft with the natives of Tahiti led to his death. This did not surprise his First Lieutenant, who knew that the natives held their possessions in common, but he was shocked to learn that Cook's body parts were later distributed as presents to all the neighboring chiefs.

A function for spikes

A fairly common artifact is a simple spike of bone or ivory, often sold with sewing implements because they look as though they could be used to make a hole in material that might become a button-hole (127). Some were turned sewing implements, coarse needles with a hole at one end, others started life as fine hooks made in Paris that later broke off, leaving a sharp point. Some were more crudely made and often had two holes through a curved bone, often a rib, with a flattened blunt point polished from use (Figure 9.2 A). Some of these had leather thongs through the holes and were labeled "Primitive Inuit tools" by a well-known auction house

(Figure 9.2 B). The correct explanation for their use came from finding their metal equivalent, rather than from imagination; a nineteenth or early twentieth century curved, pointed steel gouge with leather straps positioning the fingers to allow a firm downward strike (Figure 9.2 C, D).

Until mechanization, maize had to be stripped manually from the dried cob to obtain grains for milling. A hand-held spike was inserted and struck downwards between the grains to lever off one row at a time. Such hard work explains the need for the holes and thongs to keep the fingers in position. A firm grip on the spike was needed as it became slippery with sweat.

Considering the importance of getting maize off the cob for use and storage—farmers in the U.S. and southern Canada depended on it for their survival —it is surprising how quickly such key information has disappeared from public recollection.

The key to the interest value of small inexpensive objects lies in their iconography, the details of their historical and social context. In great paintings, this may be an understanding of the symbolism of the background. The great pearl lying over the most precious part of Queen Elizabeth I is not just an adornment but a symbol of her purity, her virginity. Great paintings are filled with such details, as the critics know well. The sum of their enjoyment is embedded in the sum of disentangled complexity, the relationships between the layers of meaning that the objects portray. Iconography may not be known, but plays the same role in the smaller, inexpensive objects described here. We may need to discover everything about

(Opposite page)
Figure 9.2. Artifacts that tell stories. A. Curved bone spike with two holes. B. A curved bone spike with a leather thong threaded through the holes suggesting how it may have been used. C. A metal spike with thongs and curved tip suggesting that tools like this were used for gouging. D. A spike being used to strip kernels from corn, the thongs ensuring a firm grip. E. The powder horn of Augustus F. Smith. F. The writing that he scrimshawed on his horn.

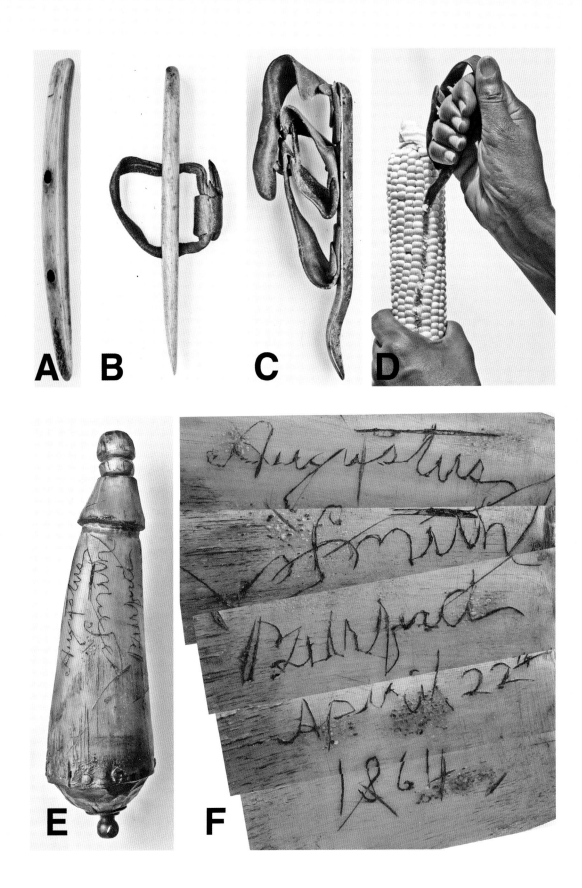

A B C D

E F

our objects before we can enjoy them. There is an urgency to this quest. Art objects have been carefully kept because of their perceived intrinsic value. Small functional objects received no such cherishing and may now be rarer than the art works. Bone and ivory wear well and may survive hard conditions, but keratin is vulnerable to insect attack. Drinking horn artworks survive, but those used by peasants showing how they used them in the local alehouse are a rarity. Millions of kilos of baleen were landed in Europe and USA in the nineteenth century, but the mass of that keratin has long since passed into the oblivion of insect guts, together with the stories that they might have told.

Augustus Smith's powder horn

Powder horns were fairly common objects in flea markets in Ontario from the 1970s to '90s. They had yet to catch the eye of antique dealers and fetched a fairly standard price of $40—$10 if you were lucky. Most were plain, but some had crude scrimshawed identifications, initials, or dates. It is unlikely that any of these scribbles were fraudulent because at that time horns had so little value. One such horn (Figure 9.2 E, F) had lettering over a roughly smoothed surface where crude polishing under the scrimshaw left several areas blistered from the heat. Although crude in the sense that it was all made with a knife and a piece of pumice stone, the maker knew what he was about. The hand carved wooden stopper topped with a solid brass ring was held in place by nails of copper to prevent static. The spout and stopper were elliptical so that a half turn kept it firmly closed. The inscription reads:

Augustus F Smith
Burford
April 22nd
1864

The lettering tells us about the writer. He carved it with a knife, probably the same one he used to cut the horn and wooden stopper. Allowing for the difficulty of using a knife, he wrote in "copper plate" script, suggesting schooling, not literacy limited to making a name in capitals. His statement is complete, he clearly wanted to say to the world, "This is mine, this is who I am," not a note to himself, "I know this is mine because this is my mark." It was not enough to say Augustus, or Augustus Smith, the F. was also important. The slips in cutting the letters suggest a child's hand without the strength of an adult. Unlike the usual brief identifications of men, there is a child-like quality to the writing: it could easily have been on the cover of a school exercise book. So who was Augustus F. Smith?

Burford Township is in Brant County, where the people have saved what they know of their ancestors in the "Brant County Ontario Biographical Sketches" (107). John Smith was born in 1733. He came to Canada from New Jersey in 1784 with Elsie, his wife, who carried one child while two others sat in baskets on each side of the horse. They had five more children in Canada. The first to be born in Canada was called Daniel (I). Daniel had seven children, the sixth being another Daniel (II). Daniel (II) became a teacher and settled in Burford township, where he taught school. He called the second of his three sons, born November 6, 1855, Augustus F. Smith. There were lots of Smiths in Brant County, but surely not many Augustus F's. A school teacher father would explain much about the powder horn inscription, the script, and its completeness. Augustus' age would explain its childlike quality, his pride in doing something that would make him an adult. Augustus would be not quite nine years old when he carved his horn. Such a boy might be thought too young to be off shooting, but we are judging him by standards of a different age. John Thurman in America wrote to Sargent Chambers Company in London, "There is not a man born in America that does not understand the use of fire arms and that well. As we have much sport … it is almost the first thing they purchase and … you can scarcely find a lad of 12 years old that does not go a gunning." Nine-year-olds were probably not far behind, looking forward to owning their first guns. What else would boys have done in that age? Perhaps his father said, "Make your powder horn, then we'll see about the gun." We may imagine Augustus making his horn in time for his birthday.

Bones as construction materials.

And Moses took Joseph's bones with him: because he had adjured the children of Israel, saying: God shall visit you, carry out my bones from hence with you.

Exodus 13:19

This injunction in Exodus gave rise to the Christian tradition of saving bones, the most easily preserved parts of the body. Such bones were sometimes worshipped. In the Chapel of Bones in Naples, skulls and bones or whole skeletons were taken from their graves once a year, dressed up and put in shrines to be worshipped, a practice banned in the 1960s. For the most part, bones were just preserved, with the exhortation ("carry out my bones") creating a serious problem of accumulation. The number of bones accumulated is enormous—the Capuchin crypt in Rome, for example, is said to be made from the bones of 4,000 monks, the Sedlec Ossuary in the Czech Republic contains the remains of 40–50,000 people, while the Catacombs in Paris store the skeletons of six million people. The problem was not confined to famous places. Churches starting off in villages found their adjacent bone-filled graveyards occupying valuable land at the center of expanding towns and cities. The accumulation of bones was made worse by waves of the Black Death. In the fourteenth century, two-thirds of the population of Europe succumbed and were buried in mass graves.

The solution to the problem of accumulation also lay in Exodus—"from hence with you." Bones were transported and used as building material for the construction and decoration of chapels. One of the first was the Church of St. Francis in Evora, Portugal, built between 1460 and 1510. Its Chapel of Bones was created by a few Franciscan monks in the sixteenth century as a practical solution to the problem. Forty-two monastic cemeteries were taking up valuable space in Evora, so they moved all the bones to a single consecrated chapel. Another example was in 1816 when Carmelite monks used the bones of 1245 of their antecedents to build the *Capela de Ossos*, in Faro, Portugal, adding a chapel and decorating their church built in 1719. They created one of the best-known bone chapels, but other chapels and ossuaries are dotted around Catholic Europe in Germany, Poland, Italy, France, Spain, Austria, and Czechoslovakia. Bone chapels were not just the prerogative of large churches. Many small, local villages, such as Alcantarilha in Portugal, solved their space problems by adding small bone chapels without florid decoration to their tiny churches (Figure 9.3). Although the bones were primarily building materials, gloss on the foreheads and ball ends of the femurs suggest that bones are still venerated, if no longer actually worshipped.

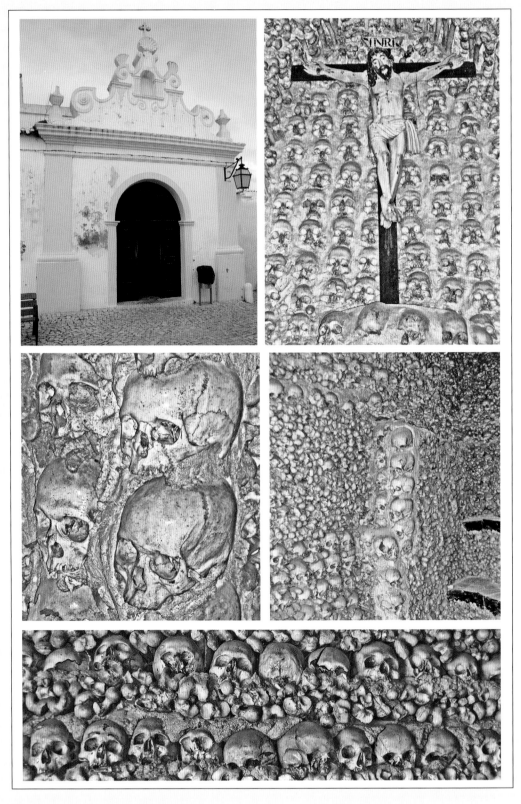

Figure 9.3. Artifacts that tell stories. Bones as construction materials. The entrance to the Bone Chapel in the village of Alcantarilha in Portugal and views of the interior.

A simple watch fob

One, two, t'ree four—Colon man
a come,
Wit' 'im brass chain a lick him belly
Bam, bam, bam.
Ask 'im for the time, an' 'e look 'im
to the sun,
Wit' 'im brass chain a lick him belly
Bam, bam, bam.

(Traditional song about the Jamaican worker who went
to seek his fortune as a laborer in Panama)

In nineteenth century England and America, the chain attached to a fob watch advertised the wealth and sophistication of the wearer. In the ten years before the First World War, Jamaicans who went to Colon to build the Panama Canal returned thinking themselves wealthy, sporting a conspicuous chain attached to a fob watch in their vest pocket. Less fortunate workers tried to keep up with the fashion of the day by wearing only the chain, hence their ridicule in the contemporary folk song. There came a reaction against this bourgeois ostentation as watches became smaller and especially as they became small enough for ladies to wear. Gold chains were replaced by discrete woven strands plaited from the hair of loved ones and they became sentimental reminders, for both male and female (Figure 9.4 A).

Darwin's Cosh

"Cosh, from the Romany Koshter,
stick or skewer: a weighted weapon
similar to a blackjack."

Webster's Dictionary

In a curious coincidence I bought a baleen cosh in Portobello market the Saturday before a Sunday visit to Down House in Kent, where Darwin lived most of his life. In the small museum of his possessions that he took with him from 1831–1836 on his "Voyage of the *Beagle*," there was a cosh identical to the one that I had just bought. It is a slender thing, 31 cms long and 8 mm wide with woven

linen baskets of lead weights at either end. It is made from eight strips cut from a baleen plate, that have been rounded to rods 2–3 mm in diameter before twisting around a baleen core (Figure 9.4 C). This gives a very springy structure: even after nearly 200 years it is easily bent through 45^0. It was the marine equivalent of the wooden coshes used by the "Bobbies" or "Peelers," the precursors of the UK police force created by Sir Robert Peel in 1829 (Figure 9.4 B). The two kinds of cosh administered very different kinds of blow. In hard coshes, the blow resulted in the sudden local release of energy into the bone, leading to skull fractures. In springy baleen coshes, the blow is spread out in space and time, allowing it to reach the brain, leading to knock-outs without fracturing the skull. Baleen coshes have the properties of the sandbags that army officers were shown how to make in the Second World War. These were soft leather bags shaped like small frying pans containing sand and lead shot in their broad end. The idea was that the platoon leader would creep up quietly behind the Nazi sentry and silently bang him on the head, but it's doubtful that this romantic notion ever happened. Baleen coshes were suited for use at sea, since their main use was in press-ganging drunks as sailors or bringing drunken sailors back to the ship. However, real marine coshes (Figure 9.24 B, C) used by real sailors were much more sturdy than Darwin's (Figure 9.4 C). Darwin's cosh was ornamental, a token of authority like an officer's swagger stick. Why would he want to take such a flimsy thing with him? The answer may be that he was conned by outfitters into believing that such coshes would be useful in self defense for the perilous trip he was about to undertake. Darwin never wrote about his cosh. He probably never showed it to Captain FitzRoy after he saw the real ones used by sailors on the *Beagle*.

Shepherd's Purse

A funny thing happened on the way to the present: history lost its model for shepherd's purses. Shepherd's purses were in a category of their own, distinct from other purses of the

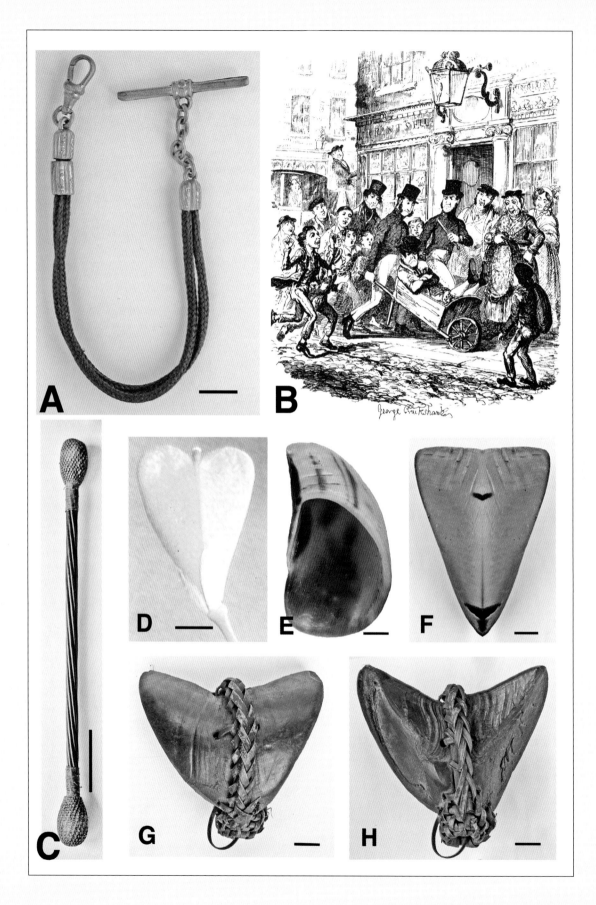

time, such as pence jugs or copper purses, which were simple bags tied with a cord, and from gold and silver purses, long envelopes protected by a flap and closed with numerous strings. All we are left with is the supposed resemblance of the seed pods of a common cruciferous weed, shepherd's purse, *Capsella bursapastoris* (Figure 9.4 D), to pouches made from hooves by shepherds. Country people in the late medieval period saw a similarity in the outline of the tiny seed pods (4 x 5 mm) to shepherd's purses (7 x 10 cms) and coined the name for the plant, formalized in 1764 by Linnaeus with his Latin binomial genus and species appellation (*capsella* = pod-like seed vessel, *bursa* = pouch, *pastoris* = shepherd).

Hooves are unlike the plant capsule in being peculiarly shaped three-dimensional structures (Figure 9.4 E), but if we put a right and left hoof together over the space leading to the bones, we can see how the profile resembles an idealized heart-shape of the seed capsule (F). Hooves were made into containers in many parts of the world. They could be hinged on one straight side and opened on the other rounded edge, or left with a hole at one end plugged with a bung, like the creation of an aboriginal Filipino craftsman who joined two hooves to make a "bottle," possibly for a shaman's store of "medicines" (Figure 9.4 G, H). Purses made from hooves by shepherds are rare and we know little of their construction other than that their outline could fit the description of the plant seed capsule.

What cutlery tells us

Never use your knife to convey your food to your mouth under any circumstances; it is unnecessary and glaringly vulgar. Feed yourself with a fork or spoon, nothing else—a knife is only to be used for cutting. ... Eat peas with a dessert spoon; and curry also (147).

A favorite theme for novelists are the changes taking place as generations strive to become middle class. Their tools are words and their sources largely their imagination. In the absence of words and visual clues, contemporary cutlery provides a kind of fossil record of the changes taking place in one aspect of daily life—how people fed themselves. Implements have followed two separate lines of development. Poorer people depended on implements made from readily available materials such as bone, for example Thomas Hardy's characters like the shepherd in *Far From the Madding Crowd* (see below under Artifacts and literacy). Richer people had metal cutlery, for example the characters in Jane Austin's novels. Their cutlery had two functions, to cut food into bite-sized pieces and to transfer these to the mouth, complicated behaviors that led to etiquette and table manners.

From the sixth to thirteenth centuries, knives, spoons, and occasional two-tined forks, were used, but knives were structurally little removed from daggers that people carried with them. Social dining for the masses of people had yet to come (18), (134). By the sixteenth century, cutlery had become more decorative. Forks acquired three or four tines. One-sided blades made knives easier to carry without a scabbard. Many from Shakespeare's time were recovered from the Thames near the entry point of an old sewer, when people lost them from their

(Opposite page)

Figure 9.4. Artifacts that tell stories. A. Human hair watch fob, late nineteenth century. These replaced the robust gold chains advertising success earlier in the nineteenth century. B. Crookshank illustration of the use of coshes by Peelers taking drunks to jail. C. Baleen cosh similar to the one that Darwin took with him on the voyage of the *Beagle*. D. The seed capsule of Shepherd's Purse that took its name in medieval times from the fancied resemblance to the purses made of two hooves by shepherds. E. A right side cow hoof viewed from the direction of the end of the leg. Hinged with its left counterpart on their straight sides, as in F, creates an openable box or purse with an outline similar to D. G, H. Binding both edges together creates a bottle from two water buffalo hooves, as in this creation by an aboriginal Filipino craftsman. Scales. C = 5 cms, D = 1 mm, all others = 1 cm.

belts as they leapt the sewer ditch. Ingram Frisar probably used a knife like that in Figure 9.6 A to murder Christopher Marlowe in a pub brawl in 1593. Two developments in cutlery tell us about the changing social environment in the seventeenth and eighteenth century. 1. Metal became cheaper, allowing more people to own more cutlery that they used at table rather than carrying it with them. 2. Designs changed with the new custom of eating as a social accomplishment.

1. From the seventeenth century, and especially from the nineteenth century Industrial Revolution, cheaper metal brought down the costs of cutlery, allowing a rich middle class to dine at table like the aristocracy. The revolution made cutlery more available, first with handles of ivory and mother of pearl, later more cheaply made of bone and antler. By the end of the nineteenth century, even lower middle class families could afford stag handled cutlery sets like those in Figure 9.5 E sold by Mappin and Webb in 1895 for as little as £3 (~ $14). By 1930, Joseph Elliot & Sons were selling stag handled sets for £1-10 (~ $7), or with ivory handles (Figure 9.5 D) for £2-17 (~ $13). We may imagine a new middle class head of the family carving the Sunday roast beef with such a set as he instructs his children in table manners.

2. This account of dining with the artist J.M.W. Turner shows how eating customs were changing, *"I have dined with him (J.M.W. Turner) at Sandycombe Lodge ... Everything was of the most modest pretensions: two pronged forks, and knives with large round ends for taking up the food; not that I ever saw him so use them, though it is said to have been Dean Swift's mode of feeding himself."* H.S. Trimmer, about 1810. Quoted in (128).

Designs changed in the seventeenth and eighteenth centuries. As dining at table became a social accomplishment, knives with valuable agate, mother of pearl, or ivory handles lost their dagger points and became scimitar-shaped with broad, rounded ends. In the 1798 Gilray cartoon, John Bull eats the French ships provided by Nelson and the British fleet with a knife having a rounded end and a fork to spear things (Figure 9.5 A). Because forks could only be used to spear food, knives 27 cms long and blades 2.5 cms wide were made to carry as well as cut. As poorer people began to dine at table, the shapes of cheaper bone and antler handled knives also changed to broad, flat blades, losing their scimitar shape and becoming parallel sided by the end of the nineteenth century. Knives were clearly conveyers for sloppy morsels, but their flatness made them inefficient (Figure 9.5 B, C). How could young ladies remain elegant while holding a loaded flat surface dripping gravy into their bosoms? Perhaps etiquette demands never to put a knife in the mouth were directed at them. However, all was not lost. Chunks of bread could be used to mop up the gravy. The book of etiquette recommends *"At family dinners, where the common household bread is used, it should never be cut less than an inch and a half thick. There is nothing more plebian than* **thin** *bread at dinner"* (147).

There seems to have been a block to designing a spoon as well as a fork to be used with the knife. Although the width of knives declined to below 2 cms by late in the nineteenth or early in the twentieth century, leaving them only useful for cutting, spoons never caught on for formal main course place settings. Perhaps it is a result of male dominance at the dining table. Knives and forks are for the masculine activities of cutting and stabbing. Spoons are reminiscent of the sick being fed slops or women eating custard, activities evoking sympathy and compassion. As a consequence, much good gravy and curry languished and continues to languish on the plate due to etiquette demanding knife and fork rather than knife and spoon.

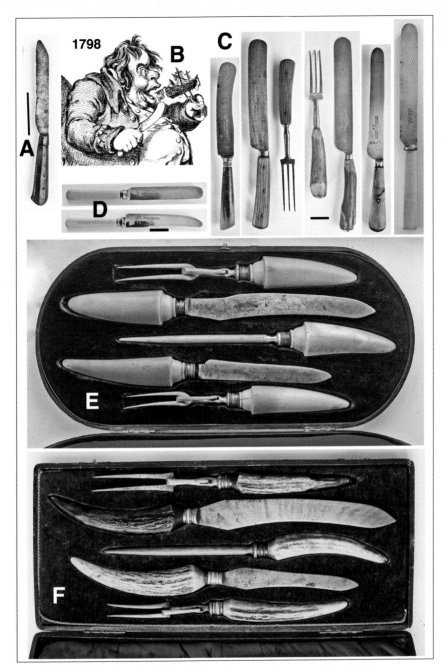

Figure 9.5. Artifacts that tell stories. A collection of cutlery. A. A knife from Shakespeare's time, about 1559, one of many dredged from the Thames presumed to have fallen from the belts of their owners as they jumped a nearby sewage ditch. The blade shape is only just removed from dagger-like. Antler handle. Cutler's mark AP. B. John Bull in an 1878 Gilray cartoon eating with a knife having a rounded end. C. The first table knives with rounded ends were distinguished by their size, as much as 27 cms long and 2.5 cms wide. From the left, handles made from: polished turned horn, bone knife and fork, antler knife and fork, turned horn, ivory. Scale = 2 cms. D. Even the first twentieth century plastic handled knives were 2 cms wide. Ivory, French ivory (plastic). Scale = 1 cm. E, F. From the mid-nineteenth to the early twentieth century, cutlery sets became popular and affordable among the middle class. E. Ivory handled set hallmarked Sheffield, 1890. Sets like this sold for as little as £2-17 (~ $13) in 1930. F. Five piece antler handled set, two carving knives, two forks, and a steel. Mappin and Webb sold sets like this for £3 (~ $14) in 1895, falling to £1-10 (~ $7) in 1930 for sets by Joseph Elliot & Sons.

Artifacts and literacy

In 1816, eighty-two miners from the north of England wrote to Sir Humphrey Davey to thank him for inventing the safety lamp that prevented explosions from "fire damp" (methane), saving so many of their lives. Only thirty-five signed their names, the rest put X's (129). Even those thirty-five may not have been able to do much more than sign. Illiteracy in the United States was just as widespread. By 1870, eighty percent of blacks and twenty percent of whites were still illiterate. We take literacy so much for granted that we have to think ourselves into a different mindset to try to understand how artifacts from 200 years ago might have been used. Ownership of artifacts was through marks, not the letters, names, or numbers that we would use now.

X's and XI patterns were the most commonly used identification marks, but images of trade skills were also used. They are most commonly found on personal things like the "bone feeding utensils" commonly known as "apple corers," babies' teething sticks, and craftsmen's identification tabs.

"Apple corers" is a general description for several types of portable feeding tools derived from hollow bones cut diagonally on the sharpened piercing end. They have been found with early human remains and are the oldest non-stone tools known. The most commonly used bones are sheep carpals and tarsals, sometimes goats or deer and sometimes other leg bones. Some were reproduced in silver, giving the idea that they were used to eat fruit by rich travelers—unlikely as anyone on a stage coach would eat the apple with one hand and toss the core out of the window. Two features lead to their real functions. 1. Made from bone, they cost nothing. Before metals were cheap enough to use, bone implements were available even to the poorest of the poor. They cost nothing, being made merely by breaking a bone in two and sharpening the end. These were not apple corers but general purpose feeding tools. 2. A hundred and more years ago,

dental hygiene was so bad that many people lost their teeth. People without teeth couldn't even bite an apple. They needed the kind of help that a tubular tool could give. Stick it into an apple or any other firm edible and suck it off the end. The rich could identify their tools by their silver ornament (Figure 9.6 A) or by scrimshawed patterns (B) as we can see in collections of elegant "apple corers" like those in the Cuming Museum, Southwark, London. The poor were illiterate and cut X's or other simple decorations on theirs (C, D).

Teething sticks are commonly found ivory artifacts with a triangular cross section, about 10 cms long and 1.5 cms wide on the long side, tapering slightly with a hole through the narrower end (Figure 9.6 E). They often hang by a ribbon or may be attached to a silver rattle. These are teething "bones." The angular edges are rounded and the flat sides indented with grooves to provide an infant with a safe but irregular surface to bite on during teething. The fanciful suggestion that the triangular cross section may symbolize the trinity and a plea for divine protection is more likely to be a consequence of the way that they were made from the cylinder of ivory at the base of a tusk (Figure 9.6 I). The X is probably just a way to get a non-flat surface to bite on, rather than an illiterate identification.

(Opposite page)
Figure 9.6. Artifacts that tell stories. Identification marks on simple eating tools. A–D. Portable tools made from sheep metatarsal or metacarpal bones (in humans, the bones between the wrist and the fingers). A. The rich man's tool with a silver ferrule, portable and used when travelling. B. A well-to-do mans tool personalized with a scrimshaw pattern. C, D. From the same household, probably illiterate, only one needing to be marked by an X. E. Teething "bone," triangular cross section. The X is probably just a way to get a non-flat surface to bite on. F–H. Craftsmen's identity tags, some perhaps indicating the particular job in hand—cutting, sawing, polishing—others perhaps used for personal recognition in an illiterate work force. F and G have no bite marks and were not used as teething bones. H have bite marks on all types of tag. Although they began life as craftsman's identity tags, they subsequently became teething "bones." I. The cylindrical base of elephant tusks were cut longitudinally to make blanks for teething "bones" and tags, explaining their triangular cross-section. Scale bar = 5 cms.

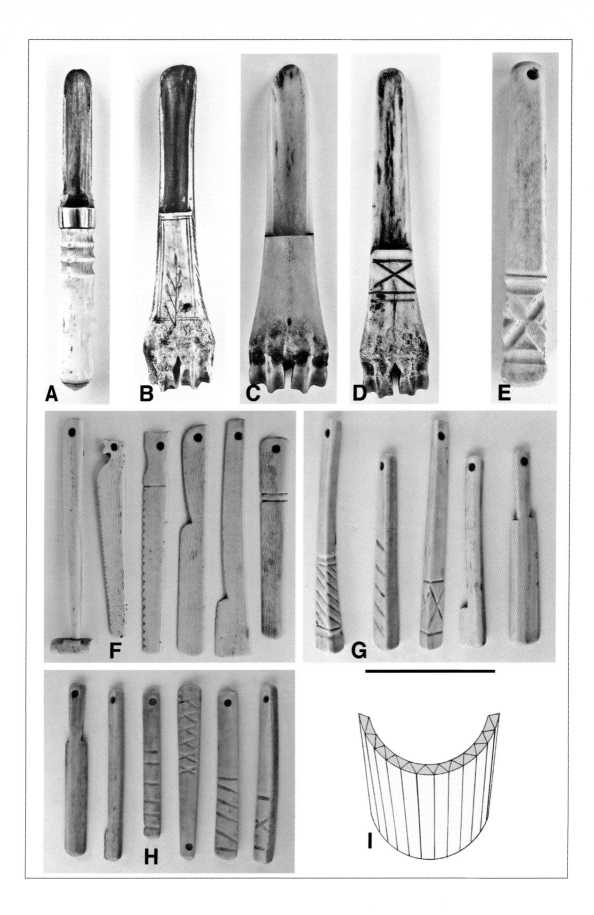

Some sticks probably started as craftsmen's identity tags. They are smaller and slimmer than teething sticks, but that may be the eventual fate of some of them, since they have tooth marks (Figure 9.6 F–H). Some are patterned like teething sticks, but most are shaped like workman's tools—saws, short, medium, and long choppers, hammers, and bat-shaped beating tools. The shapes suggest the kind of work done in an ivory or bone carver's workshop—cutting, sawing, and polishing. The bat-shaped tool is a particular mystery, resembling that used in leather making, linen batting, or snuff grinding. We know nothing of how they were used. It seems unlikely that ivory miniatures of such tool collections would be teething sticks or babies' toys. The marks suggest illiteracy. Did they hang their tag up on a board for the day to indicate they had "clocked in," where they were working, and the kind of work they were doing, the particular job in hand?

It may seem odd that all these sticks are triangular in cross-section, with none having square or circular cross-sections. The way that they were made explains their triangular, tapering form. The base of a tusk forms around a conical bone core, forming an ivory cylinder. Sections of this cylinder can be cut transversely for bracelets, but other wider sections, about 10 cms long, are most economically cut longitudinally to make 10 cm long triangular sticks (Figure 9.6 I).

9.4. Test Results

Stories Told by Figures 9.7 A—O

A is obviously a corkscrew. It is simply and delicately made with an ivory handle and silver ferrule. The metal is steel, as most are, not stainless steel, but there is little evidence to give its age. Its most striking features are its small size and the lack of right angle grip in the handle. It was not made to penetrate large corks and open large bottles. It looks feminine and was used to open very small vials of perfume before the advent of bottle caps, invented in 1892 or screw caps that were used for pharmaceuticals from the 1920s. We may imagine a lady somewhere in the nineteenth century dressing for dinner before adding the final touch from a corked perfume bottle.

B is a double lens protected by a well-worn horn folding case. The design continues to the present day, with Bakelite taking the place of horn. It is very similar to the lens that J.M.W. Turner (1775–1851) used to inspect his brush strokes. Lenses like these from the nineteenth century are frequent artifacts because of the expansion of weaving, both as a cottage and large scale industry. This one was probably used by a nineteenth century weaver to inspect the fineness of the work. We may imagine a cottage weaver standing over the loom anxiously inspecting his/her work to make sure that it had the required number of threads per inch.

C shows a pair of ivory handled steel surgical instruments. One ends in a half sphere with sharp edges, the other in three curved hooks with very sharp ends. The hooks could have been used to hold a wound open while the other instrument scraped away foreign or infected matter, but the matched shapes suggest a more specialized use as a ball extractor. The hooks could keep a pistol ball in place in the half sphere while pulling it from a wound. Was it used in battle or in duels? In either case, it projects a grim picture of probing for a deeply embedded projectile without anesthetics.

D and **E** are a comb and brush. They match one another in richness: tortoiseshell, ivory, and silver are never for the poor. Their striking feature is that they are so small and that they have handles. Could they be children's toys? Unlikely, they are not just small copies of a full size brush and comb. The handles enabled them to get near enough to stroke something equally small. They are a brush and comb for a small and neat mustache, placing them in the Edwardian period. The Victorians had facial hair that would have defeated such tools and smart young men in the First World War soon

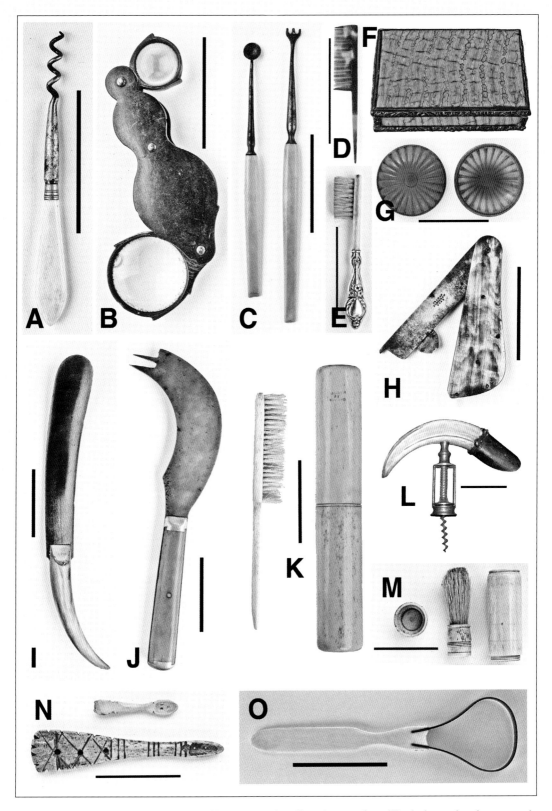

Figure 9.7. Artifacts that tell stories. A–O. Test. Imagine handling these artifacts. Think about what they are made of, what they are for, and the stories that they might tell. Descriptions in the text. Scale bars = 5 cms.

had more serious things to think about than the beauty of their mustaches.

F is a box beautifully made from slabs of tooth from an Indian elephant (See Figures 6.25, 29). It is typical of the fine eighteenth and nineteenth century Indian craftsmanship that soldiers brought back in the days of the Raj. On the obverse side of the box is a plaque saying, "The gift of I. Shields, 78th Highlanders to W.J.C." around a phoenix. We don't know who W.J.C. was, but the 78th Highlanders were one of the most distinguished regiments in the British Army. The regiment as a whole was awarded the VC in addition to the eight VC's awarded to individual officers and men. The 78th Highland Regiment of Foot were raised in 1793 by Colonel MacKenzie, Lord Seaforth, at Fort George near Inverness in Scotland and were active in many countries for eighty-eight years before disappearing as a distinct regiment. Most notably, they were active in suppressing the Indian Mutiny in 1857. "The 78th were ordered to charge and take the gun. I never saw anything so fine. The men went on, with sloped arms, like a wall; till within a hundred yards not a shot was fired. At the word 'Charge', they broke just like an eager pack of hounds, and the village was taken in an instant ..." Major General Havelock, July 17th 1857.

G is a finely made tortoiseshell box, showing how hot damp thin layers can be pressed into delicate three-dimensional shapes. Provenance suggests that it is late eighteenth century. It has a feminine look, as though it would have graced a lady's dressing table, but what was it used for? We have to think what a lady from that period might need. It was a time when the survivors of small pox were left with deep pockmarks on their faces (and elsewhere). A fashion developed with fashionable women (and men) in the court of Louis XV to cover up the marks with black patches of gummed taffeta. Even those without pock-marks fell in with the fashion and used stick-on dark spots to emphasize the beauty or whiteness of their complexions. (Is there a parallel with contemporary shaven

heads and baldness from cancer treatments?) Some of the patches were elaborate—stars, crescents, insects, and other animals—with their position forming a secret language of love and passion. The elegant lady needed a small box such as the one illustrated in which to keep her patches. **G** is a patch box.

H is a horn sheathed folding knife with a characteristically shaped blade having a short, almost half circular but pointed sharp side, opposite a flat blunt outside edge. This tool was probably used by veterinarians in the early nineteenth century. Similarly shaped tools for human use were often incorporated as part of a scalpel. Blades with this shape are phleams, tools for letting blood. In use they were placed longitudinally over a vein and given a sharp tap with a phleam mallet, resulting in a shallow cut in the vein, allowing the blood flow. The clean cut made it easy to sew up the wound with a horsehair stitch.

I is composed of a flat sheaf of horn attached by a metal tag to a handle of antler. It looks like a shoehorn, but the horn is flat and the attachment to the handle far too weak to take the strain needed to squeeze feet into shoes or cut open letters. This is an unusual artifact, probably early to mid-twentieth century. It is a spatula, probably for icing cakes and possible shaping ice cream cakes. It makes use of the physical properties of horn—poor heat conduction, low specific heat, good water repulsion, and acid resistance—all of which makes it superior to an iron blade for coating a flat surface with a warm butter, sugar, lemon juice mixture. Who thought of this invention? When did some proud housewife find that a horn blade was better than a metal one?

J is a fork-knife. After the Napoleonic wars, and even more after the American Civil War, many soldiers returned missing arms and legs. Nelson was missing an eye as well as an arm. The eye he could do little about except to use it to ignore instructions he didn't agree with. He compensated for his missing arm by using a fork-knife, an instrument that enabled him to use one hand to both cut and spear his food. Many one-armed American veterans of the Civil War used similar instruments like **J** (which is missing one prong), that enabled them to cut meat with one side of the knife and then spear it with the other.

K and **M** were used for traveling. Well preserved early toothbrushes and shaving brushes used at home are rare finds. They were usually worn out and discarded; we find only the bone handles in rubbish dumps. Travelling sets have survived much better; they were protected in cases, used while away, and stored carefully until needed again. Although military officers such as Wellington are well known for their bad teeth or lack thereof due to the privations of campaigning, later smarter officers carried sets like **K** with them and probably came home with their teeth. The first mass-produced tooth brushes were large, like this, and probably served to scrub the tongue as well as the teeth (see **O** below). Shaving brush sets are mostly Edwardian, when carefully cut mustaches and short beards requiring shaving replaced the Victorian fashion for beards. We can imagine traveling salesmen needing sets like **M**, as well as young army officers.

L is made from a boar's tooth. It is difficult to know what to do with boar upper canines other than to use them for handles. They are curved and not large enough to carve significant figures (Figures 6.15, 19), but they are good, strong ivory. **L** makes good use of the size, shape, and properties. The curve allows a good grip for the hand and the strength is equal to the task of twisting the cork out.

N is a snuff spoon. The habit of taking snuff spread around the world from the Americas almost as soon as they were discovered. It is a tribute to the addictive nature of nicotine that it spread so rapidly in spite of the difficulty of "snuffing," that is, transferring it up the nose from a pinch between the thumb and forefinger. Snuff is finely ground tobacco, traditionally made by grinding tobacco leaves between the roughened surfaces of ivory boards. Snuff can be a fine, light powder

when dry, easily blown by the wind, but it is hygroscopic and easily clumps. The objective is to get it evenly distributed on the thin mucus membranes in the nostrils. Snuff spoons have a bowl with holes so that a spoonful can be shaken to create a thin layer on the back of the hand, giving an evenly distributed cloud of particles when snuffed up the nose. Salt and pepper spoons sometimes had holes in them, but tiny perforated bowls like these would not have been useful distributors over a dinner plate.

O is a tongue scraper made from a loop of tortoiseshell on an ivory handle, probably dating from the late eighteenth century. It is difficult to imagine preferring a tongue scraper to a brush to clean the mouth. Although "tooth brushes" in some form have been used worldwide for centuries (chew-sticks even as early as 3,000 BC), they were not mass produced until the 1800s and not in general use until the second half of the twentieth century. An up and coming dandy in that early era may have been unaware of tooth brushes, preferring a tongue scraper to the early practice of rubbing the teeth with a chew-stick loaded with soot and salt. Improbable as it may seem, tongue scrapers are still produced but made of plastic. They are still part of some peoples' lives, as are many equally improbable recent fashions—high heels, nose rings, bustles, inflatable bosoms, pierced body parts, and shaved heads and faces.

9.5. Determining the Age and Origin of Artifacts

Everyday artifacts had little value, being used and passed from hand to hand without thought to where they came from or how they were made. They rarely have provenance. I have not tried to date the primitive bone tools of native peoples, which is particularly difficult. Most are nineteenth to early twentieth century, but may not have changed in style for millennia. However, some indicators can give precise and accurate age determinations.

Dating can be explicit and believable, carved or scrimshawed into the bone or ivory as in the teething ring marked Eric 1922. There is no reason to doubt the authenticity of this mark; it is not very old and does not materially alter its value. Dated whale ivory scrimshaw or powder horns are more suspect without corroborating provenance or research such as Augustus Smith's 1864 horn (Figure 9.2 E, F). Microscopic examination is a good start. Are there surface cracks that are empty of dust since they have formed since the artifact was made?

Silver hallmarks: Walking sticks, snuff boxes, and cutlery often have a silver or gold plate with initials identifying the owner and hallmarks stamped with the year letter and name of the assay office. A booklet with hallmark keys is an inexpensive but essential tool for dating. Catalogues, particularly for cutlery, can be helpful but are hard to find. Candle snuffers are usually quite old, since candles are pre-electric light (late nineteenth century), gas light (mid-nineteenth century), or even before oil lamps (eighteenth or early nineteenth century). The hallmarks on the candle snuffer in Figure 14 L give a surprising result—London, 1988, part of a silver revival. The egg spoons in Figure 9.20 O and Q give another surprise. The obvious Scotch spoon with a silver thistle was hallmarked Birmingham and the plain silver ended example was hallmarked Glasgow.

Horns and mounted trophies are sometimes stuffed with newspapers showing the country, town, and date where the work was performed. I have found horns claiming to be nineteenth century American antiques stuffed with late twentieth century Mexican newspapers.

From the mid-nineteenth century onwards, Stanhopes were sometimes inserted into simple toys and tools—needle cases, tape measures, letter openers, sold cheaply as attractions at world fairs or tourist destinations.

Stanhopes are small lenses made from glass beads that focus on a miniature photographic image on their flat side. Placing the eye close to the lens brings the image into focus, often with a date or datable event, fairground, city, tourist attraction, or celebrity. The principle behind Stanhopes goes back to Anthony van Leeuwenhoek (1632–1723) who made tiny biconvex lenses with a resolution of 1 m. Putting his eye very close to the lens allowed him to see living protozoa, sperm, and bacteria for the first time (42). Simpler, cheaper lenses were invented by Charles Stanhope (1753–1816). In 1851, J.B. Dancer used compound microscopes to produce and view microphotographs, a technique simplified in 1857 by Rene Dagron (1819–1900), who viewed microscopic pictures with Stanhope lenses. Stanhopes are used to date the artifacts in Figures 9.8 K, 9.12 D, J, and 9.14 C.

Surface wear and discoloration is often a good indication of aging. Ivory ages from white to creamy yellow. Bone may become dark brown. The feather pattern on elephant ivory, a consequence of the waved architecture, is a good indicator of natural aging. It does not appear just because the specimen is old. Mammoth ivory cut in tangential profile does not immediately show the pattern, but may show it more quickly because of lost protein. This suggests that the appearance of the feather pattern might be accelerated in elephant tusks by boiling and drying, but it is not just cracking due to drying out. Drying out can and does cause gross, deep cracks through the whole artifact. The pattern probably involves loss of protein in the surface layer through washing or sweat, as it is most obvious in well handled smooth surfaces, oiled by finger grease, and polished by use. Rough surfaces or ones that have not been perfectly polished set up other crack patterns oriented by the scratches on the surface.

The styles and kinds of datable artifacts made from the same or even different materials may give clues to similar objects that lack indicators of date.

9.6. Identifying Components Preliminary Observations

Antiquaries might find it helpful to look for an old ivory billiard ball. These are cut from whole sections of elephant tusk. Find the spot on the ball going from side to side through the center that marks the longitudinal axis of the tusk (Figure 6.45). The surface on the ball shows the ivory pattern in all transverse to tangential profiles. Sawing the ball longitudinally (it will need to be polished) displays the radial profile. This creates a beautiful and useful worry stone to compare with its bone equivalent (Figure 4.2).

Make preliminary observations of general features—shape, size, density, hardness, thermal conductivity, color, smell, and obvious surface patterns that may be a giveaway. Use a X10 hand lens to look at clean polished surfaces. Surface patterns are often most easily seen by observing reflected light mirrored from the surface. This records minute differences in depth of polishing due to variations in hardness. Does the shape or the shape of the pattern suggest the shape of the material from which the object was made? Most importantly, try to reconstruct the three-dimensional shape of surface patterns by looking to see how they vary in different planes of viewing. Look for cracks. The shape of cracks can tell much about the material. Is there lettering, a logo, or the mark of the edges of the form into which it was poured or pressed during manufacture? Are there burn marks where the object has softened, or are there pinpricks of a hot needle used by a previous investigator? Such features immediately tell you that it is plastic. Has something been eating it, leaving the surface pits characteristic of larder beetles (Fig. 7.1)? If so, it must be made of the keratin that forms hair, horn, tortoiseshell, or whale baleen. Color itself is not a very good character, as objects darken with age and surface dirt, but color often distinguishes plastics. Bright colors stand out as plastic, but most early plastic was in colors to imitate bone, ivory (off white to brown), tortoiseshell (dark and light brown), or horn (brown to black). Vegetable ivory can also be dyed any color, but the colors tend to dull as the nut turns brown with age. Swirled color patterns that you would expect from mixing liquids often distinguish plastic and glass, which is a cooled plastic.

The tooth test. Touch the object gently to the upper front teeth. Practice this with known objects and you will easily learn to distinguish the different "tooth feel" of many of them. The front teeth are usually the best, but don't use less sensitive teeth with dead nerves. A sharp crack suggests something inorganic like glass, ceramic, agate, or other stones. A gentle, dull interaction suggests softer, lighter organic materials like wood, bog oak, vegetable ivory, whale baleen, amber, horn, tortoiseshell, plastic, ivory, bone, or jet, in roughly that order of sharpness.

Feel. Whether a material feels warm or cool depends upon its thermal conductivity. If an object at room temperature (20–22°C) conducts heat away from your hand (37°C) easily, it feels cooler; if it is an insulator, conducting poorly, it feels warm. Stone, especially marble, feels cool, as do glass and most ceramics. Organic materials are insulators and feel warm.

Density. Bone has a density of 1.79–2.04, and ivory 1.7–2.05, much greater than most plastics at 1.1–1.60 (Tables 2.1 and 2.2). With a little practice it is possible to separate most plastics from bone and ivory instantly by the weight expected from their size. Recent frauds have increased the density of plastics to make them look and feel like ivory by adding lead salts (white lead—lead carbonate, used as a makeup by Elizabeth 1st to give her that white complexion).

Separating amber from plastic. Hot amber can be deformed but cold amber is brittle and fractures; hit by a hammer, it fragments into sharply edged particles. Fortunately you don't have to be quite so destructive. Look for worn edges and drilled holes where the same sharp edges are produced. Drilled plastic tends to deform; drilled amber tends to fracture, but it varies with the kind of plastic and the heat generated.

Aging. Light colored plastic tends to darken less than most natural materials, typically to the color of cheese. Damage from use causes surface deformation rather than bruising and cracking. Large cracks may form with any orientation. Some plastic tools stored in workboxes with needles may get pricks that fill with dirt, looking superficially like bone.

Mold marks. Look for joins between two halves of the mold showing up as thin, raised edges. Some plastics may be stamped with numbers or logos. Plastics can make very deceptive jet imitations because they are made from moulds of real polished stone or jet originals. They carry even the fine detail of straight line abrasive marks left after polishing.

Scratching. Some plastics are readily deformed with a hot needle, but hot needles and flames can be very destructive. Early celluloid plastics burn in a flash, as their chief component is nitrocellulose or gun cotton. Such destructive tests are rarely necessary. Even at room temperature, scratches can be informative. Scratching plastic with anything other than a very sharp needle or razor blade tends to deform the surface rather than cut into it.

Smell. A more useful reason for using the hot needle is the characteristic smell that it may produce. Scraping off a fragment for burning is a better way to get the smell. Before trying it, use some known plastic objects for practice and compare their smell with that from burning feathers or horn.

Identifying bone and ivory. Although distinguishing bone, ivory, and plastic is usually one of the easiest determinations to make, it is sometimes more difficult if the object is small, clean, and intricately but roughly carved. If it is made from a bleached long bone, the blood vessels may be hard to find on a roughened surface, even under the microscope. Cream-colored Bakelite may mimic featureless ivories like hippo incisors. Horn can also be cream-colored. The following quick, non-destructive technique will eliminate the slight uncertainty that may remain after even careful microscopic examination.

Pick a clean, smooth surface on the back or underside of the object. Touch it with the tip of a black marker pen to create a pinhead-sized drop on the surface. Use a new pen that will leave a neat drop, not an old, dry one that has to be rubbed to leave a mark. If the surface has been waxed, it may be necessary to open the clogged blood vessels and dentinal tubules by scraping with a razor blade. Wipe the drop off immediately with alcohol and observe with a hand lens or microscope. The blood vessels in bone stand out as ragged black lines, making it instantly identifiable (Figure 4.2). Ivory shows dentinal tubules as much smaller black filaments with patterns depending on orientation (Figure 6.4). Plastic has no stained substructure. Horn usually has typical brown to white concentric layers (Figure 7.6.3). Bone differs from antler in the sharp separation of laminar and osteonic layers (Figure 5.14).

9.7. Identifying the Function of Artifacts

Nothing gives more delight than success in ascribing a function to an enigmatic find. If it is a container, look for traces of something that it might have contained—salt, pepper, snuff, ink stains, or makeup. The ivory box in Figure 9.18 **H** is not a typical snuff box. Its original function may have been different, but it contained snuff and could have been used as a ladies table snuff box.

If the artifact is a fluid container, measure its volume and look in conversion tables for an equivalent unit in whole figures. Figure 9.9 **K** of a delicate ladle is a good example. It doesn't hold enough for a dash of toddy, only 8.9–9 ccs of water. This is equivalent to 2.5 fluid drams = 7.5 scruples = 150 minims, the kinds of unit used by apothecaries, the precursors to medical doctors. The probability that this is not a random association takes into account that apothecaries must have used containers like this to measure these kinds of volume. One can imagine the female apothecary in the time of Edward VI prescribing 5 grains of arsenic in 5 drams of water for his tuberculosis.

A similar approach can be informative if the artifact could have been used to measure finely divided solids. See if its volume corresponds with a known system of weights or volumes of commonly traded goods, salt, sugar, gunpowder, etc., and look for an exact correspondence (Figure 9.1 A).

Look for wear (Figure 9.2 A, B) and discoloration (Figure 9.6 B, 9.14 B) as clues to the way it may have been used.

It is impossible to illustrate, or even mention, the variety of uses for bone and ivory from the pre-synthetic plastic era. Almost every tool or article that we now use was made then, plus some with functions no longer needed or recognizable. The most interesting are those with functions that we do not immediately recognize, for they may tell us about unknown ways of life.

There were exceptionally skilled ivory workers, but in general English workshops were practical factories making a wide variety of saleable goods such as knife handles, rather than places where craftsmen were "national treasure" creating works of art as in old Japan or China. Craftsmen in nineteenth century workshops sometimes used bone and ivory indiscriminately for small items, marketing them together like the bone and ivory cigarillo holders or the page cutters/paper folders in Figures 9.8 **A, B, C.**

Envelopes are a relatively recent invention. Early letter writers obtained privacy by double folding their sheets and sealing them down with wax. Early books were sold with pages hiding their text in the folds. Adjacent pages had to be slit open before they could be read.

To deal with these foldings and cuttings, there is a class of simple tools forming a discontinuous but functionally overlapping series, from book marks to letter openers to page cutters to paper folders to the "bones" that printers used to fold sheets into flyers or multi-page sheets into stacks for book binding (Figure 9.8 **A, B, E**). Bookmarks were plain and used both for marking the page and slitting it open. Letter openers might be pointed for letter opening and flat-sided for paper folding and cutting. These common practical instruments were made of both bone and ivory.

The cylindrical shapes of bone limited what could be made. Bone objects cannot be large, at most 1.5 cms wide if they have been turned and 0.5 cms thick if made from cut sheets. Bone is most often in cylinders from which sheets (Figure 9.8 **A**) and rings (Figure 9.8 **G-I**, 9.9 **A, B, D**) were cut. Ivory is three-dimensional and does not have this limitation, except at the tusk base. The difference is illustrated by the way bone and ivory are used to make brushes. Bone slabs were not big enough to make brushes for adults, which were made from ivory. Brushes for babies and small children were usually made of bone (Figure 9.8 **D**). Even with this limitation, bones have been worked into a vast array of useful and decorative implements, illustrated below.

Whales bones are exceptional in yielding large pieces of spongy bone (Figure 9.11 **F, H**) and massive lower jaws of osteonic bone suitable for carving decorative objects (Figure 9.10 **H**). Whales are supported by the buoyancy of water and can afford to have larger, heavier bones than land animals. It is probably significant that their lower jaws are dense osteonic bone, allowing their mouths to fall open to catch krill with least muscular effort.

Naturally shaped bones and tusks as simple tools. Humans never miss a chance to make use of bones preadapted for their activities by their natural shapes and properties. Such bones may become primitive tools with little change, as in these examples.

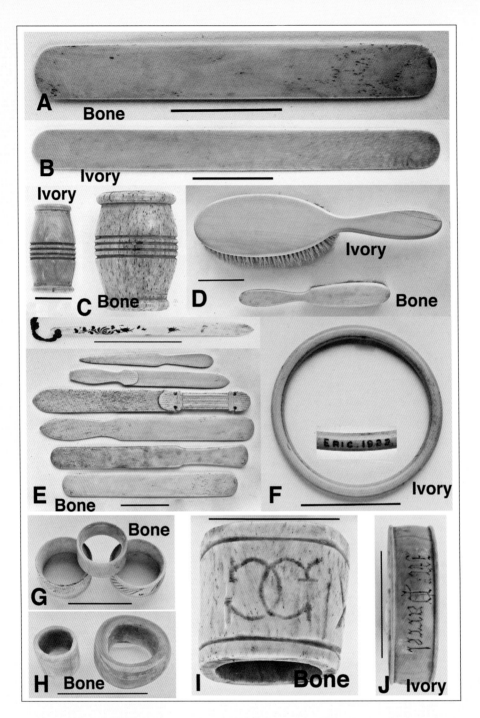

Figure 9.8. Bone and ivory were used indiscriminately for many small items. A, B. Page cutters/paper folders, larger versions were used as printer's "bones." C. Bone and ivory cigarillo holders. D. Bone and ivory hair brushes. Small brushes for children or babies were usually of bone because bones were not large enough to make full-sized brushes. E. There is a category of bone or ivory tools that form a discontinuous but functionally overlapping series from book marks (1, top) to letter openers (2, 3, 4) to page cutter/letter openers (5, 6) to letter openers/paper folders (5, 6, 7) to the "bones" that printers used to fold sheets into flyers or multi-page sheets into stacks for book binding. F–J. The cylindrical shapes of long bones and the bases of ivory tusks predisposed them to be carved into bracelets, woggles, scarf rings, napkin rings, etc. F is not a bracelet, but a teething ring inscribed "Eric, 1922." G. Napkin rings, carved and often numbered. H. "Woggles" used by Boy scouts to secure their neckerchiefs instead of tying them into knots. I. The scarf ring was owned by George Racovita, the naturalist who accompanied Amundsen on the Belgica for his exploratory expedition to the Antarctic in 1897. J. The ring used by Mr. Parrel to identify his bottle. Scale bar C = 1 cm. All others = 5 cms.

Arapaima tongues and scales. The Arapaima (*Arapaima gigas*) from the Amazon basin is the largest fresh water fish in the world, reaching 200 Kg and 4.5 meters in length. It is predatory, feeding on other fish and any small animals. The jaw contains a tongue-like bone modified as a rasp (Figure 9.9 I) used to file Guarana nuts into a fine powder to make a mildly caffeinated drink that has become the popular Brazilian equivalent of Coca Cola. Arapaima also provide nail files. Fine spicules on the surface of their scales make them perfect rasps, superior to most humanly made nail files (Figure 9.9 **H**).

Scrapers. The scapula from a seal has just the right shape to be grasped and used to scrape fat and tissue from the inside of a skin. (Figure 9.9 **A**. Inuit.). Deer ribs (**B**) and long bones (**C**) need little modification to become skin and leather working tools. Most are primarily scrapers used to remove tissue. **B1** has a serrated edge for scraping without making deep cuts; **B2** has a transverse groove to hold and tighten sinews in stitches. Modern western professions may still prefer natural bone for some purposes. (**D**) Morticians have to cut tendons and muscle to help them rearrange limbs that *rigor mortis* has set in inconvenient positions. To reduce the risk of damaging their knife blade and cutting themselves, they make their cuts against a simple tool of cow rib. Nineteenth century Ontario.

Woggles, napkin rings, and bottle labels. Sections of long bones are ready-made rings for material to be threaded through them like the diklos (Romani for scarf) of Gypsies. There was no English word to describe them until 1929 when Lord Baden Powell used "woggles" to describe the scarf fasteners created for Boy Scouts by Bill Shankley in 1923 (Figure 9.8 **H**).

Woggles were small things made for the narrow ends of scarves. There is still no word for scarf fasteners like the cow bone in Figure 9.8 I owned by George Racovita, the young Romanian naturalist who accompanied Amundsen on the Belgica for his exploratory trip to Antarctica in 1897 in preparation for his successful trek to the South Pole in 1911. The Belgica became trapped in ice for thirteen months and everyone suffered from cold and scurvy. Is it too fanciful to think that he may have carved and polished this scarf ring while trapped in the ice? The bone is in good condition, suggesting that it was not overcooked.

Victorian ladies dressed their dining tables with linens threaded through elegantly carved and turned napkin rings, a tradition that lives on in families not uglified by fast food. (Figure 9.8 **G**). Many napkin rings carry numbers from their time in seaside hotels, where they had users for the week rather than daily fresh linen.

The cylindrical shapes of the base of ivory tusks predisposed them to be carved like bones into bracelets, woggles, scarf rings, napkin rings, etc. Figure 9.8 **J** is the ivory ring used by Mr. Parrel to identify his bottle of wine or spirits. It evokes a life of sad impoverished gentility in the early twentieth century, the story of a man at the end of his days in a seaside boarding hotel, marking the daily decline in the level of his tipple as he dines alone. Figure 9.8 **F** has a more joyful note, a birth to be celebrated with an outsize teething ring, perhaps part of a silver rattle. Diligent research might reveal both their identities.

Ceremonial and decorative objects. Bacula (singular baculum), or penis bones, are long cylinders, often with a slight curve, made mainly of osteonic bone. They are present in rodents, insectivores, bats, and carnivores, but absent in rabbits, horses, elephants, marsupials, platypus, hyenas, and whales. Humans are the exception among mammals in not having a baculum, the equivalent female clitoral bone, although small ones, are present in other primates. Bacula of all kinds can be viewed in the Phallological Museum in Húsavík, Iceland. The largest baculum, 1.2 meters long, comes from an extinct walrus, the smallest, 2 mm long, from a hamster. Contemporary walrus (*Odobenus rosmarus*) have bacula up to 75 cms long. Inuit may decorate them elaborately as ooziks or ceremonial maces. The semi-fossil baculum in Figure 9.8 **E** has been polished but is undecorated.

This silver seal (Figure 9.9 **J**) made from the digit of a Jacana evokes the natural elegance of this bird that seems to stride effortlessly and elegantly over the water. Jacanas are any of eight species from the Family Jacanidae, colloquially called Jesus birds or lily trotters. Their feet with elongated toes and claws, allow them to run over the floating vegetation of shallow lakes, creating the illusion that they can walk on water.

Musical instruments. The cylindrical nature of many bones has preadapted them to be made into flutes and whistles for at least 30,000 years. This copy of a prehistoric Peruvian flute is made from a llama bone (Figure 9.9 **G**). Perhaps equally old is the use of bones for percussion like the clapper bones in Figure 9.10 **G**.

Simple spikes. Pointed bones are common artifacts with many uses that may be determined from their wear patterns or surface engravings.

Medical instruments. Dr. Peter Pfeffermann put his name on Figure 9.9 **K2**. He sold these spikes as medical probes in Vienna in the 1870–90s. Since bone cannot be sterilized, one wonders what was probed and how many infections he caused.

Marlin spikes. Spike Figure 9.9 **K4** is stamped with an anchor and perhaps with the name of a ship. It is a marlin spike used by mariners to help with all kinds of ropework—splicing, tying, and untying knots. The name comes from "marling," the word used to describe the way that twine is wound into ropes. Marlin comes from the old Dutch word merren, meaning to tie, which became marlijen, to bind, in modern Dutch. The sharp, pointy spike gave its name to the equally pointy streamlined marlin fish. Spikes like **K2** and 3 could be used to create holes in materials by moving threads without introducing the weakness caused by cutting. Sailors may have used them for making holes in sails to attach them to the rigging.

9.9. The Utility of Bone

"Any old rags, bottles, or bones."
Nineteenth century London street cry

Until the mass smelting of iron and the formulation of steel in the Industrial Revolution, metals (gold, silver, copper, tin, bronze, brass, iron) were expensive commodities restricted to the rich. Except for knife blades, objects now made of metal or plastic were made of natural materials, especially bone. Bones were

(Opposite page)
Figure 9.9. Bone tools. Bones with the right shape or properties may become primitive tools with little change. A. Seal scapula scraper. Inuit. B, C. Inuit skin and leather working tools. B made from ribs, C from deer long bone. They are primarily scrapers used to remove tissue. The top one has a transverse groove on the end on which to hold a sinew or cord as it is pulled tight. D. A section of cow rib is all that a mortician needs as a simple tool against which to cut tendons and muscle. Nineteenth century Ontario. E. Walrus bacula are used as ooziks or scepters by the Inuit. This semi-fossil baculum is polished but some are elaborately decorated to make ooziks. F. Bone is tough and stable enough to take the fine engraving needed to make rulers. G. The cylindrical nature of many bones has made them suitable to be made into flutes and whistles for at least 30,000 years. This copy of a prehistoric Peruvian flute is made from a llama bone. H and I. Prehistoric peoples seldom missed an opportunity to use the overt properties of natural materials. H is an Arapaima scale (Arapaima gigas) from the Amazon. Fine spicules on its surface make it a perfect rasp, superior to most humanly made nail files. I. Is the bony tongue of the Arapaima used as a coarser rasp especially for grating the seeds of Guarana to make the mildly caffeinated drink that has become the popular Brazilian equivalent of Coca Cola. J. This silver seal made from a digit of the Jacana evokes the natural elegance of this water fowl with its extended digits seeming to enable it to walk on water (that is on water lily leaves). K. Bones ground and polished to a sharp point are common artifacts that rarely carry clues to their many uses. Second from the top is one labeled Dr. Peter Pfeffermann who sold bone spikes as medical probes in Vienna in the 1870–90s. Since bone cannot be sterilized, one wonders what was probed and how many infections were caused. The one on the bottom is stamped with an anchor and perhaps with the name of a ship. It is a marlin spike used by sailors to help make knots. L. This elegant ladle is too small to be used for grog or punch. The bowl holds 2.5 fluid drams = 7.5 scruples or 150 minims, suggesting that it was an apothecaries measuring ladle. M. Bone resists heat and is tough enough to take the screw threads needed to join stems and pipe bowls together. Scale bars = 5 cms.

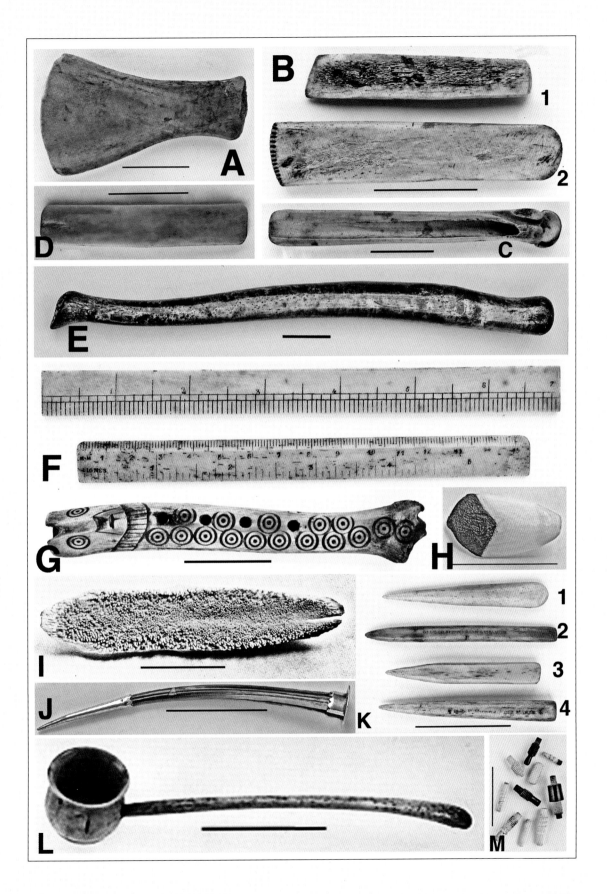

a valued raw material collected for degreasing (a valuable side commodity) and sale to the turners who passed on their scraps to be calcined for making bone china. In Britain and Europe, the bone industry was founded on the creation of everyday objects needed with the growth of cities. Bone is tough and strong (24, 46, 50, 132), and has other advantages. It is cheap, less affected by weak organic acids than iron and does not blacken like silver from contact with sulfur containing food. Its disadvantage is that it is not plastic: it cannot be bent. The presence of spaces for blood vessels prevent it from being carved with the delicate precision obtained with ivory or taking good impressions from hot steel templates. However, bone is tough and stable in flat sheets without warping and takes engraving well enough for many rulers and scales for scientific instruments (Figure 9.9 **F**) or the standard width bone mesh gauges used in lace making (Figure 9.13 **G**). It is tough enough to take the screw threads needed to join large pieces together (Figure 9.10 **A**) and to be turned into a great variety of containers, holding things from tape measures (Figure 9.13 **F**) to needles (Figure 9.13 **J**) and pencil leads (Figure 9.10 **M**). It is heat resistant and can be used to join stems and pipe bowls (Figure 9.9 **M**). Most importantly, it is tough and stable enough to make consistent, solid (Figure 9.1 **A**), and fluid measuring containers such as the elegant apothecaries ladle holding 2.5 fluid drams = 7.5 scruples or 150 minims (Figure 9.9 **L**).

Toys, games, and leisure activities

Imagine the surprise of a Victorian child opening the delicate bone cage figured in 9.10 **A**. Suddenly a "snake" pops out, rolling and quivering as if alive, behaving like a Slinky and extending about 30 cms. It is made from a nut carved into a flat, conical spiral using something like a pencil sharpener, so light that the slightest touch sets it in motion. It is also extremely delicate, which tells us how well behaved its child owner must have been for it to survive intact. The innate human reflex to fear snakes and spiders evolved from their

lethal venom, "they can kill you, therefore handle them carefully." The fear has given rise to a category of toys—model snakes—valued for the frissons that they evoke. The interlocking pieces of bone forming the snake in 9.10 **D** allow it to bend like a real snake, but the rest is up to your imagination. The terminal rattle suggests that it is American or made for the US market in the Orient.

The game in 9.10 **B** is robust, made from bone rings and iron wire by nineteenth century Romany (Gypsies), who hawked such trinkets from door to door. It is an old game with many modern versions. All have the objective of disentangling the rings from one another.

Chips like those in 9.10 **C** made it possible for self-righteous families to play gambling games without the vulgarity of money on the table. Nineteenth century. Probably Indian.

Dominos (9.10 **F**) evolved from gaming with the pairs of faces (**E**) in two dice (**I**). Antique sets on the market are often missing a few pieces. The simplest way to examine a set for completeness is to arrange them in

(Opposite page)
Figure 9.10. Bone toys, games, and leisure tools. A. Bone cage and "snake" made from a carved nut. The "snake" behaves like a Slinky. Victorian. Possibly Chinese. B. Bone ring game. The objective is to separate the rings. Victorian, English Gypsy. C. Gambling chips. Nineteenth century. Probably Indian. D. Fifty-three interlocking pieces terminating in a rattle. Nineteenth century. Rattlesnake motif suggests US or Oriental made for the US market. E, F. Domino set, bone and ebony. English nineteenth century. There are twenty-eight pieces in a complete set. Seven pieces (6+6, 5, 4, 3, 2, 1, 0), six pieces (5+5, 4, 3, 2, 1, 0), five pieces (4+4, 3, 2, 1, 0), four pieces (3+3, 2, 1, 0), three pieces (2+2, 1, 0), two pieces (2+2, 1), one piece (0+0). G. Clapper bones made from beef ribs. Nineteenth century. Quebecois. H. Cribbage board shaped like a walrus tusk but made from whale jawbone. Mid-twentieth century Inuit. I. Dice nineteenth century UK. J. Lead pencil. The point is made from soft lead, English, nineteenth century. K. Pen nib holder used for writing everywhere before the introduction of ball point pens at the end of the Second World War. This one has a Stanhope picture of Vimy Ridge, a souvenir from a visit to the battlefield just after the First World War. L. Automatic pencil holder for soft metallic lead moved forward by a screw turn. Extra leads are stored in the metal shaft. Mid-nineteenth century. M. Screw topped bone storage tube for extra leads. Scale bars = 5 cms.

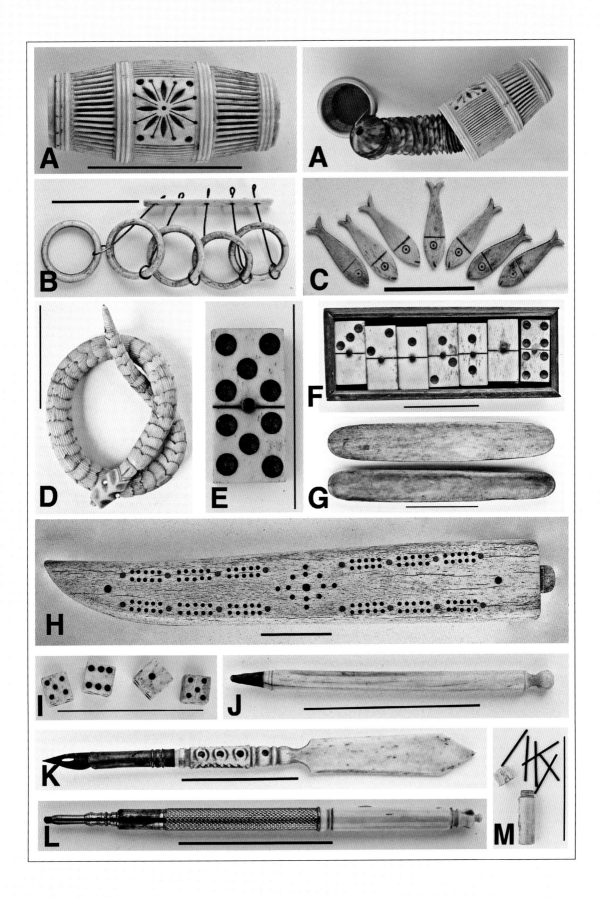

a triangle with seven at the bottom and one (0+0) at the top. A twenty-eight piece double six set should contain: there are seven pieces (6+6, 5, 4, 3, 2, 1, 0), six pieces (5+5, 4, 3, 2, 1, 0), five pieces (4+4, 3, 2, 1, 0), four pieces (3+3, 2, 1, 0), three pieces (2+2, 1, 0), two pieces (2+2, 1), one piece (0+0).

Percussion is one of the oldest and most widespread categories of musical instrument. Among the simplest are Clapper "Bones," formed from pairs of ribs clicked together between the thumb and fingers. The Clapper Bones (9.10 **G**) made from beef ribs are from nineteenth century Quebec, which has a rich tradition of clog dancing accompanied by clappers.

The tradition of Cribbage boards (9.10 **H**) being made from Walrus tusks is so strong that the Inuit copied the shape when they made them from whale jawbone. The story of Inuit carving began when Dr. Jon Bildfell went to St. Luke's Hospital in Pangnirtung, Baffin Island, on his first medical posting immediately after graduating from Medical College in Winnipeg, Manitoba. The Arctic Mission of the Missionary Society of the Church of England had only just established the hospital in 1930. While on postings from 1932–4 and 1940–42, he traded food, cartridges, and coal oil for artifacts carved especially from ivory. By the time that he left the Arctic in 1942, he had a collection of 210 sculptures now recognized as a National Treasure and the commercial foundation for an Inuit art form.

The Greeks and Romans did not gamble with six-sided dice of the kind familiar to us. Instead, they threw bones, giving the expression "to throw the bones" a literal meaning. The bones they threw were astragali (singular astragalus), the heel bones of mammals. These are roughly six-sided, but only four sides are flat enough for a stable landing. The four are unequal in stability, landing occurs on two of them about forty percent of the time and ten percent for the other two. Games were played with four bones and success was achieved according to the rarity of the combination of the four lies.

The Romans valued highly the Venus throw where each bone landed differently slightly less than four percent of the time (92). The modern equivalent are the dice in 9.10 **I**.

We still talk about pencil leads, although pencils like that in 9.10 **L** filled by lead or graphite rods from the screw topped bone storage box in **M** have been replaced by graphite in wood. Even more rarely used are the pencils with points of real metallic soft lead in **J**. This was the kind of pencil used by Jane Austin to write on the ivory tablets in Figure 9.1 **B**, and was useful for artists needing a very faint line sketch of their subject before applying paint. **L**. Automatic pencil holder for graphite or soft metallic lead moved forward by a screw turn. Extra leads are stored in the metal shaft.

Pens with nibs using ink were used for writing everywhere before the introduction of ball point pens at the end of the Second World War. Schoolboys dipped their pens in ink. Business men had fountain pens prone to leak ink on their shirts from the rubber ink reservoir connected to the nib. Gentlewomen used pens like that in **K**, with a Stanhope picture of Vimy Ridge, a souvenir from a visit to the battlefield just after the First World War.

Bone decorative artifacts

Swinging cudgels evolved into support sticks by altering the grip from a side hand grasp to vertical weight bearing by the palm of the hand. The heads of walking and support sticks could then be constructed as handles to distribute the load in many elegant ways (billiard balls, dog's head carvings, antler sections, curved horns). The simplest way to form a stick handle is to curve it like the swagger cane in Figure 9.11 **A**, made from the centrums of 138 vertebrae interspersed with eight horn rings around an iron core. Centrums are the units making the bony backbones of vertebrates. The spinal cord is dorsal to the column, not in it but protected by neural arch bones. Backbone canes are often thought to be made from snakes, but comparison of their vertebrae shows that they are made from fish

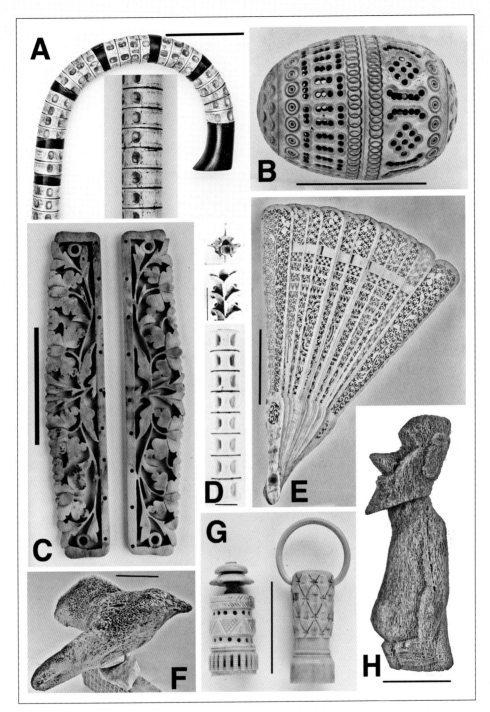

Figure 9.11. Decorative bone. A. Swagger cane made from the centrums of 138 vertebrae interspersed with eight horn rings. B. Turned and carved bone container for thimbles made in four sections, top, bottom, and two cylinders that screw together. C. Intricately carved handles closing a needlework bag. D. Comparison of backbones showing that the cane in A is made from shark, not snake vertebrae. Top, transverse, and dorsal views show snake vertebrae with neural arches and ribs attached or articulated to the centrum. Below, dorsal view of shark vertebrae with paired dorsal and ventral cavities corresponding to loosely attached neural arches and ventral ribs, matching the cane in A. E. Carved bone fan. F and H. Spongy bone of whales lends itself to simple primitive carvings like the gull (F, Inuit) and the head (H, Easter Island). G. Parasol handles show bone can be carved almost as finely as ivory. Scale bars = 5 cms.

213

(Figure 9.11 **D**). Transverse, dorsal, and ventral views show snake neural arches and ribs firmly attached or articulated to the centrum. The centrums of fish vertebrae have paired dorsal and ventral cavities corresponding to loosely attached neural arches and ventral ribs like those used to make the cane. Vertebrae in these canes come from sharks, but sharks are elasmobranchs characterized by having skeletons of cartilage rather than bone. Their vertebrae are not bone, but calcified cartilage. Swagger canes were the gentleman's delight (remember Chaplin) from late Victorian through Edwardian up to the depression era. Their curved handles allowed them to be swung and rotated vigorously in step with the walk, a practice that died out by the 1930s. They remained for decades in many hall-stands, including ours, illustrating my mother's stories of father nearly hitting other walkers with his swinging cane.

Imagine having a small, delicate object that you want to keep in a safe place. You may choose a cardboard, metal, or plastic box, multitudes of which are put into the garbage every day. Now go back 150 years to a young lady finding a place for a precious thimble that she uses every day and that might easily roll on the floor and be crushed. She stored it in a turned bone thimble container like Figure 9.11 **B**. Storage places themselves were rare and valued commodities, made to last and be admired like this one. She might keep it in a needlework bag closed with intricately carved bone handles like those in Figure 9.11 **C**. Beauty was also in fashion accessories like the bone fan in **E,** required for formal dining or visits to the theater, or in **G**, handles for the parasols to protect their complexions and young men from their seductive smiles.

The spongy bone of whales is easily carved into art forms of a different kind, rough representations of animals and human figures. Some from vertebrae are quite large, more than a meter high. The rough nature of the surface prevents signing even on genuine Inuit carvings, making attribution difficult. The gull in **F** is Inuit but without provenance

might have been carved anywhere. Similarly the head and torso in **H** is characteristic of Easter Island but unsigned.

Bone needlework tools

To prevent the warping of a bone needle's disposition, do not treat it too dryly or place it near the riling heat of the radiator.

Gertrude Whiting (140)

Needlework would have been impossible without bone or ivory made into the great variety of hooks, needles, and awls shown in Figure 9.12 (49) (127) (140).

Knitting is needlework created by connecting loops of thread using two or more straight eyeless needles like those in Figure 9.12 **A** capped to stop the work falling off at the back ends. Most wooden needles needed to be thicker to match the strength of bone. Even needles made for heavier yarns (Figure 9.12 **C**) could be thinner than their wooden equivalents. Knitters creating complex patterns used an ingenious aid to memory. Instead of counting the exact number of stitches before changing the pattern, they inserted a flat ring on the needle to remind them where to change (Figure 9.13 **C**). When pausing from her work, a knitter would stop the work falling forward off the front end with a temporary pair of caps held in place by elastic. The caps were decorative, sometimes turned but traditionally carved in the form of cow's hooves. One cow's hoof in Figure 9.13 **H** has been repaired, showing that it was a valued possession. Needles for knitting tubes such as socks were in sets of four without caps (Figure 9.12 **B**).

Crochet hooks come in every size and shape from steel points for the finest silk to heavy bone for the coarse wool (Figure 9.12 **D**). Rug hooks (**E**) need to be more sturdy. Everything about them evokes strength—the steel hooks, the short blunt bone or antler handles, and the broad brass plaques with rivets. We scarcely need a photograph of

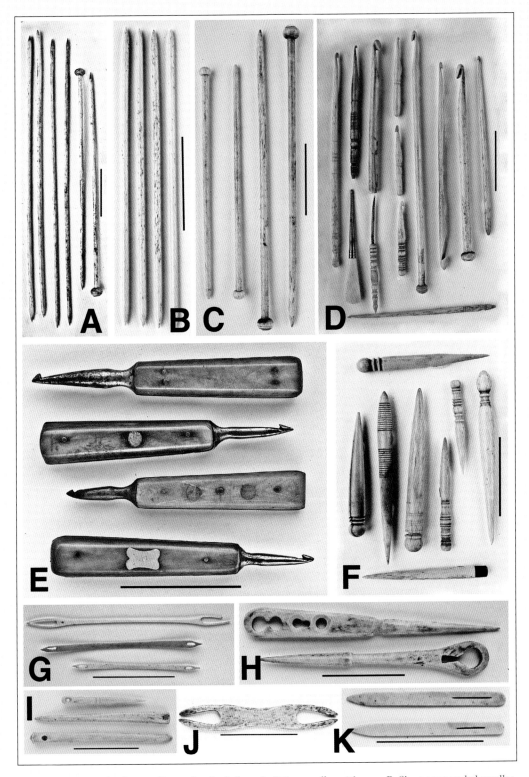

Figure 9.12. Bone hooks, needles, and awls. A. Long knitting needles with caps. B. Short open ended needles for knitting socks. C. Short thick capped needles for knitting coarse wool into slippers. D. A variety of crochet hooks. E. Rug hooks, very strong, often made from antler bone. F. A variety of bone awls. G. Fine netting needles. H. Tapestry flutes. The flute carries the thread wound around it through the tapestry. I. Coarse bone needles. J. Netting needle. K. Bodkins, needles for threading tape, ribbons, or elastic. Scale bars = 5 cms.

the hands and arms to picture the muscles needed to hook rugs. Awls (**F**), usually turned, are for making holes. Within this limitation to their shape the rings made by turning give them variety, like bar codes. (Is this where the inventors of bar codes got their idea?) Their multiple rings may make them easier to grip and to identify, but they give the impression that the turner is just showing off his art. Identification by rings is not sufficient for the instant identification needed by pillow lacemakers who decorated their bobbins with colored beads (Figure 9.13 B). Unfortunately, this extra weight coupled with the density of bone makes them too heavy, breaking the thinnest threads that have to be wound on lighter wooden bobbins. This is one of the few example where the properties of bone are surpassed by wood.

Bodkins (**K**) are simple needles for threading tape, ribbons, or elastic, or for joining materials like skin together. Netting needles extend these simple functions to create fabrics, techniques going back into prehistory that survive in the art of fishermen. All that is needed to make a fishing net was a coarse shuttle like that in Figure 9.12 **J** wound with thread. Coarse bone needles like those in **I** were used for net repair. Wet bone sheets can be bent just enough to make a shuttle (Figure 9.13 **A**). Tatting shuttles for making macramé create fabric in a similar way. Finer needle shuttles (Figure 9.12 **G**) for women's decorative materials were brought back to Europe from the East by returning crusaders in the eleventh and twelfth centuries, beginning the development of needle lace as a major activity from the sixteenth century. The width of the holes was determined precisely using mesh gauges (Figure 9.13 **G**). Flutes for weaving tapestries (**H**) function like netting needles but create patterns by carrying colored threads wound around them. The flute head is keyed to hang in the position needed for the next weave.

Needles are slippery, treacherous creatures with cat-like claws, ready to pierce and scratch and tear—sleek little polished instruments that need watching and humoring and a place of their own to be kept in. So said Gertrude Whiting (140) when describing that most important of needlework accessories, a place to store needles. In addition to eyeless needles, hooks and eyed needles, bone was used to make accessories such as places to keep them. Umbrellas were a common motif for French-made needle holders. The one in Figure 9.13 **J** has a Stanhope of the burning of the Tuileries, dating it post 1871. English needle holders were plainer examples of the turner's art. Tape measures (**D**, **F**) were essential tools in every needlework bag, requiring their own cases. **D** is made of turned vegetable ivory and bone. Although it has a Stanhope celebrating the Chicago World's Fair in 1893, it is the kind of souvenir handed out by many of the participants and is probably English.

Working in silk

Thus this renowned Honourable Dame,
Her happy time most happily did spend; …
She wrought so well in Needle-worke,
that shee,
Nor yet her workes, shall ere forgotten be.

The Prayse of the Needle,
John Taylor, 1640. (140)

Although cotton came to America in the early seventeenth century, it was banned in England until the Industrial Revolution in the 1800s to protect the wool trade. Until then, ladies worked in silk. Silk differs from other fibers in being a monofilament (like modern plastic threads), making it possible to choose the number of filaments to make any thickness of thread. Silk embroiderers separated the chosen number of silk filaments by passing skeins of silk over the serrated edge of the tool in Figure 9.13 **K** before twisting them into threads of appropriate thickness to be stored on bone silk winders, **E**. We marvel yet at the works of skilled embroiderers who built their figures by varying the thickness as well as the color of their threads.

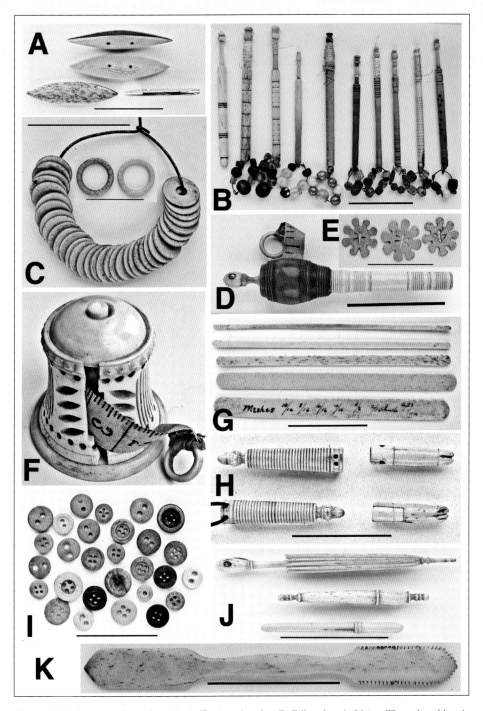

Figure 9.13. Bone needlework tools. A. Tatting shuttles. B. Pillow lace bobbins. The colored beads identify the threads used to create complex lace patterns. C. Knitting spacers. The discs are threaded onto the needle to mark particular changes in pattern. Inset: bone curtain rings for comparison. D. Bone and vegetable ivory tape measure with a Stanhope celebrating the Chicago World's Fair, 1893. E. Bone silk winders. F. Tape measure and case. G. Set of mesh gauges. H. Two pairs of needle sheaths. Elastic threaded through the sheaths held them on the needle ends, stopping the knitting from falling off the needles while not in use. A cow's hooves were a common motif. I. A range of bone buttons. J. French needle holders were often carved in the form of umbrellas like this one with a Stanhope of the burning of the Tuileries dating it post 1871. The other two are examples of the turner's art. K. Silk thread maker. Skeins of silk passed over the serrated edge to divide them for twisting into threads. Scale bars = 5 cms.

Bone toiletry and fashion

People's use of everyday objects tell us much about their lives—toiletry for the intimate details, fashion for the outward show, both affected by industrial changes. Turning the English industrial mills to cotton weaving from wool stimulated laundering. Unlike wool that shrinks, cotton changes little with washing. Cotton fabrics also created a need for more bone buttons, Figure 9.13 **I**, but they had the disadvantage of disintegrating when the laundry was boiled (bones are boiled for soup). The problem was solved by making detachable buttons that allowed shirts to be washed without their buttons, and studs that allowed collars to be detached and washed more frequently than shirts (Figure 9.14 **G, K**). Although bone buttons were replaced by mother of pearl and plastic, the practice continued for the first half of the twentieth century, surviving still in black/white tie and some tuxedoes with collars.

Few fashions are more discretely showy than white chamois leather gloves, *de rigeur* for the social occasions of Victorian ladies until recent times. They presented a problem in that their whiteness showed dirt and they had to be washed, making them shrink. To enlarge them enough to be wearable again, they needed to be stretched, preferably while still damp, using bone or ivory glove stretchers (Figure 9.14 **A, B**). The extent of the fashion, from royalty who still wear gloves on "walk abouts" to working class Sunday attire, is attested by the many nineteenth and twentieth century advertisements for glove washing soap and the abundance of stretchers that have survived.

Some tools seem too neat to be real. Did some Edwardian lady or male dandy really pick their teeth and clean the wax from their ears with the tool in Figure 9.13 **C**? Or did they buy it on a whim because it looked like a good idea? And why have three picks to choose from? **D** and **E** are just as neat but clearly functional, variants on the need for small brushes to stroke the mustache. Did the mustache need brushing? Probably not, but one can imagine the dandy anticipating the feel of a light touch on his upper lip.

The very small cut throat razor (**F**) has a feminine look to it, suggesting intimacy in a ladies boudoir. It is stamped (made in) Germany. Without any more information, we might not be able to guess at its provenance or function, but it is also stamped in English VOM CLEFF a well known cut throat razor blade maker, and CORN RAZOR, telling us what it was for. Women in their cramped shoes suffered from corns and certainly cut them in private but it could have been used for corns by any sex.

The eyebrow tweezers in **H** would certainly have graced a ladies dressing table. We recognize these tweezers because plucking eyebrows is still done, but we are no longer so preoccupied with ear-wax. We don't have personal ear-wax removers like **I** and **J**, because we are now surrounded with things that will function just as well. The frequency of survival of tools for particular purposes may be a deceptive indicator of the frequency of the need for their function. Ear-wax removers may have survived because of their lack of use as we turned to paper clips and twists of tissue, etc.

A candle snuff (Figure 9.14 **L**) and a shoe "horn" (**M**) are both tools that have survived with limited utility. Candles are only used for special intimate occasions and candle snuffs have become "high traditional," decorative rather than functional. Shoe horns are in decline as the sale of close fitting shoes has declined in competition with elastic backed casual wear, but long handled horns continue to be needed with the increasing number of stiff-backed seniors.

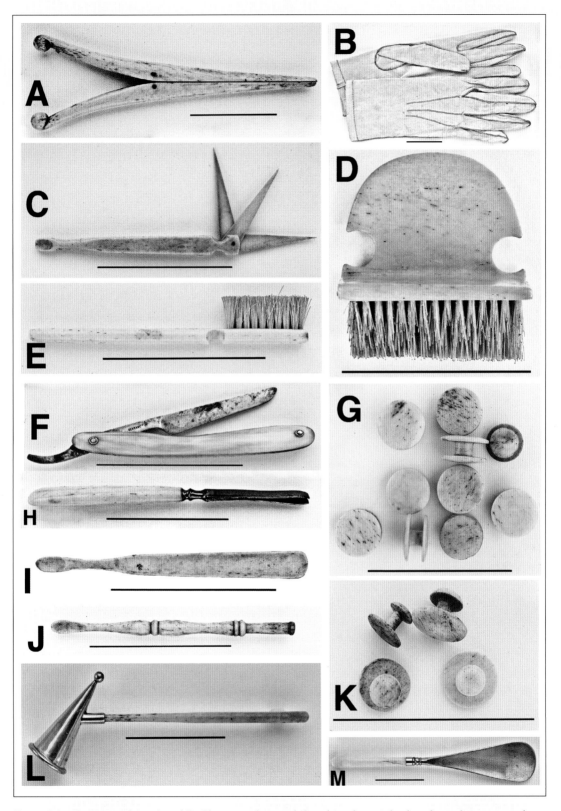

Figure 9.14. Bone in toiletry. A and B. Glove stretchers and the white chamois leather gloves they were used on. C. Combined tooth pick and ear wax remover. D and E. Moustache brushes. F. Bone handled cut throat razor. G. Replaceable ladies shirt buttons. H. Eyebrow tweezers. I and J. Ear wax removers. K. Men's front and back studs used to attach replaceable collars to shirts. L. Candle snuff. M. Shoe "horn". Scale bars = 5cms.

Bone culinary tools

Even when metal became cheap enough for general use, bone continued to be used for many culinary tools where salt, acid, and sulfurous compounds corroded metal. In the nineteenth and first half of the twentieth century, two tined bone forks (9.15 **A**) were shipped with dessert fruits from around the world. The handles were turned and often painted with brightly colored enamel that fell off easily. Forks 2–4 from the left came with crystallized ginger from Hong Kong. Forks 2–7 from the right are from Japan. The center fork is not turned but flat backed, carved and painted with Kris Kringle (Father Christmas) for the German or Dutch Christmas markets, or perhaps carved locally. Unpainted forks, or some that lost their paint, came from Egypt and North Africa with boxes of dates. Since bone resists vinegar, they often graduated for use as pickle forks. Scottish egg spoons (9.15 **B**) were sometimes distinguished by having a hollow for salt at the tip of the handle. The depression might be on either face of the handle, but the smaller depression on the rear face is more elegant. Bone was a practical and popular material for children's cutlery, softer, less sharp, and less likely to damage teeth or cut the lips and tongue. This child's fork and spoon (**C**) were probably made as souvenirs to commemorate the consecration of St. Ann de Beaupres, *La Nouvelle Basilique*, Quebec, in 1934. The original church was burned down in 1922 and rebuilding begun in 1924. The fork has a Stanhope depicting the rebuilt church. The sulfur in egg yolk blackens silver and reacts with iron, so until stainless steel became available (post 1914), egg spoons were made from bone (**D**). Both Scotland and France (Boulogne) had bone carving industries and made spoons with no stylistic differences that I know. Mustard spoons (**E**) can often be recognized by their yellow brown staining. Salt corrodes most metals and salt spoons (**F**) were often made from bone. They sometimes dipped either the handle or the bowl into the mustard. Salt spoons were originally shaped like fairly large shovels, a shape that survived in later diminutive salt spoons (**G**). Marrow spoons (**H**) were sometimes made of bone. Traditional piecrust cutters (**I**) had corrugated bone wheels with turned boxwood handles.

In Egypt, China, and South East Asia, bone was more important as an ivory substitute for making more decorative objects. Ivory remained the main carving material in India, where the Hindu religion made animal bones hard to get.

(Opposite page)

Figure 9.15. Bone had culinary uses where salt and acid corroded metal. A. Dessert fruits in the 19th and first half of the 20th C were shipped from around the world with turned two tined bone forks. B. Scottish egg spoons were often distinguished by having a hollow for salt that may be made on either face of the handle. C. Childs fork and spoon with Stanhope depicting St Ann de Beaupres, La Nouvelle Basilique, Quebec. D. The sulfur in egg yolk blackens silver and reacts with iron so before stainless steel egg spoons were made from Bone. Both Scotland and France (Boulogne) had bone spoon industries. E. Mustard spoons can often be recognized by their staining. F. Salt corrodes most metals and salt spoons were usually made from bone. They were sometimes dipped into the mustard either with the handle or the bowl. G. Salt spoons were originally shaped like fairly large shovels, a shape that survived in later diminutive salt spoons. H. Marrow spoons were sometimes made of bone. I. Traditional piecrust cutters had corrugated bone wheels. Scale bars = 5cms.

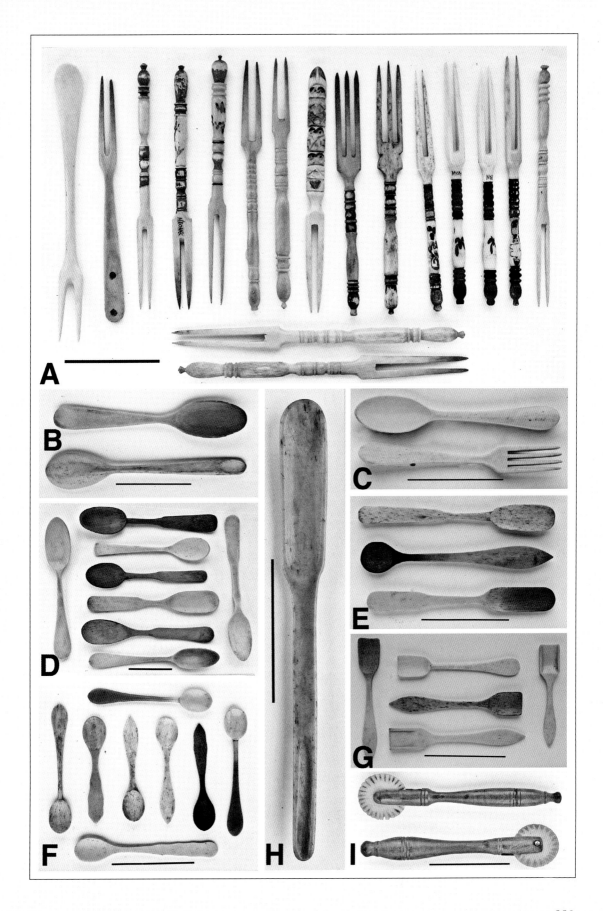

9.10. The Utility of Ivory

"Passing by Smithfield I went to see some workmanship of that admirable artist Reeves, famous for perspective and the turning of ivory. May 10th 1652".

John Evelyn, Diarist, 1620–1706

In Europe, London was the center of the ivory trade, with much carving done in Boulogne. In eighteenth century America, tusks were brought as ballast from Africa to Connecticut, where ivory carving developed in the part of Essex County that became Ivoryton. In 1789, Phineas Pratt owned an ivory workshop there, making combs and many women's items. Although most ivory in the world is elephant, that from other animals may be a local speciality, even far afield from their habitats. In 876 BCE Ashurnarsipal II took tribute in walrus tusks from the conquered cities of Tyre, Sidon, and Byblos in what is now Lebanon. The origin was often not important. In the Eastern Arctic, *Tuugaaq,* the Inuktitut word for ivory, includes both walrus and narwhal. The Cantonese used hippo ivory from Africa for their specialties, elephant bridges and arched landscapes. In the late eighteenth and early nineteenth centuries, hippo ivory was used in England and France specially for making false teeth.

The properties of ivory allow carving in exquisite detail (19, 78). For the finest carving, a Chinese or Japanese master retreated to a dark cabin pierced by a small hole that restricted illumination of the workpiece to a fine beam of sunlight. The ivory was soaked in water long enough to soften it without causing damage by extracting the collagen, or for the most intricate objects, like the meshworks of fans, the carving was done underwater. The result might be a miniature three-dimensional masterpiece or an intricately patterned box lid like that in Figure 9.16 **A** that has tracery less than 1 mm wide. Fine work like this is cut from sheets oriented to the length of the tusk. Orientation of the tusk was important as cracks initiated by cuts tend to be longitudinal. Equally fine is the workmanship on the edge of a turned ivory plate cut from a transverse tusk section (Figure 9.16 **F, G**). Art objects like these deserved and were made for discriminating collectors. Almost as good are the perfectly carved but cheap ivory brooches made for export (Figure 9.16 **C, D, E**). A far less justifiable use of ivory was the carving of minute elephants for tourists in India, feat of craftsmanship though it may have been. Young boys carved elephants so small that 100 could fit into a seed from the red sandalwood tree, *Adenanthera pavonina* (Figure 9.16 **B**). These cheap souvenirs were sold up to the mid-twentieth century, after which the size increased until there was only room for twelve in a seed. As a result of the boys suffering such inhumane long hours of close up work that they became blind, minute carving was eventually banned.

(Opposite page)
Figure 9.16. Ivory's properties make possible the carving of exquisite detail. A. Chinese box top. Much of the tracery is below 1mm wide. B. The Indian masterpiece of 100 carved ivory elephants in a seed from the red sandalwood tree (Adenanthera pavonina) with carved elephant stopper. C – E. Chinese ivory broaches made for export. Not as finely carved as A, but still very fine. F, G. A Chinese plate turned to a thickness of 1mm from a tusk cross section, decorated and with a finely carved periphery.
Scales, A, F = 5cms, all others 1cm.

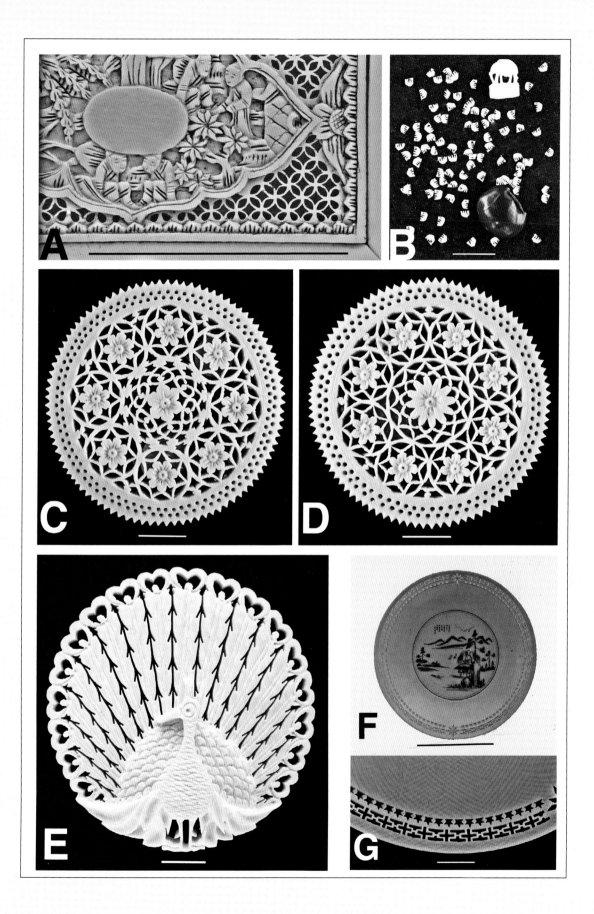

Ivory carving goes back into prehistory, predating even cave paintings as the first human art form (121). The stability of ivory allows the finest scratches to carry pigment, a property made use of in rulers and scales for scientific instruments (Figure 9.17 **A**), and in scrimshaw (Figure 9.18 **E, J**). Scrimshaw is the art of illustrating by filling scratched lines on an ivory surface with pigment (89). The same technique by Inuit was formerly called engraving, reserving scrimshaw for the same kind of work done by Yankee sailors, but the terms are now interchangeable. Inuit from the Bering Sea incised geometric and linear designs on their possessions two thousand years ago (111). The tradition, perhaps modified by contact with Russian traders, continued in the seventeenth and eighteenth centuries. The techniques were picked up by whalers in the nineteenth century to give rise to the now familiar scrimshaw, particularly on sperm whale teeth. All that sailors needed was a nail ground to a knife point for the engraving and a candle flame to fill the lines with carbon black. They had plenty of free time to develop their skills, beginning by pricking out the outlines of female beauties through newspaper illustrations, but the talented soon developed their own images, some raucous, even pornographic, others scenic of ships and coastlines. Genuine old scrimshaw are now collector's items, valuable enough to encourage forgeries. Edward Burdett, the first recorded whaler scrimshaw artist, decorated the ivory handles on a knife and fork that sold recently for $60,000.

The problem of determining whether a work is genuinely old and valuable is further complicated by the popularity of scrimshaw carving as a modern art form. Work from a skilled contemporary artist that has passed through enough hands to lose its modern provenance may be hard to distinguish from an old piece.

Figure 9.18 **E** demonstrates the problem associated with scrimshaw that lacks provenance (other than its acquisition in about 1960 in this case). It is genuine in the sense that it is on a natural whale tooth, probably a killer whale. It has subject matter and a carving style that could be nineteenth century. Microscopy shows nothing to give it away as a modern forgery. It may have been made in the mid-twentieth century by a local artisan for tourists at a time when his labor was cheap and whale teeth readily available, much like the sailors with time and teeth on their hands a hundred years earlier. In a sense, that makes it genuine scrimshaw in that it was not made as an antique copy for a big profit. But might it be 150 years old and judged to be a valuable antique? Probably not, as the workmanship does not suggest the endless time invested by a sailor on a long voyage. This brings us to the shaky ground of connoisseurship, where belief replaces rational deduction. The connoisseur may be right, but there is no rational yardstick by which the belief in the value of the carving style and subject matter can be measured.

"All her teeth were made in the Blackfriars, both her eyebrows in the Strand, and her hair in Silver Street." in *Epicene*, 1609, by Ben Jonson (1572–1637). The toughness of ivory has long made it an essential raw material for making accessories such as false teeth, buttons, studs, and piano keys. Human teeth were a valuable source of ivory. There were enough teeth gathered from the dead in the battle of Waterloo to make dentures for half of Europe. They were expensive. Toughness made ivory useful for tool handles of all kinds, especially high value items like the

(Opposite page)
Figure 9.17. The utility of ivory. A. The stability of ivory coupled with fine engraving made it suitable for making rulers and these map surveyors tools. B. Toughness made ivory useful for tool handles like this knife sharpener. C. Strength, even in thin rods made ivory useful for this Victorian speciality, a back scratcher. D. Socks are knitted with three or four needles. Traditionally one or two of the needles were held in place by a bunch of cock's feathers tied to the waist or in a bone or ivory device stuck in the belt like this very rare one made from walrus ivory shown here. E. The variety of carving for Victorian cutlery handles. F, The ivory handle for a louse comb, showing that the Victorian upper class were not immune to louse infestations. G, An ivory holder for a lancing needle and the storage of hypodermic needles, part of a doctors bedside kit. H. A real penknife, the tool used to re-cut the writing quill as it became worn. Scales = 5cms.

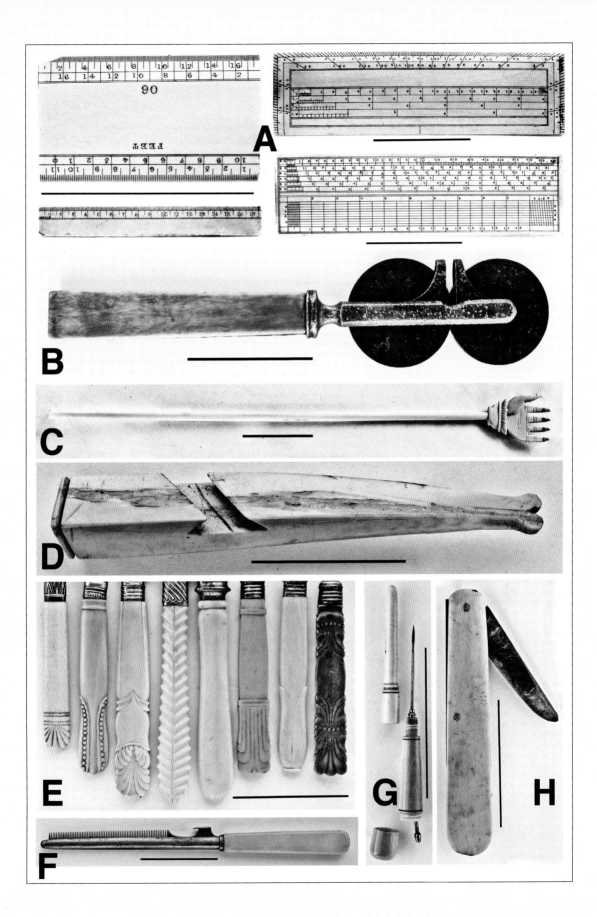

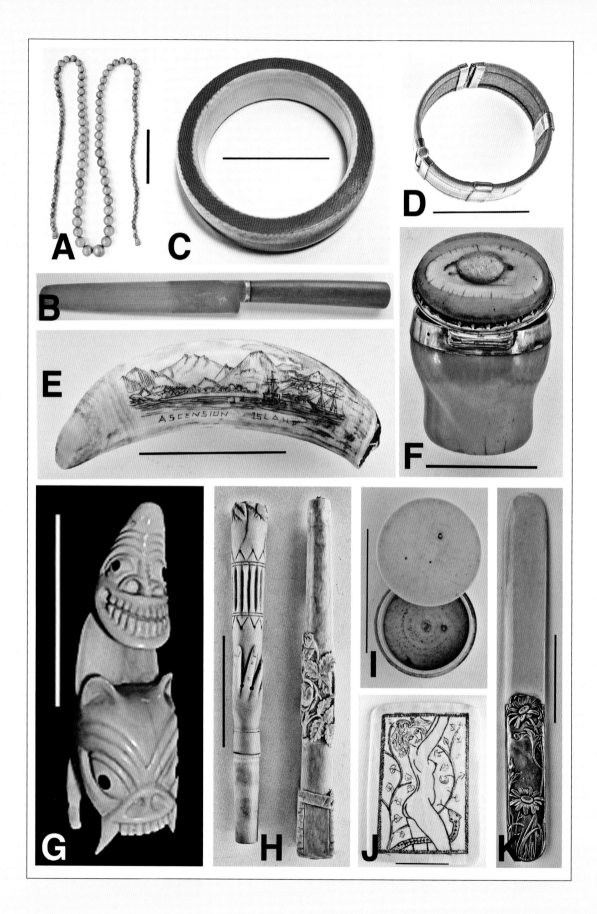

ivory handle for a louse comb (Figure 9.17 **F**) and a knife sharpener in Figure 9.17 **B**. The comb was developed to deal with the louse *Pediculus humanus capitis,* a subspecies of the common louse infecting hair of the head. The ivory handle of the louse comb tells us that it was expensive, for upper class Victorians. The ivory handle also tells us that it was on show: if it were to be hidden away it could have been made from less expensive bone, wood, or metal. This implies that head louse infestations were commonplace, not occasions of shame, evidence of dirt or insanitary lifestyle, but everyday events to be coped with even in the best of families. There is something else about this particular device; it had a lever to withdraw the teeth into the holder, forcing the lice off the comb, presumably when it was held over the fire. It conjures up the picture of a maternal figure, mother or governess, combing children's hair by the fire where the lice are conveniently incinerated.

Knives in Victorian times were wrought iron or carbon steel at best, prone to rusting. They were maintained in two ways. The edge was sharpened using tools like that in Figure 9.17 **B**, where the blade was run between two sharp-edged hard steel circles. The rust on the blade surface was polished off on knife boards, flat pieces of wood covered with pumice—fine particles of volcanic glass from ground pumice stone, the solidified remnant of frothed up obsidian lava. This repeated surface fine polishing removed the rust and gave a high polish. These two treatments caused the original broad blades with rounded

ends to survive only as paper thin pointed blades.

Ivory as a raw material played a big part in the expansion of the cutlery industry that came as part of the Industrial Revolution. Blades needed handles, lots of handles, first of ivory, later of bone and antler. Handles were beautifully carved in great variety. Some were stained green (Figure 9.17 **E**).

An event in human evolution that rarely receives comment is the development of the human arm in a way that prevents the fingers of most people from reaching the upper center of the back. Being tool users, humans invented an instrument to remedy the deficiency—the back scratcher—found throughout the world, but is it necessary any longer? Although back scratchers were common household implements in earlier times with a last gasp in the Victorian era, they are rare in present day homes or workplaces. Two interrelated factors may have had something to do with the change, replacing woolen underclothing with cotton and the ubiquity of body lice (*Pediculus humanus corporis*). Until the early 1800s, wool was the usual material for underclothing. Wool was itchy, difficult to wash without shrinking, and an ideal habitat for body lice. Dirty wool and lice demanded body scratching. The introduction of easily washed and less itchy cotton undergarments through the nineteenth century lowered the louse population, reducing the need to scratch and the requirement for back scratchers, now a Victorian relic, a collector's item attesting to the strength of ivory, even in thin rods (Figure 9.17 **C**).

Knitting is not just a gentle fireside occupation for women with time to spare. Working women may knit while walking or transporting bundles on their heads. To do this, they need something to hold the needles in place. Traditionally, one or two of the needles were held by sticking them in a bunch of cock's feathers tied to the waist. More sophisticated tools of bone or ivory like that in Figure 9.17 **D** were also stuck in the belt to hold the needles. **D** comes from Cumberland

(Opposite page)
Figure 9.18. The utility of ivory. colored & decorative Ivory. . A & B. Necklace and knife handle stained with copper arsenate. C. Indian single piece ivory armlet stained pink. D. Hinged Indian ivory anklet colored pink mainly from wearing over stained skin. E. Modern Scrimshaw, probably about mid 20th C. F. Snuff box. Elephant ivory sides with walrus ivory top and bottom, possibly 17thor 18thC. G, Greenland Tupiluk. H, Parasol handles. I. Snuff box. J. Modern Scrimshaw by the author about 1960, homage Eric Gill. K. Paper knife with silver Art Nouveau handle, Austrian, early 20th C. Scales, I = 1cm, all others = 5cms.

in the north of England and is made from walrus ivory. Needles could rest sideways in the slot and firmly in a hole in the square end. Wool could be secured by twisting around the slot in the square end.

Many doctor's black bags contained tools turned from ivory or stored in ivory containers. Figure 9.17 **G,** part of a doctors bedside kit, tell us about past medical practice. There is a turned cap protecting a lancing needle with the handle also functioning to store hypodermic needles. He may have been able to sterilize the needles in boiling water, but the ivory handle of the lancing needle would limit sterilization to alcohol, if he had any.

> *"Bartleby did an extraordinary quantity of writing ... copying by sunlight and by candle light ... he wrote on silently, palely, mechanically."*
>
> "Bartleby the Scrivener"
> Herman Melville, 1853

Eventually Bartleby would do nothing in the office and when asked to copy uttered those memorable words, *"I prefer not to."* Melville gives his famous description of the operation of a Wall Street office 160 years ago, writing, copying, preparing legal manuscripts, without mentioning the key tools—ink and pens or quills, and how they were made and used. The office may have had metal nibs that were just coming into use but more probably Bartleby would have needed a pen knife for cutting feathers into quills. The tedium of preparing quills from feathers escaped Melville's observation, it was too commonplace, but perhaps it was the boredom of such repetitive activities that drove Bartleby to "prefer not to." Pen knives were once an essential part of a writer's equipment used to cut the quill needed before writing could begin. The writer or scrivener or copier had to cut a quill from a large goose feather. This required a sharp knife to make a diagonal cut to the base and a vertical longitudinal cut to separate the cut end. We now use the appellation "pen knife"

to describe a variety of folding knives without thought to the origin of the name. The "real" pen knife in Figure 9.17 **H** has one blade protected in a slit in a single piece of ivory twice its length.

Ivory and bone are easily stained any color with synthetic dyes but the custom never caught on because of the discovery of plastics and aniline dyes at about the same time, the 1870s. It became unnecessary to change the color of ivory when plastics could be made in any color. A limited industry for coloring ivory with synthetic dyes, especially red and green, was centered in Hyderabad, India. Traditional techniques for staining ivory pink and green date from an earlier time. Indian ivory bracelets like that in Figure 9.18 **C** are pink from contact with *alta*, a Hindi word for the red dye used to stain the feet, especially at marriage. The original natural dye was from juice of the Red Sandalwood (*Adenanthera pavonina*) (44) but has been replaced by synthetic aniline dyes. The green copper arsenate stain of the ivories in Figure 9.18 **A, B** was obtained by mordanting in copper sulfate followed by sodium arsenate.

> *"... a fine snuff rasp of ivory given me by Mrs. St. John ..."*
>
> November 1st 1711
> Jonathan Swift 1667–1745

The snuff that he made by rasping tobacco leaves into a fine powder might have been stored in the ivory table snuff box in Figure 9.18 **F**. The silver is unmarked and cast; the top and bottom are walrus ivory and the sides follow the natural shape of an elephant's tusk, oval in cross section. It is interesting that the first Meissen ceramic table snuff boxes adopted this shape as though copying the ivory, although it is much easier to model clay with a circular cross section.

The Greenland Inuit tupilak in Figure 9.18 **G** is a fearsome creature, as it is meant to be. Not all tupilak were like this. The tupilak of the Iglulik and Caribou Inuit were invisible ghosts and those of the Copper Inuit were like the Christian devil. The Greenland Inuit were different; they made **objects** that they cast into the sea with instructions to harm their enemies by their magical properties. Shamans originally made them from bone, skin, hair, sinew, or the corpses of children, giving them power and life by ritual chanting. The ritual didn't always work: tupilak could come back to destroy their maker if the enemy had greater magical powers. When Europeans became interested, the Inuit carved tupilak of ivory from sperm whale, narwhal, and walrus or antler from caribou that they could sell to tourists.

For the lovers of Art Nouveau, it is still possible to find small, affordable ivory creations such as parasol handles or paper knives made at the turn of the nineteenth century (Figure 9.18 **H, K**).

9.11. The Utility of Horn

"Whereas there has been a horrid and detestable Conspiracy formed and carried on by Papists and other wicked and traitorous persons for Assassinating his Majesties Royall person in Order to Incourage an Invasion from France to Subvert our Religion Laws and Liberties, Wee the Master Wardens Assistants and other Members of the Company of Horners of London whose names are hereunto Subscribed doe heartily sincerely and solemnly Profess Testifie and Declare That his Majesty King William is Rightfull and Lawfull King to these Realms ..."

Oath of association of the Horners Company, 1696. (37)

The King William referred to is William III, his wife Queen Mary II having died two years earlier. Such support for the King was part of a reciprocal relationship. Horners needed Royal Statutes like the one Edward IV gave them in London in 1465 and the twenty-seven page long Charter from Charles 1st signed by Wolseley in 1638. Among other things, the charter gave the Horners a monopoly free from competition, decreeing "... no stranger ... should buy any English horns unwrought ... within the city ... or within twenty-four miles ... of the city ..."

The Horners guild represented a skilled and rich artisan trade class long before the nineteenth century developed its wealthy industrial classes. Horn, even more than bone, anticipated plastic in its properties more than any other natural material. It came in chunks, sheets, and natural shapes that lent their form to make functional objects, and it was cheap and readily available. Almost anything could be and was made from horn. It preceded plastics in the diversity and ubiquity of its uses, beautifully illustrated by F. J. Fisher (37) and Paula Hardwick (100 different horn objects (53)). The problem facing the collector is how to date and attribute finds that almost always lack provenance. The descriptions given in Figure 9.19 and 20 must be viewed in this light. They are only possible, probable, incomplete, and perhaps wrong, but they are a beginning for others to criticize and build on.

Horn's natural shape lent itself for use as containers, particularly ready-made drinking vessels. Figure 9.19 A shows a drinking horn used by Kikuyu in East Africa until the middle of the twentieth century. Such traditional complete horns made clumsy drinking cups, suitable for passing around in ceremonies or lying empty on the great table, but inconvenient baggage to pack for a rough journey. The voyageurs, French Canadian fur traders from the beginning of the seventeenth century, transported ninety-pound bundles of furs by canoe to Montreal and the East Coast from progressively further distances in the interior. They needed a cup they could carry easily and dip in the water while paddling. Their solution was to cut off cow horns about 5 cms from the base and cover the wound with tar to help healing. After about two years, the cut surface repaired itself with new horn. When cut off, it made a

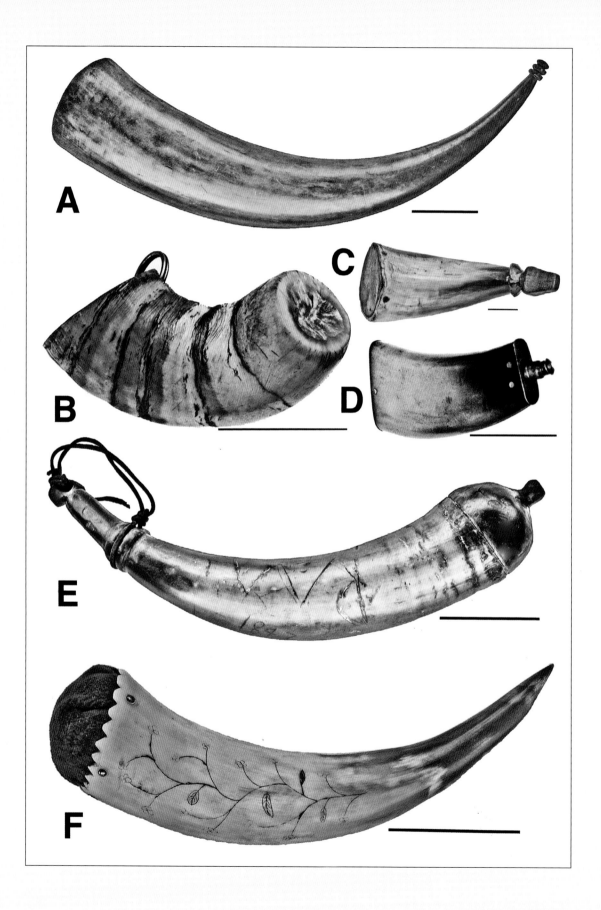

convenient short cup that could be hooked to the belt (Figure 9.19 B). Powder horns (Figure 9.19 E) could be slung around the shoulder, but were also clumsy. Shorter powder horns that could slip into a pocket were made by cutting a short segment, flattening it, plugging one end (usually with wood), and putting a nozzle, often of metal, on the fine end (Figure 9.19 D). Small horns were used for lead shot, not powder (Figure 9.19 C). The natural shape was also helpful in making whistles, like the football referee's whistle in Figure 9.20 F. They had a mellower tone than the metal whistles that came after them and the inclusion of a pea in the chamber could give them a warbling note. The long, curved form of horns was a natural shape for them to become musical instruments, such as the Shofar, blown in synagogues at Rosh Hashana and Yom Kippur, or secular horns blown for their strident notes in war and the chase. The favorite mounts of cavalry officers were remembered on their death by converting their hooves into mementos—inkwells or engraved silver paper weights—for the officer's mess (Figure 9.20 A). Country farmers, prone not to waste good material, turned cow horns into coat racks and the legs of foot-stools. Stuffed and covered with fabric, horns and hooves made elegant pin-cushions (Figures 9.19 F, 20 B, C, D), but why was all the material in such strident shades of red?

(Opposite page)
Figure 9.19. The utility of horn. A. Drinking vessel made from whole horn. Kikuyu, central Africa, mid 20th C. and earlier. B. Voyageurs water cup, Quebec. 18th to 19th C. C. Small horn for storing lead shot, 19th C. Ontario. D. Flattened horn with metal closure for powder. 19th C. Ontario. E. Powder horn, 19th C. Upper Canada. F. Horn pin cushion. 19thC. Ontario. Scales, C = 1cm, all others 5cm.

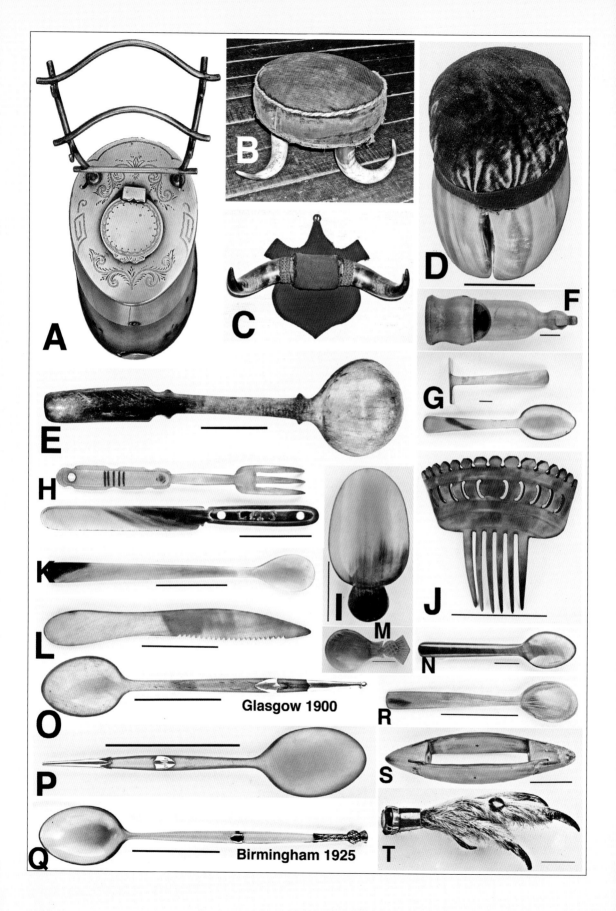

A

B

C

D

F

G

E

H

I

J

K

L

M

N

O

Glasgow 1900

R

P

S

Q

Birmingham 1925

T

At the beginning of the Industrial Revolution, buffalo and cow horns were a major industrial raw material used to make superior handles for cutlery (Figure 9.5 C). The tips are solid enough to carve very chunky beads and rings in three dimensions (Figure 9.21 B, C). Sheets could be cut and formed into many kinds of spoons, forks, combs, and paper cutters (Figure 9.20), illustrating the ways of life of the times. They all have stories to tell. Thistle decorations denote Scotland, but the egg spoon with a thistle was made in Birmingham while the one with a silver ball was made in Scotland. Also, why did some of them end in a silver spike, is there something about eating eggs that has been forgotten? The knife and fork (H) were inlaid with mother of pearl, but fell on hard times, losing some of the inlay and suffering crude red sealing wax filled carving identifying them as the property of LMS, the London Missionary Society (or conceivably but unlikely the London, Midland, and Scottish railway). The LMS operated abroad from London. Were these implements to teach the foreign heathen table manners as well as Christianity? The properties of horn allow it to be used at opposite ends of a scale of toughness to delicacy. Shuttles for weaving wool into coarse fabrics take a constant battering that few materials other than horn can take (Figure 9.20 S). At the other end of the scale, horn is the perfect material for a babies' spoon and pusher, it takes a fine polish, making it easy to clean, is light with no sharp edges, and it is not discolored by eggs (Figure 9.20 G). The early twentieth century fashion for teaching babies to feed themselves with a spoon and pusher may have passed, but these delicate objects have survived better than today's table manners.

(Opposite page)
Figure 9.20. A. Hoof with brass cover for inkwell and pen rack. 19th c. English. B, C, D, Ontario 19th c. cottage furniture using horns. B. Foot-stool supported on cow horn legs. C. Cow horn coat rack. D. Cows foot pincushion. E. Punch ladle, Early 19th C English or Scottish. F. Referees whistle, similar in design to current metal soccer referees whistles, late 19th to early 20th C. G. Spoon and pusher, a child's first eating utensils, English, Edwardian. H. Horn Knife and Fork with mother of pearl inlay (3 missing). Crudely incised L.M.S. and III &IIII. I. Flour or apothecaries scoop. J. Ornamental hair comb. K. Caviar spoon. L. Serrated letter/page opener. M. Tea caddy spoon. N. Salt spoon. O. Egg spoon with knobbed silver end hall marked Glasgow, 1900. P. Egg spoon with silver spike end. Q. Egg spoon with thistle silver end hall marked Birmingham, 1925. R. Egg spoon, Scottish, 19th.C. S. Shuttle for weaving coarse wool into fabric for Yurts, 19thC Chinese Turkestan. T. Grouse pin with cairngorm (smoky quartz). 19th. C Scottish. Scales, F, G, N, T = 1cm, all others 5cm.

Sheets of horn take exquisite detail from hot steel engravings. Techniques for printing from steel engravings invented at the beginning of the nineteenth century were applied to horn sheets, with heat replacing ink to give shallow three-dimensional pictures like those in the two buffalo horn table snuff boxes in Figure 9.21 A. They were made in a style typical of Sheffield from 1815 to 1835 (53). Many were engraved by one of three Wilsons: Jonathan, William, and William's son—William Junior. The one engraved "Tallyho" on the top and lyre, book, plough, and parchment motif on the bottom are signed plain Wilson. The box with a top of cupid and roses motif and the words:

> *"Cupid once, upon a bed*
> *Of roses, laid his weary head.*
> *Luckless urchin, not to see*
> *Within the leaves a slumbering bee.*
> *The bee awak'd with anger wild.*
> *The bee awak'd and stung the child"*

And a grape leaf motif on the bottom, is signed W. Wilson J., presumably a son.

The mourning broaches in Figure 9.22 are more deeply impressed, giving three-dimensional images, not just two dimensional patterns. Mourning brooches were made from pressed buffalo horn made darker by black enamel. They became popular in Queen Victoria's prolonged mourning period (the rest of the century) after Prince Albert's death in 1861. In spite of their somber aspect, they are beautiful in their own right and deserve their revived popularity as accent pieces to modern dress. The knife handle (Figure 9.22 A), celebrating the battle of Waterloo in 1815, is intermediate between the fine shallow craftsmanship created by Wilson in the table snuff boxes (Figure 9.21 A) and the three-dimensional pressed horn brooches.

The various ways that horn can make containers by molding after heat softening and by carving is illustrated by the six snuff boxes in Figures 9.21 D–I. Scottish snuff mulls use the natural shape of sheep horns, often decorated

(Opposite page)

Figure 9.21. The utility of horn. A. Horn takes very fine detail as in these steel engravings on table snuff boxes: "Tallyho" Signed by Wilson, 1830, with the bottom having a Lyre, book, plough, and parchment motif; the second box has a cupid and roses motif, "Cupid once, upon a bed of roses, laid his weary head. Luckless urchin, not to see within the leaves a slumbering bee. The bee awak'd with anger wild. The bee awak'd and stung the child" engraved by W. Wilson J. The bottom has a grape leaf motif. B, C, Horn tips are solid enough for small three-dimensional carvings like this ring and bead made from African buffalo horn in mid 20th C. Kenya. Horn becomes plastic when heated. D – E show six ways that horn can be moulded to make containers such as snuff boxes. D. Scottish snuff mulls use the natural shape of sheep horns with silver trim decorated with cairngorm (citrine quartz) or agate as here (two small banded agate cabochons). The softened horn has been tightly coiled. E. A rare form, possibly 19th C American uses sheets of horn in stacks. Layers of horn form an oval cylindrical box opened through a hinged side lid. F. Two heat softened horn sheets have been pressed around oval moulds and riveted together with a hinged lid inserted on one side. Probably 19th C Scottish. G. A cow hoof has been fitted with a lid made from the pad from another hoof. Probably also 19th C. Scottish. H. A moulded box with an engraved lid depicting Christ carrying the cross. Engraved JESUS IMPRIMANT SA SAINTE. French, about 1820. I. Box made from two horn sections moulded into ovals that fit tohether with top and bottom inserts and a silver shield. Scottish, 19th C. All scale = 5cms.

234

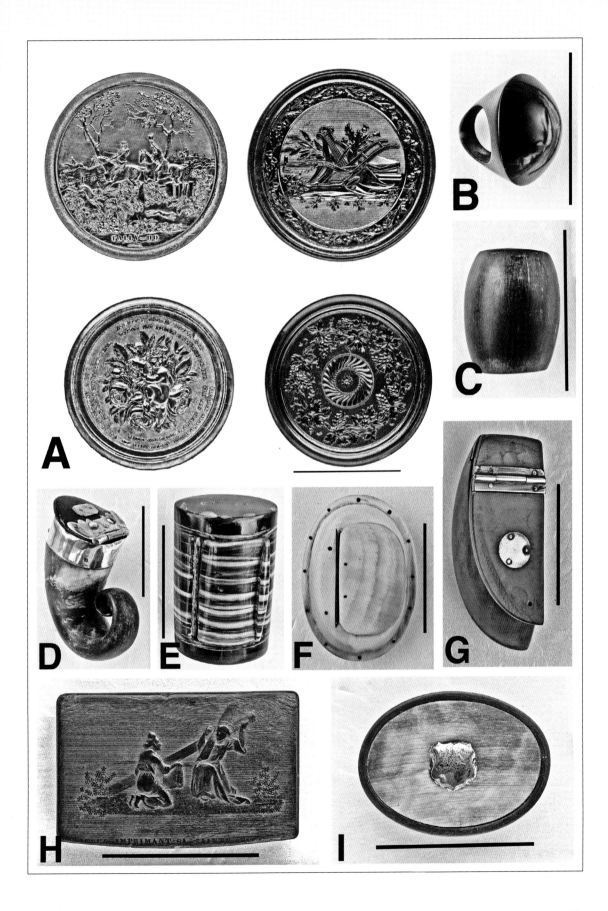

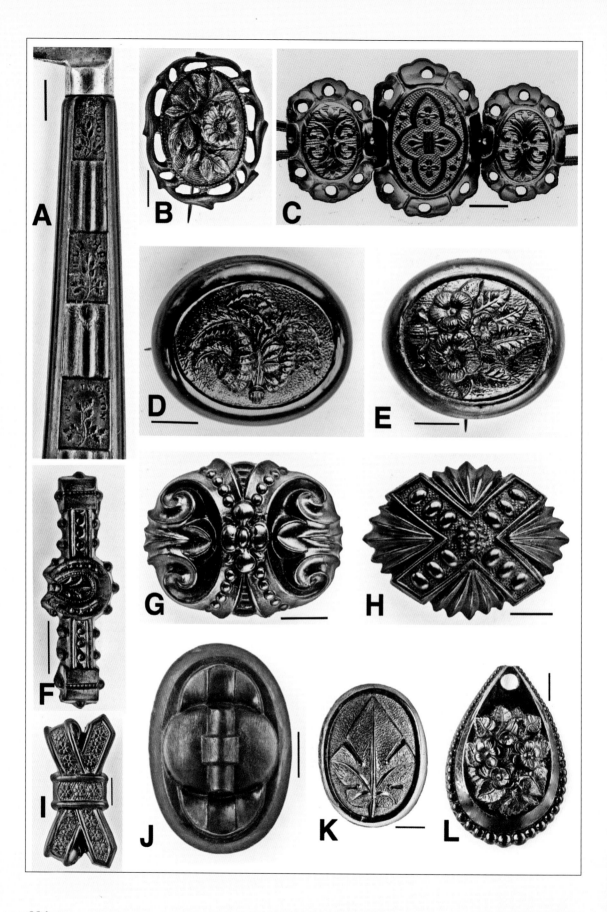

with silver trim and facetted cairngorms (citrines or smoky quartz) or cabochons cut from agates found in local streams. Layers of horn are sometimes stacked up to make three-dimensional structures that can then be hollowed out, as in the snuff box (E). In F, two horn sheets have been softened around oval molds, riveted together, and a hinged lid inserted on one side. Cow hooves are ready made boxes, if a little peculiar in shape, only needing a lid for closure (G). Example I is made like a pill box. It is formed from two horn sections molded into ovals to make a top and bottom that fit together. H is a typical French box, with a molded and carved lid depicting Christ carrying the cross. It is engraved *JESUS IMPRIMANT SA SAINTE.*

(Opposite page)
Figure 9.22. Pressed horn. A. Pressed horn knife handle celebrating the battle of Waterloo in 1815. Three panels are marked "Waterloo, Blucher, Wellington" around sprays of oak leaves. B – K. Mourning broaches typical of Victoria's reign after the death of Prince Albert in 1861. C. Bracelet from the same period. L. Ornament from a coach horse pulling a hearse that has been modified into a pendant. All scales = 1cm.

9.12. The Utility of Hair

The history of hair and wool used to make felt and textiles is dealt with on easily accessible websites and will not be repeated here. The diversity of other uses of hair is less well known. The hair of family members had an intimate value for the creation of memorials. A touching activity of ladies in the Victorian era was their artistry in the arrangement of different colors of hair from their near relatives (Figure 9.23 A, B, D). Memorials led to an industry devoted to purely decorative artwork (9).

Among the least attractive objects that appear commonly in flea markets are containers for hair, circular boxes covered by a wide funnel into which a lady stuffed the leftovers from her hair brush before retiring. Why didn't she just toss them in a wastebasket if she wanted to stop them becoming dust bunnies? The reason is that she wanted the hair for her jewelry creations. Hair that had fallen out after brushing had the advantage of being long; hairs only fall out at the end of their life span, making this a much better collection than that snipped off by her hair dresser. Presumably, she also traded hair so that her collection could be multicolored. The contents of her hair box were the raw material for the creation of elaborate vases of hair flowers, framed light boxes of hair wreaths or more intimate twists within sentimental lockets and broaches. She may also have had the skill to weave and knot hair earrings, perhaps the most difficult and elegant of Victorian crafts, beautifully described and illustrated by Bell (9).

Not all hair work was so decorative. There can be few monuments to the absurdity of human taste greater than the fashion of wearing wigs that developed in seventeenth century Europe from periwigs functioning to cover baldness. It presumably began in imitative flattery of a bald aristocratic ruler trying vainly not to look his age. However it started, it was a major movement spreading throughout the Western World that did not decline until the nineteenth century, still surviving as a head dress distinguishing barristers and judges pleading cases in senior courts of English Law (Figure 9.23 E). In spite of their absurdity, wigs are returning to fashion, albeit in a different form. The adornment of women's heads with other peoples' hair, largely from India, is now a multibillion dollar industry.

The properties of natural hair have never been surpassed by synthetics for many kinds of brush, from those used in the finest painting to the largest shaving brushes (Figure 9.23 F). At the other end of the scale, elephant and giraffe hair are so coarse that individual strands can be made into bracelets (Figure 9.23 G). In cows' stomachs, the conditions that favor the bacterial digestion of cellulose also lead to the softening of hair that has been trapped in balls until it fuses together into a horny mass. Such hairballs are interesting natural objects that show the plasticity of keratin (Figure 9.23 C). The hair of New and Old World porcupines has independently evolved into different kinds of spiny quill (Figure 7.7.2), demonstrated in the very different ways that they have been used to decorate boxes (Figure 9.23 H, I).

The availability of horsehair influenced the design of household furniture. Prior to the nineteenth century, it was luxury enough to have a hard wooden bench to sit on, but with a population of 8 million horses in U.S. and 21.5 million in U.K. there was an abundance of horsehair and stuffed furniture became possible. Benches became sofas and chesterfields, oak wingback seats became easy chairs.

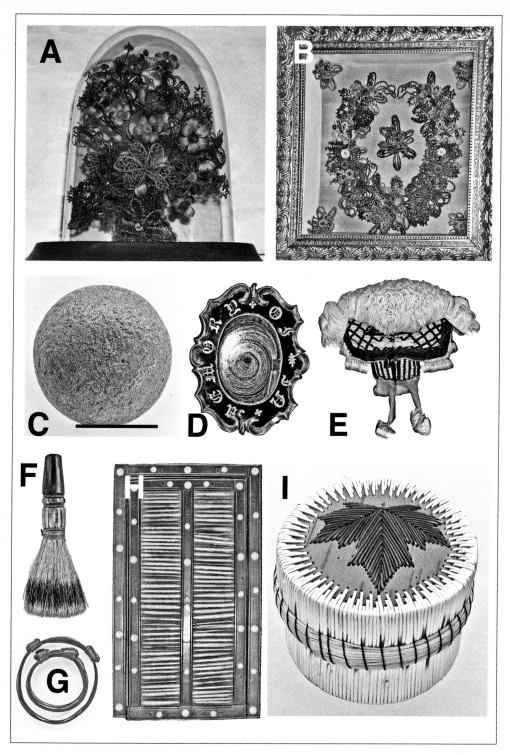

Figure 9.23. The utility of hair. The hair of family members was often used to create memorials. This lead to the creation of purely decorative hair art work. A. Decorative flower display protected by a glass dome. B. Framed box containing hair wreath. 19th C. Canadian. A plague scare in the early 1900s caused many hair wreaths to be burned. C. Hair ball from cows stomach. D. Decorative broach containing locks of hair in memoriam or as love tokens. 19thC. English. E. Barristers wig made from white horse hair. English20thC. F. Barbers shaving brush made from badger hair. 19thC. English. G. Bracelets of elephant hair, Kenya, Mid 20th C. H. Box decorated with African porcupine quills. 19thC. South African. I. Birch bark box decorated with American porcupine quills. Mid 20thC Amerindian. Scale = 5cm.

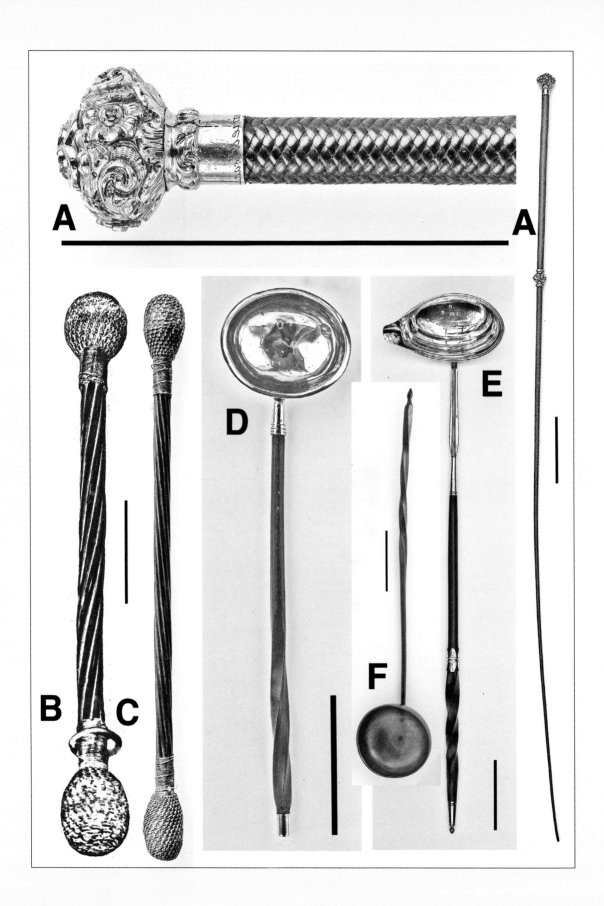

9.13. The Utility of Baleen

"All in general wear gowns loose in the back, with a kirtle and close upperbody, of silk or light stuff, but lately the French sleeves born out with hoops of whalebone, and the young married gentlewomen no less than the virgins show their breasts naked."

Fynes Moryson, An Itinerary (1617), quoted in (106)

The "hoops of whalebone" above were whale baleen, commonly but inaccurately known as "whalebone." The whalebone misnomer came about because breastplates and stays were originally made from whalebone, the bone from the lower jaw of baleen whales. It was a valuable commodity, coming in large pieces of solid osteonic bone ideal for the creation of stiffeners in ladies dresses, scrimshawed breastplates, and especially in Victorian and Edwardian times, the strips to make the stays for ladies' corsets. But baleen's lightness and elasticity made it more suitable for outlining the form of delicate structures. Unlike bone that was used for its rigidity, baleen could be deformed into new shapes that kept their elasticity. Baleen can either be extremely elastic, giving coshes and riding whips their whippiness, or after heating and twisting can become stiff, as in the handles of ladles.

The riding whip in Figure 9.24 A, made by Swaine & Isaac, London, whip makers to royalty from 1835–1846, the time of William IV (1830–1837) and Victoria (1837–1901) has survived for nearly 200 years. It is 65.5 cms long with a gold-formed cap and a good grip from a delicately woven basket handle of baleen filaments. The length of the whip is made from 25 filaments embedded in matrix protected by linen basketwork. It is beautifully made for the very upper class. It is impossible to handle it without a quick flick at the air to enjoying its whippiness. It could have been Queen Victoria's. One can imagine it in her young hand whipping the air and stinging the horse's flank at a gallop.

Baleen's elasticity made it ideal material for making coshes (see above, 9.3.3 D. Darwin's Cosh). Sailors made them from thick baleen filaments twisted around a core of filaments twisted with an opposing orientation, both held together at each end by woven linen baskets containing lead weights. Riding whips and coshes are both constructed from filaments, separated from matrix when thick or functioning as a unit when very fine and left in their matrix. The separation increases elasticity by allowing filament movement relative to one another. On the other hand, thick strips can be made rigid after being allowed to set in a stretched position, obtained by twisting heat-softened baleen. The rigid baleen ladle handles in Figures 9.24 D–F have been made in this way. These were made when baleen was still a rare commodity at the end of the eighteenth century, before industrial whaling. The similarity between the horn and silver bowls is striking. Presumably the horn, cheap and readily available, came first.

(Opposite page)
Figure 9.24. The utility of baleen. A. Riding whip with a Gold-formed cap marked Swaine & Isaac, London. They were whip makers to his majesty from 1835-1846 (William IV 1830-1837, Victoria 1837-). The whale baleen has 25 filaments left within matrix at the tip covered by linen basketwork on the length and baleen filament basketwork on the handle. Total length 65.5cms. B. Sailors cosh made from thick baleen filaments twisted around a core of filaments surmounted at each end by woven linen baskets containing lead weights. C. Baleen cosh, 31cms long, identical to the one carried by Darwin on the Beagle. It is made from much thinner baleen filaments with smaller lead weights than B. D. Gravy Ladle, 15.3cms long, 13.2cms baleen. Hall marked London, 1805-1806. E. Punch ladle, 35.5cms long, 10+2.5cms silver, 23cms baleen. Hall marked London, E. Morley, 1799-1800. F. Horn and baleen punch ladle, English, 18thC. Scales = 5cm.

9.13. The Utility of Tortoiseshell

T'u-p'l or tortoiseshell is used in Chinese medicine to "open up meridians and activate the lo passageways." A barefoot doctor's manual. If that doesn't work, try *Ti-lung* (earthworms).

Apart from its use in Chinese medicine, tortoiseshell is the ideal material for making small, expensive decorative objects. Its colors and patterns are beautiful in their own right. Background colors range from yellow to olive brown, blotched patterns from orange brown to deep yellow brown to black—the full range of colors that melanin can make. The blotched melanin pattern can be bleached to give translucent or cloudily transparent yellow brown sheets. It is tough and takes a high polish. Heat softens it for molding and pressing into complex shapes. Surfaces can be fused by heat and pressure to make scutes into rings, stacks of thin scutes into blocks, and many small scutes into larger sheets. Its one fault is its sensitivity to heat: it burns easily as a result of friction in careless polishing. Its great disadvantage is that its use threatens the survival of the animal that gives rise to it—the hawksbill sea turtle, *Eretmochelys imbricata.*

A problem for the collector is to establish age and origin.

Tortoiseshell is chemically similar to horn, almost pure keratin, but with a finer grain that allows fine silver or gold decorations to be forced into the surface in the art of appliqué (Figure 9.25 A–C). The technique involves forcing hot metal into the tortoiseshell surface. The metal may be a complete pattern, as in the small brush (B), complex patterns of differently shaped metals as in the snuff box lid (A), or bead-like patterns made by the distribution of tiny gold caps in the hair clip (C). The hair clip shows the principles of fine appliqué work. Round ended steel tools were hammered into gold spheres (or thin gold sheet) to make tiny bowl-shaped hemispheres. These were then laid out with their sharp edges down and forced into the tortoiseshell.

The patch boxes and the platter in Figures 9.7 G, and 9.25 D, E, show the versatility of tortoiseshell for molding. Scutes were heated and flattened into flat sheets that were then shaped on hot templates and allowed to cool with their new form. The bangle in Figure 9.25 F is not a section of cow's horn but a sheet of tortoiseshell that has been bent and joined to itself by heat and pressure. It may have been made from the thick scutes of the ventral plastron, many of which lack dark pigmentation or the melanin may have been bleached.

Lorgnettes were invented in the eighteenth century by George Adams (senior), but became fashion items, jewelry rather than spectacles. The lenses in the lorgnette (Figure 9.25 G) are firmly held by tortoiseshell that has hardened around them after being softened to fit. The lenses themselves are weak, as would be expected if they functioned as a fashion accessory rather than as spectacles.

Tortoiseshell takes a finer finish and cracks less easily than horn, making it the preferred material for expensive toilet accessories like the tongue scraper in Figure 9.7.O, the Edwardian mustache brush and comb (Figure 9.25 H, I), or needlework tools like the fine steel darning hook (Figure 9.25 L), of the kind used by Victorian gentlewomen to repair socks in the drawing room where men might be present or their underwear in the privacy of their dressing rooms. Scutes also provided sheets large enough for the elegant backs of brushes like the set of clothes and hair brushes with gold monograms (Figure 9.25 K).

Tortoiseshell is resistant to weak acids and does not soak up and stain with oils like wood, making it ideal for salad servers (J). These salad servers also show the extreme contrast possible between background and blotched color pattern, almost black against the brightest, lightest yellow.

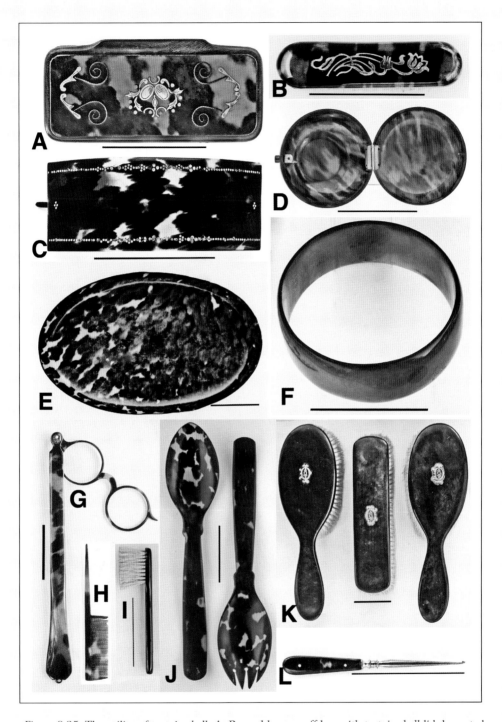

Figure 9.25. The utility of tortoiseshell. A. Pressed horn snuff box with tortoiseshell lid decorated with gold and silver pliqué. Late 18th to early 19thC French. B. A small tortoiseshell backed brush with silver pliqué. Pigs bristles. The tortoiseshell curls around the brush body. Circa 1900 Edwardian style. C. Tortoiseshell hair clip with gold pique. D. Pressed tortoiseshell hinged patch box. Early 19thC English. E. Tortoiseshell platter made from a large dorsal scute like that in Figure 7.4.1E. F. Arm bangle made by joining the ends of a strip from a ventral scute, the ones most often free from dark patterns. G. Lorgnette and spectacles. The lenses are weak enough to suggest that lorgnettes were worn more for show than function. Early 20thC English. H, I. Moustache brush and comb, Edwardian, Early 20thC English. J. Salad servers. Early 20thC English. K. Clothes brush and hair brush set with gold monograms. Late 19th or early 20thC English. L. Fine steel darning hook. 19thC English. Scales = 5cm.

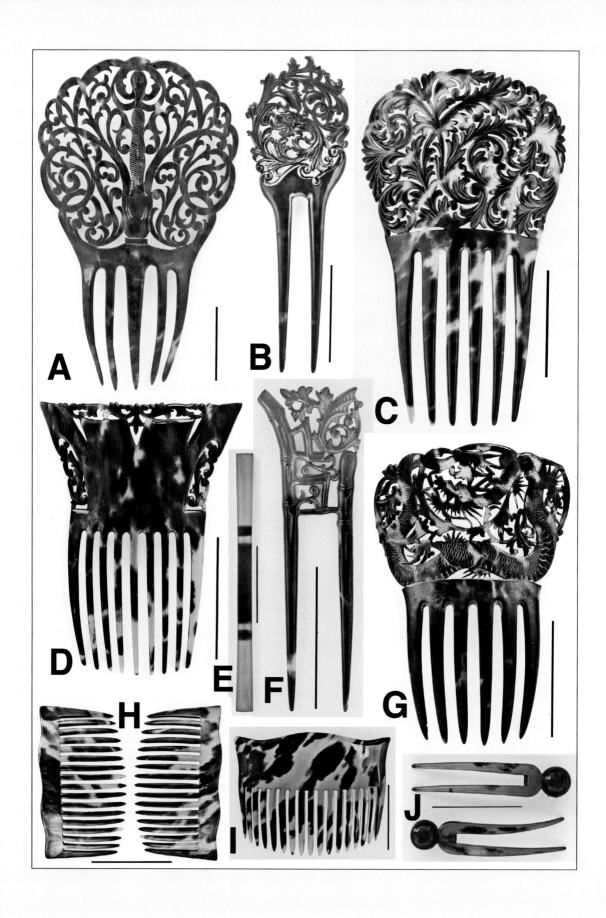

For beautiful hair ornaments, tortoiseshell is prime material (Figure 9.26), outdoing horn (Figure 9.20 J) for its color, polish, and stability. Since the hawksbill sea turtle has a worldwide distribution, tortoiseshell carving industries for export sprang up around the world wherever the craft was introduced. In the absence of provenance, this makes dating and determining the origin of particular artifacts very difficult. Bachman for instance (6), in a beautifully illustrated book, gives no origin for twenty combs figured and comes no closer than 6/20 circa 1850 and 7/20 circa 1887.

There were two main design and fashion influences: Oriental, particularly Chinese and Japanese, and Spanish, spreading through their colonies to the Caribbean and Mexico. Those with Spanish influence may be found everywhere. Mayans, for example, were skilled carvers and polishers of tortoiseshell, having learned their craft from the Spanish. Chinese and Japanese carved tortoiseshell can also be found worldwide.

Back hair combs had an ornamental area above the comb teeth that were inserted at the back of the head. Barrettes, also called hair-slides, hair clips, or bobby pins are functional as well as ornamental, being used to clip locks of hair in place anywhere on the head. Tortoiseshell hairpins are decorative U-shaped hair fasteners less efficient than their simple unobtrusive utilitarian metal equivalent.

One of the simplest and most elegant hair ornaments are Japanese *kogai*. They are sticks of any material around which long locks of hair are wound so that the head of a traditional Japanese beauty may be surmounted by several curving tresses, each with *kogai* emerging at their own angles. The *kogai* in Figure 9.26 E is a composite made from several overlaid ventral plastron scutes. The pattern in ventral scutes is sometimes banded rather than in separate spots, which allows the matching of the dark bands from several layers as in this *kogai*. It was probably inserted below a few strands on one of the main tresses to show off the centrally located pattern. The hairpins in J are equally Japanese in their simplicity. They are almost uniformly yellowish brown, just forks surmounted by spheres made by fusing several layers together.

Japanese hair combs are often easily recognized by their pleasing lack of symmetry, as in the pins B and F. At first glance, the pin in F might be taken for a fragment from a large comb, indeed it was sold as such for a trivial amount by a dealer. However, it is complete and perfectly proportioned. Combs probably made in China for the export market were also often asymmetrical (Figure 9.26 C, G). Symmetrical combs (Figure 9.26 A, D, H, I) are closer to the Spanish tradition.

(Opposite page)
Figure 9.26. Tortoiseshell, the prime material for beautiful combs and barrettes. A and D, symmetrically patterned decorative hair combs, possibly Spanish or Mexican, 19thC. B, F, asymmetrically patterned decorative hairpins, Japanese, 19thC. C and G, asymmetrically patterned decorative hairpins, Oriental, perhaps for European market. E. Kogai, Japanese hair ornament, pattern made by matching the dark regions in several overlain scutes, 19thC. J, simple hairpins with composite end balls made from several overlain scutes, Japanese, 19thC. H and I, Simple decorative combs, 19thC. Scales = 5cm.

9. 14. The Utility of Rhinoceros Horn

I shall not presume to discuss the carving in China and Indonesia of horns of the Asian rhino into decorative cups (21, 22), many of which are on display in the Chester Beatty Museum in Dublin, Ireland, or their beautiful early European equivalents. These are some of the greatest artworks of all time. This book is about more utilitarian artifacts such as walking sticks and riding crops from the longer horns of African rhinos that have been less well described.

Rhino horn sticks are often confused with those made from bovine horn because side views of sheets (bovine) are hard to distinguish from side views of filaments (rhino). The following features illustrated in Figure 9.27 distinguish A rhino horn, from B bovine horn. 1. Rhino horn is often at least partly of an attractive yellow brown color, recognizable at a glance (C–F). 2. African rhino horn (at least from the middle of the nineteenth century) was available in longer lengths than is possible in bovine horn. Rhino horn walking sticks with a curved handle may be made from only one or two lengths of horn (C–F). Bovine horn sticks may need three or six pieces as well as a handle. African zebu and Texas longhorn cattle may have long horns but they are thin walled, unsuitable for stick making. Sticks require a solid rod at least 1 cm in diameter that only occurs for a few centimeters near bovine horn tips. 3. Cross sections of the ends of rhino horn sticks show uniform fields of filaments in transverse profile, difficult to see by eye but visible with a microscope. In contrast (A enlargements), the ends of bovine horn sticks show easily discernible eyes from which the horn sheets radiate (B enlargements). There may be several eyes near the tip, but usually only one further down. If the stick has been cut from one side of the horn, the eye may appear as a longitudinal streak along the length. 4. Sticks with handles carved from the base of the rhino horn (C) show filaments in side view continuous with those in the length of the horn (C enlargement).

9.15. The Utility of Feathers

... I gyve unto my wief (Anne Hathaway) my second best bed with the furniture, ...
The Last Will and Testament of William Shakspere, Obiit April 23, 1616

At first, this seems a trivial bequest, but in those times, even in middle class families, the feather mattresses, pillows, and quilts were often their most valuable possessions. The mattresses were stuffed with the down from ducks and geese. The most expensive pillows and quilts were made from the lighter down of eider ducks, becoming known as "Eiderdowns." Until the advent of plastics, ducks and geese were an important part of farming, and the gathering of down from the nests of eider ducks was on an industrial scale.

Down insulation is rated by fill power, a measure of "fluffiness." It is the volume of air in cm^3 per gram of down. Higher fill power means more air pockets and better insulation. It ranges from about 900 cm^3/g for the highest quality down to 175 cm^3/g for feathers. Insulation in most outdoor equipment ranges from about 230–520 cm^3/g. If well cared for, it retains its fluffiness up to three times longer than do most synthetics.

(Opposite page)
Figure 9.27. Rhinoceros horn sticks and their difference from Bovine horn. A. Rhino horn curved when softened by heat. Inserts, end views of handle. The transverse structure of the filaments is often difficult to resolve without high resolution. B. Bovine horn for comparison with rhino horn. The eye is usually very distinct in transverse profile. C. Rhino horn with handle carved from whole horn rather than bent. Transverse profile of the handle then shows the filament structure in lateral view. D, Riding crop circa 1830 made by the kings whip maker, more decorative than functional. E. Walking cane made from an exceptionally long horn. F. English riding crop mid 19th C. Rhino horn is often distinguished from bovine horn by its attractive yellow brown color and long lengths. Note the one or two piece construction. Scales, A = 5cm, enlargements = 1cm and 1mm. B = 5cm, enlargements = 1cm and 1mm. C - F = 5cm.

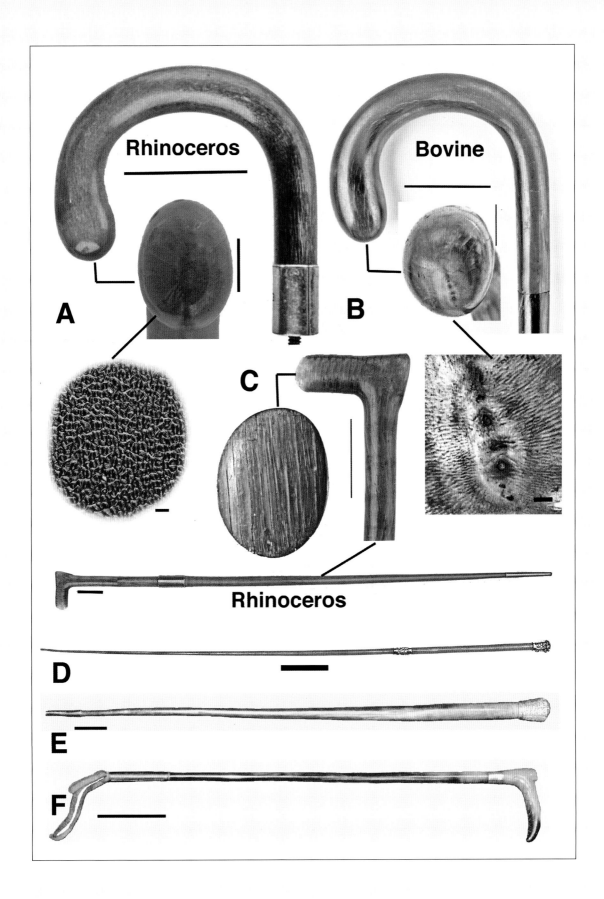

247

Most insulating material now comes from synthetics and from domestic duck and farm-goose down. Ducks descended from the wild mallard (*Anas platyrhynchos*), domesticated for thousands of years for their meat, eggs, and down, have given rise to more than thirty breeds. Many more have come from the Muscovy duck (*Cairina moschata*). Domestic geese had an additional reason for their domestication in Europe as the source of writing quills. They have dual origins from the descendants of Greylag geese (*Anser anser*) and the wild swan goose (*Anser cygnoides*).

The Common Eider duck, *Somateria mollissima*, still provides the best quality down. It nests along the northern coasts of Europe, North America, and Siberia. The soft, warm nest lining made from down plucked from the female's breast was harvested for filling pillows and quilts. Eiderdown harvesting continues as "wild farming" in Iceland, Scandinavia, and Siberia, with a sustainable yield of about 20 gms of high quality down per nest and no harm to the birds.

Another use of feathers is in decoration, from New Guinea tribesmen, to the pre First World War fashion boom, to the stage extravaganzas of Las Vegas, brilliantly described by Thor Hanson (52). Part of the success of feathers as decoration lies in their brilliant colors. The colors are of three kinds (Figures 7.10.1, 2), pigments that they manufacture, like the brilliant reds of the Cardinal, relocated pigments captured from those in the diet—the delicate pinks of flamingos, and physical colors due to diffraction—the greens and blues of the peacock eye.

The cylinders of thin, tough keratin forming the rachis of flight feathers preadapted them for use as quill pens. Any large flight feathers could be used, but in the early nineteenth century most came from geese that were reared for their quills as much as for their meat and down. According to Hanson (52), one London stationer had annual sales of six million quills in the 1830s. But quills were awkward writing implements compared with metal nibs, little suited to the booming mass literacy later in the nineteenth century. With education came universal reading and especially day-to-day writing, that evolved from local recordings with lead pencils on ivory, chalk on boards, quills, and ink on vellum to mass communication using metal nibs and ink for letter writing on paper.

Chapter 10
Curating, Restoring, and Repairing

Curating means looking after a collection to maintain it in its original condition. Curiously, although it looks like a familiar word, a verb with a self evident meaning, it does not exist in the dictionary. Restoration involves bringing an artifact back to its original condition. Repairing is the process of replacing or putting back together broken parts to recreate or copy the original condition. A newly acquired treasure may require anything in this continuum of treatments, from nothing to total breakup and reassembly. The important decision is how much to change and to know when to stop.

The first principle, like that of Hippocrates in medicine, is "do no harm." Anything done should be reversible if possible, because we never know how the usefulness of some future technique may depend on how well we have cared for something now. Who would have predicted the wealth of information in the DNA of old bones, for example. Remember that we are curators, looking after a piece of art or craftsmanship for a future generation.

The second principle is "do not deceive." The objective is to restore an artifact to its previous state without compromising the normal consequences of aging. Where repairs have to be made, they should be as discrete as possible, but not elaborately hidden. The result should improve the appearance, beauty, and even utility, but not be aimed at increasing market value. Its true age may be emphasized, but should not be exaggerated to make it out to be something that it is not.

All natural materials are soft relative to man made materials, other than some plastics. Although some (bone and ivory) may contain apatite (hardness 4) and hydroxy-apatite, their mean hardness is only about 2 1/2. Even mother of pearl is limited to 2 1/2–4, its main component being aragonite (hardness up to 4). Organic materials may be tough, meaning that they are hard to break, but their softness makes them easy to scratch. They may be cleaned with a soft brush but be extra careful using a paint brush. Use a brush with the bristles set in plastic or quill rather than metal. One slip and metal gouges a furrow in your prize.

The softness of organic materials also makes them easily worn down. Never use any motor driven wheel, even of soft bristles, to clean a delicate pattern. A rotary brush on a motor tool can strip the pattern from a piece of pressed horn in seconds. Clean any patterned surface by hand with a fine brush.

Be patient. Adopt the medical doctor's rule, if in doubt, do no harm: take no radical steps until you have thought of all the consequences. Be prepared to leave some things on the workbench for months while they change their shape, harden, or the glues polymerize.

Some firm *do nots*: Do not use quick fixes like modern varnishes that polymerize to give an admirably resistant and glossy surface, but one that is insoluble and impossible to remove. Similarly do not use olive oil on dull tortoiseshell to increase its luster. Olive oil penetrates nicely but it goes rancid, smelly and opaque.

Do not use power tools and abrasives to polish a surface. A nylon brush on a rotating head can destroy the delicate pattern on a pressed horn snuff box in seconds, causing hundreds to thousands of pounds or dollars in lost value.

Do not try to polish metals at the same time as the natural materials, such as bone or ivory in which they are embedded. Silver, copper, or iron particles removed in the polish penetrate bone and ivory causing an ugly black stain that is virtually impossible to remove. Cover the object with masking tape before polishing the metal. Cover the metal with tape while polishing the natural material.

Do not use hot ovens to dry out an object.

Curating. There are two stages to curating artifacts—cleaning them and keeping them in good condition.

Brief and occasional exposure to water, water with detergent or soap, alcohol or acetone will do no harm to plain natural materials. Simply wipe the surface as clean as possible with a cotton swab. Solvents will evaporate before they have had time to dissolve surface lipids. Water can be wiped off before it has had time to cause local swelling. Wipe it lightly so as not to force surface grime into the cracks or into the empty blood vessels of bone. Scrubbing with a tooth brush is alright to remove grime from valleys in robust carved surfaces. Scrimshaw, dyed, or painted surfaces require special treatment.

The keeping stage of curating aims to prevent deterioration due to the loss of water and solid components that leads to shrinkage. All natural materials are hydrated to some extent. Most are strongly hydrophilic but with time two things happen: some proteins denature and become hydrophobic and other proteins are washed out. Both cause shrinkage with dehydration, leaving tiny surface cracks and larger, deeper ones.

Microcracking can be prevented by keeping the surface hydrophobic, that is making it repel water. Many lipids—hydrophobic wax, oil, and grease molecules—will do this, but not all are suitable. The ideal lipid is liquid enough to penetrate but thick enough not to leak out, colorless, inert (does not smell or react with other molecules) and stable over time (does not change to become sticky or ineffective). Olive oil should not be used because it goes rancid, as do many animal fats and unsaturated vegetable oils. Mineral oils tend to be too liquid. Linseed oil is unsaturated and oxidizes,

polymerizing to a sticky mess. A minimal amount of warm beeswax is good as are some natural oils beloved by woodworkers—walnut oil, teak oil. After cleaning, rub with wax and/or oil, making sure that everywhere has been covered. Leave it for a day to sink in and then rub off all the surplus. A simple treatment like this should be enough for several years. One of the best treatments is daily handling. The skin grease that comes from daily handling and a nose rub is excellent.

The most important objective of curating is to prevent the formation of large, deep, damaging cracks. The cold, dry winters of northern countries with central heating can be especially damaging. I once had a very large hippopotamus tusk, quite an old one, that I put on the mantlepiece in a Canadian winter. Near Christmas I was in a nearby room when there was a loud blast. A neighbor, thinking it was a gunshot, came to the door to see if I was alright. The tusk had exploded into several pieces: the tensions set up by the excessive dryness had their final release as the tusk flew into several large fragments.

Controlling the climate is often the only way to prevent deep cracking. Storage should be at a uniform humidity if at all possible. It's nice to have treasures on display, but in some climates and when they are not being looked at, keep them in ziplock bags.

One of the most destructive kinds of cracks develop from the differential expansion of metal that is part of the object. Iron tangs of plated cutlery rust, converting the iron to iron oxide, which occupies more space and almost always cracks the handle, especially if it is ivory. Bone and horn are a little more tolerant. Cutlery should never be washed in water, which penetrate the handle and causes the tang to rust. If there is any sign of rust in an ivory handle, consider preventing cracks by the reconstruction below under repairing. Silver tangs give no problem because their surfaces form only thin films of oxide or sulfide.

Store out of sunlight and artificial light that generates ultraviolet rays. Prolonged exposure to ultraviolet destroys the collagen in bone and ivory and the conchiolin in mother of pearl, so that they become exceedingly brittle. Be careful with functional objects like handles and sewing needles. They may already have become brittle from breakdown of the protein component that gives them their toughness.

Restoring. With age, the cracks in some materials, especially horn and tortoiseshell, fill with air, separating the sheets composing them. This may give them ragged edges and reflective surfaces like cracked glass. A simple treatment for damage localized to a few small spots or edges is to apply a tiny drop of crazy glue. It will penetrate and fill the air pockets. The surface can then be sanded down and repolished.

If the whole object is cracked and the layers separated, then a more drastic treatment is needed that requires patience but the results are worth it. Horn spoons, for example, can be restored to a beautiful condition. The need is to fill the air spaces with a medium that will polymerize to become colorless, transparent, and hard. Some of the new synthetics infiltrate well and can be polymerized by exposure to ultraviolet light. Linseed oil is more readily available and will do as well but will take much longer. Thoroughly clean and dry the object and sand any very rough edges. Infiltrate with the oil (or other reagent) preferably in a vacuum oven. If the object is in a plastic bag, it is possible to submerge it while using very little oil. Lower the pressure while the object is under the liquid and allow it to bubble until all the air has been exhausted. Then let the pressure return very slowly. Wipe all of the oil off using several changes of paper towel. The more oil that is left, the harder it will be to clean the surface later. Now expose the piece to the air and wait patiently for several months. Finally, finish with a very fine sanding and repolishing.

Repairing. The most destructive cracks occur in the ivory handles of iron cutlery and walking stick handles. As the iron rusts it swells until the pressure is released by longitudinal cracking. Bone and horn are a little more forgiving but once rust has started cracking is inevitable. Handles are often beautifully carved and saving them is worth the effort. The cracks cannot be forced together with outside pressure even after softening in water; the extra material inside has to be removed first.

The metal tangs of cutlery were glued into the handle with shellac mixed with a filler such as ivory shavings. The first step is to loosen the shellac by soaking in alcohol or acetone. After an hour the shellac should have softened enough to allow the tang to separate from the handle. Immediately clean out the hole in the handle using a drill of the same diameter as that originally used and soak the handle in fresh solvent. Old shellac dissolves to make a brown varnish that will stain the cracks permanently if the initial loosening step is allowed to go on too long. After an extended soak in clean solvent, thoroughly clean the handle, especially the crack itself. Make sure no dark dust specks or hard grains are left in the crack to disfigure the repair or to prevent the edges from closing. Then leave it in the water for a day or more. The ivory will swell slightly in water, filling much of the crack (and sealing dirt in position if you have left any). Water also softens the ivory, making it plastic enough to force the cracks together. Wipe off the water and allow it to dry for a few minutes. Allow a drop of crazy glue to flow down the hole, so that it gets pulled into the crack from the inside. Now cover the crack with a thin strip of adhesive tape to prevent the glue from sticking to the rubber. Bind the handle with about a foot of surgeon's rubber tubing, fastening the ends with a metal bulldog clip (heavy elastic bands can be used but elastic rubber tubing as used by carpenter's is available at their supply houses). Pull the rubber very tightly to put the maximum, even pressure on the pieces that are to be forced together. This will force the ivory back into its original shape. It can now be allowed to rest for a week or more for the ivory to adjust to its new/old shape. All that remains is to put the handle and metal back together using epoxy glue, clean up, and re-polish.

Toolbox. The essential tool for an antiquarian is a X10 or X15 magnifying glass to look at things held in the hand under varying light. I carry mine everywhere. It is also useful to have a pair of X3 "Granny glasses" to get a close up view of objects displayed behind glass.

Useful tools and supplies. The author has been fortunate to have a lapidary workshop and a biological laboratory to work in, but nothing as elaborate is really needed. The following list of tools is enough to do everything mentioned in the book, from making objects to collecting and studying them.

Acetone.

Alcohol.

Beeswax.

Crazy glue.

Drill and drill bits.

Dubbin or similar soft colorless polish.

Epoxy cement, 5 minute and ordinary 24 hour hardening.

Glass jars with secure lids, some tall and narrow to hold minimal amounts of solvent around knives, for example.

Loup, X10 or X15, to be carried with you everywhere.

Microscope, binocular stereomicroscope with lamp. The only requirement is that it should have a large depth of field to give plenty of workroom. It should not be an expensive instrument as you may get the viewing plate wet and dirty when cleaning and polishing delicate pieces.

Optivisor, X3 and X7 for use in the workshop.

Granny glasses, X3 to get a close up view of objects displayed behind glass at shows and for easy magnification of pieces being studied or worked.

Paper towels.

Plastic bags, assorted with ziplock closures.

Razor blades.

Rotary tool on a flexshaft, Foredom®, or similar, together with small rotary tools for cleaning, sanding, and polishing.

Vice, small table vice.

Wastebasket.

Workshop procedures. Polishing organic materials is not like polishing metals or gemstones where surface is smoothed by local melting to achieve the final polish. Such a treatment can burn, brown, and crack an organic surface. Bringing up the luster on smoothly ground organic material is more like burnishing, pushing the surface together, squeezing it into smoothness sometimes with the help of wax or finger grease.

Polishing and cleaning horn, tortoiseshell and amber. Do not use high speed rotating tools to clean or polish. The heat generated will soften and burn the surface, removing patterns or creating a crust that has to be ground away to restore a polishable surface. Use a handheld toothbrush or polishing pad. Keratin is a very poor conductor of heat, which is why it feels warm to the touch. For this reason use hand tools wherever possible. If you must use electric tools, use pads more than three inches in diameter, preferable wet, and hold the work piece in one hand and the tool in the other to reduce the pressure and resulting friction. When cutting and polishing the edges of a piece of tortoiseshell, make sure that the long face is parallel to the wheel movement. If the edge is presented at right angles to the wheel movement, it will vibrate and chatter, causing cracks and even wrench the specimen out of the hand.

Making a feather quill. Cut off the tip of the base of a large feather with a razor blade and scrape off the outer dried epidermis. Dip the smoothed end in a glass of water for a day or two to soften it. With fine scissors cut one side open for about 1.5 to 2 cms from the base. Cut the quill diagonally with a razor blade to a point split into two where the first cut ends. Cut across the tip to give the minimum width of the lines to be made.

Carving "barley corn" twisted handles. Cut a sheet of paper into a right angle triangle. Twist it around the blank handle and trace the edge of the hypotenuse on the bone with needle pricks to mark out the spiral. Cut into the handle along the needle pricks, sand, and polish.

Replacing broken scales on cutlery handles. It is difficult to drill holes in replacement scales exactly matching those in the steel tang. Prepare two blank replacement scales slightly wider than the tang. Grind flat surfaces to match the metal. Attach one to the metal with any thin glue. Drill holes in the scale through the metal tang. Glue the second scale in place and drill its holes through from the other scale and tang. Insert the rivets, shape, and polish the scales.

On Oils and Waxes. Infiltration of surface pores and airspaces with oils can be a simple and effective first step in artifact preservation, preventing the accumulation of dirt and allowing the very slow drying out that prevents local buildup of stresses causing cracks to form. We therefore need to know something about the oils and waxes suitable for preserving artifacts. An ideal oil or mixture for preservation will 1) penetrate (that is it will not be too viscous), 2) it will cross-link with the artifact, stabilizing it in three dimensions to prevent uneven contractions and cracking, and 3) the component that is not involved with cross-linking will evaporate, leaving no sticky mess.

Mineral oils are mainly long chain hydrocarbons (Figure 12.1). The longer they are, the less volatile and more viscous they become, until they change from being oils to waxes such as those used in candles. Very short chain oils may evaporate at room temperature while hard waxes may be stable over geological time. Their characteristic is that they are unreactive, they are just carbon chains covered over with nothing but hydrogen's. This means that they will do no harm to anything that they are applied to but will remain extractable or liable to evaporate if they are short enough chains. This means that liquid hydrocarbons are useful as carriers for more viscous oils. They can help a viscous oil or wax to penetrate and then leave it behind when they evaporate.

Natural oils also contain long hydrocarbon chains, but they are not inert; they have a variety of other groups that make them reactive, becoming chemically part of the artifact through cross-linking with it. Chief among these reactive groups are double bonds in the hydrocarbon chain itself. These are easily broken, leaving the chain intact but with two bonds now linking the chain to molecules in the artifact (or other chains). Linseed oil is a good example, with many double bonds. In a sealed can, the double bonds may remain unbroken for years, but exposed to air and light they quickly oxidize into a sticky mess that gradually solidifies. It is used by carpenters as a slow setting varnish that ultimately cross-links oil and wood into a gleaming brown solid. It should be used very sparingly and then only if you are prepared to wait for months for the reaction to be complete. Other natural oils contain ketone groups (these give butter its flavor), alcohols, and aldehydes, giving many other scents and flavors. All are more reactive than plain hydrocarbons and may harden to preserve the specimen but also give it a characteristic smell. A common remedy advocated on *Antique Road Shows* to bring back the shine on worn surfaces of tortoiseshell is a smear of olive oil. This will cover over the dullness but it will also go rancid, leaving it with a rank oil smell. It is far better to use some of the oils developed by carpenters for the job, such as walnut oil or teak oil. These will penetrate, cross-link, and evaporate. Silicone oils should never be used. They prevent other treatments and are impossible to remove.

Caring for ivory beads. The smaller an object, the smaller the tensions that can build up in it due to uneven shrinkage. Hence beads are less prone to serious cracking than large carvings. Never-the-less, the humidity fluctuation between wearing and storage can introduce problems that are easily preventable. Put two or three drops of oil (see above) on a pad of cotton wool or lint and work it in until it is evenly distributed and invisible. Run the string of beads gently through the pad each time you wear them or about once a year. If you can see oil on the bead surface it is too much. Over the years the oil will slowly infiltrate the surface giving it a translucency that changes the dead white of new ivory into a natural ivory color. Store the pad with the beads in a ziplock plastic bag. Keep this bag inside a second bag. The objective is to create a constant environment minimizing changes in temperature and humidity. Ivory can withstand low humidities without damage if they are constant and not suddenly presented, but exposure to the alternating extreme summer and winter humidities present in many houses can be very damaging. If your house has the low humidity of a summer desert or a northern air-conditioned winter, put a pad damped with water inside the outer bag.

Bleaching bone. Be circumspect in using wild "found" bones that might carry mad cow disease, elk wasting disease, or rabies in their dust. Degrease fresh bones before bleaching by washing with detergent in a dishwasher. Ideally use uncooked bones with their proteins fixed in position with formaldehyde or glutaraldehyde to keep as much collagen in place as possible. Fresh bone is often colored a dull grey to purple from blood left in the blood vessels that darkens with age to black, giving bone an ugly, dirty look. Exposed blood vessels also tend to collect dust. Soaking in dilute Chlorox® or Javex® bleach removes the discoloration but such strongly alkaline solutions also destroy the bone by dissolving proteins. A few hours in dilute hydrogen peroxide (3%) is a safer treatment. It is better to rough out the shape of something being made before bleaching rather than treating a large block of bone for the time needed to bleach the interior. Fill the blood vessels by polishing with wax after bleaching.

Specimen for bone recognition. Antiquaries might like to make themselves an aid for bone identification. Save the next bone from a cut across a beef shank. Poke out the marrow and cut out a thick piece with two lengthways cuts. Sand all the surfaces smooth and flat and add a few more edges and rounded ends to copy the many orientations that you may find in an antique. Leave it to soak in a jar of Indian ink for a week. Wash all the surplus ink off, let it dry, then buff it and polish with a little wax. You now have a specimen that when viewed with a hand lens will demonstrate the patterns in any carved bone. You will also have made a beautiful worry stone to carry in your pocket forever.

Chapter 11

Glossary

Words used to describe natural materials extend from the medical and biological literature to prehistory, antiquities, old technology, and the art world. Many are esoteric but used and defined here because the reader may find them in the literature.

Angang gading: Hornbill "ivory" is the keratin beak of the helmeted hornbill (*Rhinoplax vigil*) carved in South East Asia, especially Java and Japan.

Antlers: External projections from the parietal bone of the skull of deer, typically having three layers, a laminar bone shell, cortex of osteons, and spongy bone core.

Alicorn: The horn of the unicorn. Use of alicorn obviates the need for the ugly, redundant expression unicorn horn.

Anatomy: The study of the structure of organisms, the naming of their component parts.

Beam: The trunk of an antler that bears lower tines protecting the head and peripheral point tines that engage those of the opponent.

Bands: See growth bands.

Bark: The name used by ivory workers for cementum, the softer derivative elephant tusk equivalent of tooth enamel.

Basic multicellular unit (BMU): The collection of cells involved in creating secondary osteons in bone remodeling (Martin and Burr 1989a; Parfitt 1994).

Black coral: One of about 230 species of the Order Antipatharia prized for its hardness, durability, and fine polish.

Bog Oak: Wood preserved by tannins in quaternary bogs from Ireland popularized by Queen Victoria for carved mourning broaches.

Bolster: The strengthening shoulder between the blade and the handle of a knife that takes the strain when stress on the handle is transferred to the blade during cutting.

Bone: A compartment containing calcified collagen lamellae, the form of which depends upon the pattern of infolds around vascular elements.

Bolster: Thickened metal between the tang and the blade in cutlery. Can be applied metal or part of the blade.

Bone compartments: The flat stacks (laminar) or cylinders (osteonic) of bone separated from one another by vascular compartments.

Burr: See coronet.

Cachalot: The sperm whale, *Physeter macrocephalus.*

Cancellous bone: See spongy bone.

Cap: The protective fitting on the end of the handle in cutlery, often of metal. It may be attached to the tang.

Capillary network sheets: The vasculature between bone laminae.

Cartilage: Translucent in compressible connective tissue coating joint surfaces.

CDJ: See the Cementum-Dentine Junction.

Celluloid: Thermoplastic material soluble in alcohol used as an ivory and bone substitute. Although made from wood cellulose, it is really the first of the synthetic plastics patented by the Hyatt brothers in U.S.A. in 1869. Its manufacture is based on "Parkesine" invented by Alexander Parkes in 1840. Trade names include "Ivorine," "Ivoride," and "Xylonite."

Cement: The tissue that secures a tooth in the jawbone. Not to be confused with the cementum, which is a layer.

Cement sheath: The boundary of uncertain composition and permeability that separates secondary osteons from their surroundings.

Cementum: The enamel layer over most exposed ivory and in teeth below the gum line continues as a softer derivative, the cementum. In some ivory (hippopotamus, *Gomphotherium*, the tips of immature walrus and elephants) regions of enamel and cementum are continuous on the exposed tusk. Not to be confused with cement, which is a tissue.

Cementum-Dentine Junction: The peripheral region of a tusk where the first layers of both cementum and dentine arise. It may be smooth or ridged affecting the shape of dentine and cement patterns on each side.

Chattesina: Work from north Italy where bone and ivory is inlaid in wood.

Choil: The chin of a metal blade just below the bolster.

Choil: The indentation at the base of a blade that allows sharpening without scratching the bolster or haft.

Ciborium: Cup-shaped receptacle.

Circumferential lamellae: Lamellae at the endosteal and periosteal surfaces surviving from stacks of laminae after the loss of their capillary network sheets.

Circumferential system: Laminae and/or lamellae at the endosteal and periosteal surfaces surviving from stacks of laminae after varying degrees of loss of their capillary network sheets.

Collagen: The characteristic vertebrate polymer protein building block for structures that are often calcified, but within the body metabolic pool (i.e., alive).

Complete helicoids: The structure achieved when parallel fibers form sheets that stack above one another in such a way that the orientation of the fibers changes in a regular manner from sheet to sheet is a helicoid. A complete helicoid results when the fibers have changed their orientation through a full 180°.

Coronet: The crown-shaped ring of bone formed by an antler towards the completion of growth at its base above the junction with the pedicle. Also called the Burr.

Curls: In their progression from the core to the periphery, changes in the direction of some dentinal tubules (pigs) are transverse as well as radial, making them curls rather than waves, distinguishing them from waves aligned in laminae within the same radial axial plane.

Dentinal tubules: The main oriented component of dentine are cylindrical tubules with a hollow core easily penetrated by stain. They may be straight, curly, or form regular sine waves (Fig. 4 **B, C**). In the dentine of most teeth they are widely separated in a less stainable matrix, but in ivory they may align in laminae (Fig. 4 **D–H**). Within laminae, dentinal tubules can stack parallel to those in adjacent laminae or change their orientation in a regular way in waved arrays (Fig. 4 **I, J**).

Dentine: Ivory dentine is composed of dentinal tubules about 5 mm in diameter, in a matrix of 5–20 mm particles embedded in a harder ground substance.

Dermis: The inner layer of the skin derived in embryology from the mesoderm.

Dimensions: 1 meter, m = 100 cms, 1 cm = 10 mm, 1 mm = 1,000 mm, 1 mm = 1,000 nm (1 nm = 10 A in old units no longer used).

Dudgeon: Wood, usually boxwood, used to turn the handles of knives and daggers.

Enamel: A hard outer enamel layer covers the surface above the gum line in most teeth, but not in ivory tusks where it is replaced by cementum.

Endosteum: The layer of cells, connective tissue, and blood vessels lining the inner face of hollow bones.

Endosteal surface: The inner surface of hollow bones facing the bone marrow.

Epidermis: The outermost epithelium providing an interface between multicellular organisms and their environment.

Epiphyseal plate: The circular transverse bone plate that separates the cartilage ends of a long bone from the laminar bone of the shaft.

Epithelium: Cells forming a continuous sheet as in the epidermis covering the body.

Ferrule: A ring or cap, usually of metal, to hold the components of a stick or handle together and/or protect the end.

Ferrule: The metal collar between the bolster and the handle in cutlery or the metal tip to a walking stick.

Finial: The decorative end to any rod-shaped structure such as a handle.

Forks, serving: Two pronged forks used at least as early as the thirteenth century, first for holding meat while cutting, and more decorously, for transferring sweet-meats to the mouth.

Forks, Table: Three or four pronged forks used to transfer food from the plate to the mouth from the mid- to late seventeenth century.

Ground substance: The material around matrix particles that makes some regions such as growth cylinders and the walls of Schreger columns harder.

Growth bands: The complex layers deposited asynchronously at an angle to the forming face in the banded ivory of hippopotamus canines to distinguish them from the concentric synchronously deposited cylindrical growth layers found in incisors.

Growth layers: The layers deposited in sequence from the outside to the inside of a tusk. They represent previous activity at the forming face. The layers are usually cylinders parallel to the forming face, but may not always indicate synchronous deposition (see growth bands). Growth layer has been used in preference to growth ring or line to emphasize their three-dimensional nature.

Growth rings: A common but loosely used descriptor for transverse profiles of the layers deposited sequentially at the forming face of rod-like structures such as bones, teeth, or horns.

Haft: The handle of a cutting instrument such as a knife.

Haversian system: The older word for groups of osteons (American journals) or osteones (British journals). Secondary osteon (Currey 1982).

Helices: Helices can be right handed as in a keratin ⟨ helix where the thread moves away from the observer as it twists up and to the right (the motion of turning a screwdriver to the right to force the screw forward) or left handed as in the keratin three stranded rope, where the thread moves away from the observer when it twists down and to the left (the motion of turning a screwdriver to the left resulting in the ejection of a right handed screw or forward motion for a left handed screw).

⟨ Helix: The conformation of polypeptides stabilized axially in a right handed helix such as a keratin ⟨ helix.

Helicoidal architecture: The structure achieved when parallel fibers form sheets that stack above one another in such a way that the orientation of the fibers changes in a regular manner from sheet to sheet to achieve a rotation through 180° (Fig. 6.33).

Horn: The covering of hard keratin over paired, permanent bony outgrowths from the skulls of Bovidae (cattle, goats, and antelopes) and the similar but semi-permanent structures of pronghorn antelopes.

Horn eyes: In transverse profiles of the tips of bovine horns the relic of the bone core appears as one or a few eyes, in caprines as multiple eyes and hundreds in the musk ox.

Hornbill "ivory:" Also known as Angang gading in Java is the keratin beak of the helmeted hornbill (*Rhinoplax vigil*) carved in South East Asia, especially Java and Japan.

Inro: Traditional decorative medicine boxes balanced by netsukes on the sash of Japanese gentlemen.

Interstitial lamellae: Derived from laminar bone, filling some of the space between osteons after the loss of capillary network sheets.

Ivory: The dentine of large teeth and tusks composed of tubules, particles, and matrix forming a concrete-like structure. The featureless matrix corresponds to the cement, the particles, correspond to the pebbles, and the dentinal tubules are the reinforcing rods. All are made of proteins such as collagen, variably calcified. If calcification is like that in bone, complex polysaccharides interface between the proteins and bone minerals such as hydroxylated calcium phosphate (hydroxyapatite).

Ivory black: Ivory or bone are heated until all the organic components turn to carbon. This is then finely ground to make the main component of the best black inks.

Ivory components: There are three components. 1. Dentinal tubules about 5 mm in diameter with a spacing of 10–20 mm are sharply defined by the stain that leaks into their hollow cores. 2. Particles 5–20 mm in diameter present in all ivory are most easily seen in narwhal dentine but are easily overlooked because of their weak staining. 3. Matrix in which the tubules and particles are embedded.

Ivory pearls: Concretions in the core of teeth, such as those in the tusks of hippos, pigs, walrus, orca, and sperm whales. Growth is from the inside to the outside, like pearls. Most have radial dentinal tubules, but they are lacking in others, such as walrus.

Jagger: A tool for jagging, that is, for making a rough, jagged mark in a surface such as leather.

Jambiya: The Arab dagger with a short, curved blade adapted for slicing; it is most prized when the handle is made from rhino horn.

Japanned: Painted black.

Jet: Fossilized *Araucaria* wood from Jurassic marine deposits, most notably from Whitby, Yorkshire, England, but also from around the world.

Jigged bone: Bone carved and dyed to look like antler as in some stick and cutlery handles.

Keratin: The characteristic protein building block outside the body metabolic pool (i.e., dead) deployed by vertebrates for protection from the environment in skin, horns, scales, hair, feathers, and nails.

Kern: The tip of a quill pen.

Lamella: A layer formed from oriented fibers that may change their orientation layer to layer (Fig. 6.33). Change in orientation may be through 180° to create a helicoid. Lamellae may be parallel to the forming face as in insect cuticle and horn, or radial as in proboscidea or angled to radial as in hippopotamus ivory (Fig. 6.4).

Lamellae: Bone layers in both laminar and osteonic bone consist of a 20–50 mm thick layer of collagen fibers on which calcium salts may be deposited. The fiber orientation varies, often changing from lamella to lamella like the layers in plywood or interspersed with non-lamellar orientations. The orientation determines the different kinds of bone (woven, parallel fibered, lamellar, fibrolamellar) described at the ultrastructural level by: Weiner, et. al. 1999; Currey 2002; and others.

Laminae: Layers formed from 4–20 lamellae making up primary bone. Laid down between capillary network sheets and surviving as interstitial lamellae between osteons and in endosteal and periosteal layers.

Laminar bone: Primary bone made from laminae.

Latten: An alloy consisting of about 3 parts copper to 1 part zinc with about 2% iron. Commonly used as a filler between the hard steel and soft handles of cutlery.

Left handed spiral: A spiral that moves from left to right away from you like that made by the surface grooves in a narwhal tusk.

Marine ivory: Hard bone from the long bones of marine mammals, such as whales. It is a term to be avoided, as it is misleading and used for a dishonest purpose. If it were to mean anything, it would refer to the teeth of walruses, sperm whales, and the narwhal, but these ivories are better and more clearly defined using their proper specific names—walrus ivory, etc. Marine ivory is used by dishonest dealers to describe bone objects with a marine provenance to increase their value by suggesting that they are made from a kind of ivory. Bones from marine mammals have an especially rich blood supply. When their vascular compartments have blackened with age, the striking contrast between white bone and dark vascular compartments give them a special beauty of their own. Although the term "marine ivory" sounds grand in the mouth of a dealer, they are schilling bone.

Matrix: The material in which dentinal tubules are embedded, consisting of particles 5–20 mm in diameter in a ground substance varying in hardness and staining (Fig. 4 **A**).

Matrix bands: Concentrations of matrix in radial/longitudinal bands twisted clockwise, opposite to the twist of the cementum in narwhal tusks.

Medullary bone: Bone around the central cavit of long bones containing many cavities where blood cells form.

Melanocyte: Cells located at the junction between the epidermis and dermis that are characterized by producing melanin in melanosome granules.

Melanosome: Intracellular granules of melanin produced by melanocytes that they may transfer to epidermal cells.

Mesoderm: One of three main layers of cells developing between the ectoderm and endoderm in the vertebrate embryo.

Lamina: Laminae are axial sheets of laterally aligned dentinal tubules. The dentinal tubules may have various orientations within the plane of the lamina (Fig. 4 **B–J**).

Morphology: The science interpreting the structure of organisms, why they are as they are.

Morse ivory: Marine ivory, such as that from a walrus tusk.

Mother of pearl (MoP): The nacreous shell of the pearl oyster. MoP became common in fish knife handles from the 1880s.

Mousing: The hot pre-polishing (glazing) of bone that gives off a smell reminiscent of mice.

Netsukes: Because rich new middle class men in the Tokugawa period were not allowed jewelry, they took to wearing netsuke, highly decorative toggles balancing their personal possessions on the other end of a cord slung through the sash. They were first made in ivory by Yoshimura Shuzan of Osaka in the early eighteenth century Kyoho era.

Nerve channels: Many tusks such as those of the narwhal, the lower incisors of hippos, upper canines of pigs, and the tusks of elephants have nerve channels radiating out diagonally from the pulp cavity.

Odontolite: The name given to semifossil mammoth or walrus ivory that has become colored, usually blue or green, from the mineral rich soil in which it has been embedded.

Okimono: Carvings intended to ornament the alcove (*tokonoma*) decorating the principle Japanese living room. Larger than netsukes, they were made from the first half of the eighteenth century.

Osteoblast: Cell concerned with bone deposition.

Osteoclast: Cell concerned with bone resorption.

of a knife or razor. 2. The horny plates into which stiff epidermal keratin sheets are divided to provide flexible coverings in reptiles, birds, and some mammals

Scale tang: The steel sheet bearing scales on each side that creates cutlery handles.

Scaliola: Dyed Italian marble.

Schreger columns: The columns are the basic repeating unit stacked circumferentially and radially to produce the Schreger pattern, not to be confused with the Hunter-Schreger bands in enamel (Espinoza and Mann 2000).

Schreger lines: The pattern seen in transverse profiles of proboscidean tusks that forms a series of crossed helices beginning at an acute angle to the surface below the cementum and ending in a more obtuse angle at the center of the tusk. Differences in angle separate African from Indian elephants (Trapani and Fisher 2003) and elephants from mammoths (Espinoza and Mann 2000).

Schreger pattern: The pattern made by the Schreger lines in transverse profiles of proboscidean tusks.

Scute: A scale or bony plate protecting an animal as in the covering of some turtles. The common usage is confusing, being applied to both bone and horny coverings. In this book, scute has been restricted to bone plates with "tortoiseshell" coverings being referred to as keratin scales.

Segments: In elephant ivory waved dentinal tubules aligned in radial/axial stacks form radial laminae grouped into segments.

Shagreen: A kind of leather characterized by the pattern left after removing the enamel denticles from the skins of sharks and rays, especially that of the Cowtail Stingray.

Sheets: Sheet is a general term for fibers aligned laterally into flat layers as in Fig. 1. Lamina is the term for the sheets of dentinal tubules stacked axially one above the other in the length of an ivory tusk.

Shell: A general term to describe surface layers of tubular structures structurally and functionally distinct from the cortices below them.

Skein: Skein is a general term for the association of dentinal tubules into strands rather than laminae. It occurs particularly with the curled or wavy dentinal tubules of pigs, where the abundant matrix may allow associations other than close packed laminae.

Spongy bone: Also called cancellous bone, it fills the core of bones such as ribs and vertebrae and the spaces at the ends of long bones. The basic structure is the same as that in compact bone, differing only in its arrangement in rods and sheets that cross or surround spaces containing marrow and blood vessels.

Stainless steel: Developed by Thomas Brearly of Firth and Sons, Sheffield. The first forged blades were introduced in 1914.

Strength: The minimum stress, force per unit area in tension or compression, needed to cause a fracture.

Swage: An ornamental grooving or mold.

Tang: The extension of a metal tool used to secure it to its handle. The Whittle or knock-on tang was a spike inserted into the handle. Through and pin tangs extended to the end of the haft where they were secured. Pin tangs largely superseded whittle tangs by the 1850s.

Thermoplastic: A plastic material such as celluloid that can be reshaped by reheating it after it has set.

Thermoset: A plastic material such as Bakelite that cannot be melted and remolded after it has set.

Thirled: Pierced with a hole or holes.

Tines: The projections terminating in points on antlers. Those closest to the base pointing forwards are brow tines, the second set are bez tines and the third trez, all others are points.

Tortoiseshell: The inappropriately named "Tortoiseshell" consists of ® keratin plates lying above the bone carapace of the marine hawksbill turtle *Eretmochelys imbricata*.

Totipotent: Cells such as stem or embryonic cells that can develop into any part of an adult.

Toughness: A measure of the energy required to break a material.

Trabecular bone: A derivative of spongy bone with the addition of fibers, spicules, or elongated cavities. Derived from the Latin for "small beam."

Tropocollagen: The intracellular precursor for extracellular collagen in bone, ivory, and connective tissue.

Tusks: Elongated teeth adapted to resist lateral deformation.

Undercutting: The removal of softer components during polishing causes undercutting, the projection of harder materials above the surface. Hard ivory components, like some growth bands, the walls of Schreger columns, and at a finer level dentinal tubules, reveal themselves by projecting above polished surfaces.

Unicornum falsum: False alicorn, ivory tusks of the narwhal.

Unicornum verum: True alicorn, mammoth tusks dug from the earth.

Vascular compartment: The compartment containing capillary networks or osteonic blood vessels and connective tissue, separated by an epithelium from the bone compartment.

Vegetable ivory: Endosperm from the tagua nut, *Phytelephas macrocarpa*, Family Arecaceae.

Vellum: The skin from almost any mammal, commonly calves or sheep, but even from pigs, horses, and camels, prepared to take writing or printing ink. The most highly prized is made from the unborn calf fetus.

Volkmann's canals: The radially oriented spaces with blood vessels connecting capillary sheets and to a lesser extent, osteons. They are often diagonal to the long axis.

Vulcanite: Double bonds in rubber molecules form crooked chains, giving rubber its elasticity. Hard, black vulcanite is created when these double bonds are broken by hot sulfur.

Waves: In their progression from the core to the periphery, some dentinal tubules (elephants, banded hippo ivory) are curved in waves within the same laminar plane, distinguishing them from the curls of pigs.

A note on grammar in scientific reporting

Science media writers and commentators often make grammatical errors irritating to scientists.

One of these concerns the binomial system for labeling organisms. All organisms are grouped into genera (singular genus) and species, something like a surname and a Christian name. A genus is a collection of species sharing some similar characteristics. A species is a group of organisms described by a unique set of characteristics. To show that the words used are not part of normal descriptive English, they are written in italic with the genus capitalized and the species in lower case for example, *Escherichia coli*.

A second usage that journalists have difficulty with concerns bacterium (singular) and bacteria (plural). Bacteria are a group of single-celled organisms that have not separated their genetic material from the rest of their cell contents. Bacteria can be used without a definite article—e.g., "bacteria may cause disease," or with "the" as in "the bacteria in rotten food may cause disease." Bacterium is singular and requires a definite article, e.g., "the bacterium was *E. coli*," or "a bacterium was the cause."

	1 meter (m)	1 centimeter (cm)	1 millimeter (mm)	1 micrometer (µm)	1 nanometer (nm)	1 Angstrom (Å)
1 meter (m)	1	$100\ (10^2)$	$1,000\ (10^3)$	$1,000,000\ (10^6)$	10^9	10^{10}
1 centimeter (cm)	$10^{-2}\ (0.01)$	1	10	10^4	10^7	10^8
1 millimeter (mm)	$10^{-3}\ (0.001)$	$10^{-1}\ (0.1)$	1	10^3	10^6	10^7
1 micrometer (µm)	$10^{-6}(0.00001)$	10^{-4}	10^{-3}	1	10^3	10^4
1 nanometer (nm)	10^{-9}	10^{-7}	10^{-6}	10^{-3}	1	10
1 Angstrom (Å)	10^{-10}	10^{-8}	10^{-7}	10^{-4}	10^{10}	1

Read across for the dimensions equivalent to the units in the left hand column. Read down for the dimensions equivalent to the units in the row across. The symbol Å for Angstrom should not be used but is given here because it is still to be found in older papers and many textbooks. Useful reference points: keratin filaments are about 10 nm in diameter, collagen fibers 100 nm, and dentinal tubules 10 *µm*. Osteons are about 250 mm in diameter and their vascular compartment about 50 mm.

Chapter 12
References

*"Come, and take choice of all my library,
And so beguile thy sorrow."*

Titus Andronicus, IV i 34
William Shakespeare

1. Alexander, C. (2003) *The Bounty*. Penguin Books London.

2. Alibardi, L., Sawyer, R.H., (2002) "Immunocytochemical analysis: analysis of B keratins in the epidermis of chelonians, lepidosaurians and archosaurians." *J. Exp. Zool.*, 293:27–38.

3. Alibardi, L., Toni, M., (2006) 9 *Tissue and Cell* 38:53–63.

4. American Cetacean Society (2010) Whale Fact Sheet. American Cetacean Society.

5. Anon. (1977) *A Barefoot Doctor's Manual.* Cloudburst Press, Madrona Publishing, Seattle Washington.

6. Bachman, M. (1998) *A Collector's Guide to Hair Combs, Identification and Values.* Collector Books, a division of Schroeder Publishing Co., Paducah, Kentucky.

7. Baden, H.P. (1970) "The physical properties of Nail." *Journal of Investigative Dermatology*, 55:115–122.

8. Baker, C.S., Cipriano, F., Palumbi, S.R. (1996) "Molecular identification of whale and dolphin products from Commercial markets in Korea and Japan." *Molecular Ecology* 5:671–685.

9. Bell, C.J. (1998) *Hairwork Jewelry.* Collector Books Paducah, Kentucky.

10. Berger, J., Cunningham, C., Gawuseb, A. A., Lindeque, M. (1993) "Costs and short term survivorship of hornless black rhinos." *Conservation Biology* 7:920–924.

11. Bertram, J.E.A., Gosline, J.M. (1986) "Fracture toughness design in horse hoof keratin." *J. Exp. Biol.* 125:29–47.

12. Bertram, J.E.A., Gosline, J.M., (1987) "Functional design of horse hoof keratin: the modulation of mechanical properties through hydration effects." *J. Exp. Biol.* 130:21–136.

13. Bloom, W., Fawcett, D.W. (1975) *A Text Book of Histology.* W.B. Saunders, Philadelphia.

14. Bonn, T., Yates, B.C. (2002) "Identification guidelines for Shahtoosh and Pashmina," *Service USFaW* (ed), vol M-02-81. National Fish and Wildlife Law Enforcement Ashland, Oregon, USA.

15. Bragulla, H. (2003) "Fetal development of the segment-specific papillary body in the equine hoof." *J. Morphology* 258:207–224.

16. Brear, K., Currey, J.D., Kingsley, M.C.S., Ramsay, M. (1993) "The mechanical design of the tusk of the narwhal" (*Monodon monoceros*:

Cetacea). *J. Zool.* London 230:411–423.

17. Brown, S.G. (1976) Modern whaling in Britain and the north east Atlantic Ocean. *Mammal Rev.* 6:25–36.

18. Brown, B. (2001) *British Cutlery. An illustrated history of design, evolution, and use.* Fairfax House, York.

19. Burack, B. (1984) *Ivory and Its Uses.* Charles E. Tuttle Company Rutland, Vermont, Tokyo, Japan.

20. Burton, M. (1965) *Dictionary of the World's Mammals.* Sphere Books, Aylesbury.

21. Chapman, J. (1982) "Chinese Rhinoceros horn carvings and their value as dating tools," *Oriental Art* 28:159–164.

22. Chapman, J. (1982) "The use of manipulation in Chinese Rhinoceros horn cups," *Arts of Asia* 12:101–105.

23. Chen, P. Y., Stokes, A.G., McKittrick, J. (2009) "Comparison of the structure and mechanical properties of bovine femur bone and antler of the North American Elk (Cervus elephas canadensis)," *Acta Biomaterialia* 5:693–706.

24. Currey, J.D. (2002) *Bones: Structure and Mechanics.* Princeton University Press, Princeton and Oxford.

25. Currey, J.D., Brear, K., Zioupos, P. (1994) "Dependence on mechanical properties on fiber angle in narwhal tusk, a highly oriented biological composite," *J. Biomech.* 27:885–897.

26. Darwin, C. (1874) *The Descent of Man.* H.M. Caldwell Co., New York, Boston.

27. Darwin, F., Seward, A.C. (1903) *More Letters of Charles Darwin.* Vol 1. D. Appleton & Co., New York, pp. 195.

28. Debruyne, R., Chu, G., King, C.E., Bos, K., Kuch, M., Schwarz, C., Szpak, P., Gröcke, D.R., Matheus, P., Zazula, G., Guthrie, D., Froese, D., Buigues, B., Marliave, C., Flemming, C., Poinar, D., Fisher, D., Southon, J., Tikhonov, A. N., MacPhee, R.D.E., and Poinar, H.N. (2008) "Out of America: Ancient DNA Evidence for a New World Origin of Late Quaternary Woolly Mammoths," *Current Biology*, Volume 18:1320–1326.

29. Dobson, J. (1952) "Pioneers of Osteogeny, Clopton Havers," *Journal of Bone and Joint Surgery—* American Volume 34 B:702–707.

30. Edlin, H.L. (1969) *What Wood Is That?* Penguin, London.

31. Enlow, D.H., Brown, S.O. (1956) "A comparative histological study of fossil and recent bone tissues. Part I," *Texas Journal of Science* 8:405–443.

32. Enlow, D.H., Brown, S.O. (1957) "A comparative histological study of fossil and recent bone tissues. Part II," *Texas Journal of Science* 9:186–214.

33. Enlow, D.H., Brown, S.O. (1958) "A comparative histological study of fossil and recent bone tissues. Part III," *Texas Journal of Science* 10:187–230.

34. Ernst, C., Lovich, J., Barbour, R., (1994) *Turtles of the United States and Canada.* Smithsonian Institution Press, Washington and London.

Osteocyte: Bone cell formed by the incorporation of an osteoblast into the bone matrix (Aarden et al. 1994).

Osteoid: Preosseous tissue, lamellae before ossification.

Osteon: A cylinder of concentric lamellae around a tubular space containing blood vessels. Primary osteons form at the periosteal surface of bones nearing maturity and lack a cement sheath. Secondary osteons are a replacement of laminar bone forming around blood vessels derived from capillary networks (Currey 1982), or the basic multicellular unit (BMU) in bone remodeling (Parfitt 1994). They have a cement sheath.

Palmate antlers: Some antlers, such as those of moose, have their tines supported on a flattened beam like the fingers on the palm of a hand.

Particles: The "pebbles" 5–20 mm in diameter cemented by ground substance that gives the ivory matrix a concrete-like structure.

Pearl-like concretions: The roughly spherical concretions of dentine found in the core of many teeth that are the main component of walrus tusks. In some teeth they have dentinal tubules, but not in the walrus.

Pedicles: Knobs on the frontal bone of the skull of deer from which the antlers grow.

Peculiars: as in "the Queen's peculiars." Skeletal remains usually interred in a religious edifice such as Westminster Abbey.

Pedicles: Projections from the frontal bone of the skull forming the base from which antlers grow.

Periosteum: The layer of cells, connective tissue, and blood vessels that protects the outer surface of bones.

Peripheral ivory: In proboscideans peripheral ivory below the cementum has a waved architecture. The waves become shallower towards the core.

Phleam: Scalpel with leaf-shaped blade made to cut into a vein for blood letting. Used with a mallet to give a sharp tap to cause a sharp clean cut. Handle often of bone, ivory, or wood.

Plastics: Vulcanite, Ebonite from 1839. Gutta percha, from 1843. Bois Durci, made from heated compressed wood flour, egg albumen and blood, made from 1855–1875. Crayford ivory, Fictile ivory, Xylonite, Celluloid, from the 1870s. Bakelite, Ivorine, and Xylo from the 1920s.

Pricker: Bodkin used by monks to prick parchment to mark lines or areas for illustration.

Pyx: A small box.

Rack of antlers: A full set of antlers, consisting of the collection of tines emerging from the antler beam, is called a rack.

Right handed spiral: A spiral that moves from right to left away from you like that made by the inner dentine grooves in a narwhal tusk.

Ricasso: The unsharpened part of the of blade just above the guard or handle on a knife or sword.

Rondel or Roundel: Material in the form of rings or disks that can be stacked together around a core to form a handle or rod.

Seahorse teeth: Tusks of the hippopotamus.

Scale: 1. Each of the two plates of material used to form the outside of the handle

35. Espinoza, E.O., Mann, M-J. (2000) *Identification Guide for Ivory and Ivory Substitutes.* World Wildlife Fund & Conservation Foundation Richmond, Virginia USA.

36. Espinoza, E.O., Mann, M-J, LeMay, J.P., Oakes, K.A. (1990) "A method for differentiating modern from ancient proboscidean ivory in worked objects," *Current Research in the Pleistocene* 7:81–83.

37. Fisher, F.J. (1936) *A Short History of the Worshipful Company of Horners.* Galleon Press, G.B. Cotton & Co. Ltd., Croydon.

38. Fouche, F.J., Kotze, D., Louw, I. (2003) "Fingerprinting of ivory and horn through the application of nuclear analytical techniques," *Journal of Radioanalytical and Nuclear Chemistry* 257:109–112.

39. Freund, T. (1995) *Objects of Desire. The lives of antiques and those who pursue them.* Penguin Books, New York.

40. Fudge, D.S., Szewciw, L.J., Schwalb, A.N. (2009) "Morphology and Development of Blue Whale Baleen: An Annotated Translation of Tycho Tullberg's Classic 1883 Paper," *Aquatic Mammals* 35:226–252.

41. Fudge, D.S., Winegard, T., Ewoldt, R.H., Beriault, D., Szewciw, L., and McKinley, G.H. (2009) "From ultra-soft slime to hard alpha-keratins: The many lives of intermediate filaments," *Integrative and Comparative Biology*. 49(1):32–39.

42. Gall, J.G. (1996) *A Pictorial History, Views of the Cell.* American Society for Cell Biology, Bethesda.

43. Geist, V. (1998) *The Deer of the World, Their Evolution, Behavior, and Ecology.* Stackpole Books.

44. Golchale, S.B., Tatiya, A.U., Bakliwal, S.R., Fursale, R.A. (2004) "Natural dye yielding plants of India," *Natural Product Radiance* 3 228–234.

45. Goldberg, W.M., Hopkins, T.L., Holl, S.M. Schaefer, J., Kramer, K. J., Morgan, T.D., Kim, K. (1994) "Chemical-Composition Of The Sclerotized Black Coral Skeleton (Coelenterata, Antipatharia)—A Comparison Of 2 Species," *Comp. Bioch. Physiol. Biochem. Mol. Biol.*, 107:633–643.

46. Gordon, J.E. (1978) *Structures, or Why Things Don't Fall Down.* Plenum Press New York.

47. Goss, R.J. (1995) "Future directions in antler research," *Anat. Rec.* 241:291–302.

48. Gross, J., Lapierre, C.M., Tanzer, M.L. (1963) "Cytodifferentiation and macromolecular synthesis," Locke, M. (ed) *The Twenty-First Symposium, The Society for the Study of Development and Growth,* Vol 21. Academic Press, Asilomar, California, p 274.

49. Groves, S. (1966) *The History of Needlework Tools and Accessories.* Country Life Books, Feltham, Middlesex.

50. Halstead, L.B. (1974) *Vertebrate Hard Tissues.* Wykeham Publications, London and Winchester.

51. Hanotte, O., Bradley, D.G., Ochieng, J.W., Verjee, Y., Hill, E.W., Rege, J.E. (2002) "African Pastoralism: genetic imprints of origins and

migrations," *Science* 296:336–337.

52. Hanson, T. (2011) *Feathers, The Evolution of a Natural Miracle.* Basic Books, Perseus Books Group, New York.

53. Hardwick, P. (1981) *Discovering Horn*. Lutterworth Press.

54. Hieronymus, T.L., Witmer, L.M., Ridgely, R.C. (2006) "Structure of White Rhinoceros (*Ceratotherium simum*). Horn Investigated by X-ray Computed Tomography and Histology With Implications for Growth and External Form," *J. Morphology* 267:1172–1176.

54B. Hill, G.E., R. Montgomerie, C.Y. Inouye, and J. Dale. (June 1994) "Influence of Dietary Carotenoids on Plasma and Plumage Color in the House Finch: Intra- and Intersexual Variation," *Functional Ecology* (British Ecological Society) 8 (3): 343–350.

55. Horwitz, L.K., Tchernov, E. (1990) "Cultural and environmental implications of hippopotamus bone remains in archaeological contexts in the levant," *Bulletin of the American Schools of Oriental Research* 280:67–76.

56. Iizuka, H. (1994) "Epidermal turnover time," *Journal of Dermatological Science* 8:215–217.

57. Jenyns, R.S. (1981) *Chinese Art.* Phaidon Press Ltd., Oxford.

58. Johnson, S. (1784) *Collected Letters of Samuel Johnson.* 25th March 1784, p. 144.

59. Katz, D.A. (2005) *Hair Analysis.*

60. Kim, K., Goldberg, W.M., Taylor, G.T. (1992) "Architectural and Mechanical Properties of the Black Coral Skeleton (Coelenterata: Antipatharia): A Comparison of Two Species," *Biol. Bull.* 182: 195–209.

61. Knudtson, P. (1998) *The Nature of Walruses.* Greystone Books, Vancouver/Toronto.

62. Krocher, E.K. (2007) "Skull of *Orcinus orca*," Schaedel Senckenberg museum Frankfurt am Main. Modified from Photograph. In: license hccolb-sde (ed) Wikimedia Commons. Licensed under the Creative Commons Attribution— Share Alike 2.5 Generic.

63. Krondl, M. (2008) *The Taste of Conquest.* Ballantine Books, New York.

64. Krzyszkowska, O.H. (1988) "Ivory in the Aegean Bronze Age: Elephant Tusk or Hippopotamus Ivory?" *The Annual of the British School at Athens* 83:209–234.

65. Lambert, O., Bianucci, G., Post, K., de Muizon, C., Salas-Gismondi, R., Urbina, M., Reumer, J. (2010) "A new raptorial sperm whale from the Miocene epoch of Peru," *Nature* 466:105–108.

66. Larsen, W.J. (1993) *Human Embryology*. Churchill Livingstone, Inc., New York.

67. Leach, DaO, L.W. (1983) "Ultrastructure of the equine hoof wall secondary epidermal lamellae," *Am. J. Vet. Res.* 44:1561–1570.

68. Lentz, T.L. (1971) *Cell Fine Structure.* W.B. Saunders, Philadelphia.

69. Ley, W. (1959) *Willy Ley's Exotic Zoology.* Viking Press, New York.

70. Li, C., Suttie, J.M. (1994) "Light

microscope studies of pedicle and early first antler development in red deer (*Cervus elephas*)," *Anatomical Record* 239:198–215.

71. Li, C., Suttie, J.M. (2000) "Histological studies of pedicle skin formation and its tranformation to velvet in red deer (*Cervus elephas*)," *Anatomical Record* 260:62–71.

72. Locke, M. (2004) "Structure of long bones in mammals," *Journal of Morphology* 262:546–565.

73. Locke, M. (2008) "Structure of ivory," *Journal of Morphology* 269:423–450.

74. Locke, M., Dean, R.L. (2003) "Vascular spaces in compact bone," *The American Biology Teacher* 65:701–707.

75. Locke, M., Kiss, A., and Sass, M. (1994) "The cuticular localization of integument peptides from particular routing categories," *Tissue & Cell* 26:707–734.

76. Lopez, B. (1986) "The Narwhal," *Arctic Dreams: Desire and Imagination in a Northern Landscape.* Scribners & Sons. Republished in *By the Light of the Glow-worm Lamp,* Alberto Manguel, Plenum Press, New York.

77. Lott, D.F., Greene, H.W. (2003) *American Bison: A Natural History.* University of California Press.

78. Lowdon, J. and Cherry, J. (2006) *Medieval Ivories and Works of Art, The Thomson Collection at the Art Gallery of Ontario.* Skylet Publishing, Toronto.

79. Lutz, P.L., Musick, J.A. (1997) *The Biology of Sea Turtles.* CRC Press, Boca Raton, Florida.

80. Lynch, L.J., Robinson, V., Anderson, C.A. (1973) "A scanning electron microscope study of the morphology of rhinoceros horn," *Aust. J. Biol. Sci.,* 26:395–399.

81. Manguel, A. (1996) *A History of Reading.* Random House of Canada Ltd., Toronto.

82. Martin, E., Vigne, L. (2002) "Yemen's centuries old rhino horn trade," *Columbus Zoo and Aquarium Report.*

83. Martin, E.B., Martin, C.B. (1982) *Run Rhino Run.* Chatto and Windus, London.

84. Martin, R.B., Burr, D.B. (1989) "The formation of secondary osteons," *Structure, Function and Adaptation of Compact Bone.* Raven Press New York, pp. 105–142.

85. Martin, R.B., Burr, D.B. (1989) "The historical development of concepts surrounding the structure and function of bone," *Structure, Function and Adaptation of Compact Bone.* Raven Press New York, pp. 1–17.

86. Martin, R.B., Burr, D.B. (1989) "The microscopic structure of bone," *Structure, Function and Adaptation of Compact Bone.* Raven Press New York, pp. 18–56.

87. Mathews, J.L., Martin, J.H. (1971) *An Atlas of Human Histology and Ultrastructure.* Lea and Febiger, Philadelphia.

88. McKenna, M.C., Bell, S.K. (1997) *Classification of Mammals Above the Species Level.* Columbia University Press, New York.

89. McManus, M. (1997) *A Treasury of American Scrimshaw.* Penguin Studio, New York.

90. Messenger, S.L., McGuire, J.A. (1998) "Morphology, Molecules, and the Phylogenetics of Cetaceans," *Systematic Biology* 47:90–124.

91. Milner-Gulland, E.J., Beddington, J.R. (1993) "The exploitation of elephants for the ivory trade: An historical perspective," *Proceedings of the Royal Society of London Series B Biological Sciences* 252:29–37.

92. Mlodinov, L.M. (2008) *The Drunkards Walk, How Randomness Rules Our Lives.* Pantheon Books, New York.

93. Muller, H. (1998) *Jet Jewelry and Ornaments.* Shire Publications Princes Risborough, Buckinghamshire.

94. Naderi, S., Rezaei, H-R., Pompanon, F., Blum, M.G., Negrini, R., Naghash, H-R., Balkız, Ö., Mashkour, M., Gaggiotti, O., Ajmone-Marsan, P., Kence, A., Vigne, J-D., Taberleta, P. (2008) "The goat domestication process inferred from large-scale mitochondrial DNA analysis of wild and domestic individuals," *Proc Nat'l Acad Sci U. S. A.* 105:17659–17664.

95. Neme, L.A. (2009) *Animal Investigators*. Scribner, New York.

96. Nemoto, T. (1959) "Food of baleen whales with reference to whale movements," *Sci. Rep. Whales Res. Inst.* 14:149–190.

96A. Nweeia, M.T., Eichmiller, F.C., Hauschka, P.V., Tyler, E., Mead, J.G., Potter, C.W., Angnatsiak, D.P., Richard, P.R. , Orr, J.R., Black, S.R. (2012), *Anatomical Record*, 1–11.

97. Ogle, R.R., Fox, M.J. (1999) *Atlas of Human Hair Microscopic Characteristics.* CRC Press, Boca Raton.

98. Owen, R. (1840–45) "Odontography; treatise on the comparative anatomy of the teeth; their physiological relations, mode of development and microscopic structure in the vertebrate animals," *Hippolyte Bailliere*, London.

99. Parakkal, P.F., Alexander, N.J. (1972) *Keratinization A Survey of Vertebrate Epithelia.* Academic Press, New York & London.

100. Paral, V., Witter, K., and Tonar, Z. (2007) "Microscopic examination of ground sections—a simple method for distinguishing between bone and antler?" *International Journal of Osteoarcheology* 17:627–634.

101. Paris, E. (1995) *End of Days.* Lester Publishing, Toronto.

102. Perrin, W.F., Myrick Jr., A.C., et al. (1980) "International whaling commission report. Report of the workshop." Perrin, W.F., Myrick, Jr., A.C. (ed) Cambridge, pp. 1–50.

103. Perrin, W.F., Wursig, B., Thewissen, J.G.M. (2008) *Encyclopedia of Marine Mammals.* Academic Press, Elsevier Burlington, San Diego, New York, London.

104. Peters, A., Leech, L., Lincoln, B., Marshall, J., Walker, A., Hughes, L. (1989) *The Encyclopedia of Wood.* Quarto Publishing, Oxford.

105. Pilgram, T., Western, D. (1986) "Inferring the sex and age of African elephants from tusk measurements," *Biological Conservation* 36:39–52.

106. Pritchard, R.E. (2000) *Shakespeare's England, Life in Elizabethan and Jacobean Times.* Sutton Publishing Limited, Thrupp, Stroud, Gloucestershire.

107. Project G. (2000) "Brant County, Ontario Biographical Sketches," *Coordinator BC* (ed) Canada Biographical Sketches. www.rootsweb.com/~onbrant/bioburf.htm.

108. Quammen, D. (2006) *The Reluctant Mr. Darwin.* W.W. Norton, New York.

109. Raubenheimer, E.J., Bosman, M.C., Vorster, R., Noffke, C.E. (1998) "Histogenesis of the checkered pattern of ivory of the African elephant (*Loxodonta africana*)," *Archives of Oral Biology* 43:969–977.

110. Raubenheimer, E.J., Brown, J.M.M., Rama, D.B.K., Dreyer, M.J., Smith, P.D., Dauth, J. (1998) Geographic variations in the composition of ivory of the African elephant (*Loxodonta africana*). *Archives of Oral Biology* 43:641–647.

111. Ray, D.J. (1996) *A Legacy of Arctic Art.* Douglas and McIntyre Ltd., Vancouver.

112. Reid, D.G., Duer, M.J., Murray, R.C., E.R. W. (2008) "The Organic-mineral interface in teeth is like that in bone and dominated by polysaccharides: universal mediators of normal calcium phosphate biomineralization in vertebrates?" *Chemistry of Materials.*

113. Roca, A.L., Georgiadis, N., Pecon-Slattery, J., O'Brien, S. (2001) "Genetic evidence for two species of elephant in Africa," *Science* 293:1473–1477.

114. Rolf, H.J., Enderle, A. (1999) "Hard Fallow Deer antler: a living bone till antler casting?" *Anatomical Record* 255:69–77.

115. Rookmaaker, L.C. (1983) *Bibliography of the Rhinoceros. An analysis of the literature on the recent rhinoceroses in culture, history and biology.* A. A. Balkema, Rotterdam.

116. Ryder, M.L. (1962) "Structure of Rhinoceros Horn," *Nature* 193:1199–1201.

117. Sanders, E. (1937) *A Beast Book for the Pocket*. The University Press, Oxford.

118. Sims, M.E. (2010) "Unusual appearance of Schreger-like pattern in Hippopotamus amphibius ivory: Wildlife forensics investigation of a netsuke," *Forensic Science International* 200:19–20.

119. Sinkankas, J. (1981) *Gemstone and Mineral Data Book.* Van Nostrand Reinhold Company, New York.

120. Society AC (2010) Whale Fact Sheet. American Cetacean Society.

121. St. Aubyn, F. (ed) (1987) *Ivory, A History and Collectors Guide*. Thames and Hudson Ltd., London.

122. St. Aubin, D.J., Stinson, R.H., Geraci, J.R. (1983) "Aspects of the structure and composition of baleen, and some effects of exposure to petroleum hydrocarbons," *Can. J. Zool.* 62:193–198.

123. Szewciw, L.J. (2010) *The Structure*

and *Biomechanics of Whale Baleen Alpha Keratin.* Graduate Studies, M.Sc. University of Guelph, Guelph, p. 13.

124. Szewciw, L.J., Kerckhove, D.G., Grime, G.W., Fudge, D.S. (2010). "Calcification provides mechanical reinforcement to whale baleen a-keratin," *Proc. .Roy. Soc.* B 277(1694).2597–2605.

125. Thomason, J.J., Biewener, A.A., and Bertram, J.E.A. (1992) "Surface strain on the equine hoof wall in vivo: implications for the material design and functional morphology of the wall," *J. Exper. Biol.* 166:145–165.

126. Thompson, D.A.W. (1942) *On Growth and Form.* Cambridge University Press, Cambridge.

127. Thompson, H.L. (1997) *Sewing Tools and Trinkets, Collector's Identification and Value Guide.* Collector Books, Schroder Publishing Co.

128. Thornbury (1877) *Life of Turner.*

129. Thorpe, T. (1896) *Humphrey Davy, Poet and Philosopher.*

130. Trapani, J., Fisher, D.C. (2003) "Discriminating proboscidean taxa using features of the Schreger pattern in tusk dentin," *Journal of Archaeological Science* 30:429–438.

131. Virag, A. (2012) "The histology and importance of the unique structure of proboscidian ivory," *Journal of Morphology* in press.

132. Wainwright, S.A., Biggs, W.D., Currey, J.D., Gosline, J.M. (1976) *Mechanical Design in Organisms.* Edward Arnold Limited, London.

133. Waldo, C.M., Wislocki, G.B., and Fawcett, D.W. (1949) "Observations on the blood supply of growing antlers," *American Journal of Anatomy* 84:27–62.

134. Walton, C. (1999) "The art and evolution of Cutlery. A Goldsmiths' Company Exhibition," Goldsmiths' Company, Goldsmith's Hall, London, p. 56.

135. Ward, R. (1907) *Records of Big Game.* Rowland Ward Ltd., Piccadilly, London.

136. Weiner, S., Arad, T., Sabany, I., Traub, W. (1997) "Rotated plywood structure of primary lamellar bone in the rat: orientations of the collagen fibril array," *Bone* 20:509–514.

137. Weiner, S., Traub, W., Wagner, H.D. (1999) "Lamellar bone: Structure-function relations," *Journal of Structural Biology* 126:241–255.

138. Weisbrod, A.V., Shea, D., Moore, M.J., Stegeman, J.J. (2000) "Organochlorine exposure and bioaccumulation in the endangered northwest Atlantic right whale (*Eubalaena glacialis*) population," *Environmental Toxicol. & Chem.* 19:654–666.

139. Whitehouse, A.M. (2002) "Tusklessness in the elephant population of the Addo Elephant National Park, South Africa," *Journal of Zoology* 257:249–254.

140. Whiting, G. (1971) *Old-time Tools & Toys of Needlework.* Dover, New York.

141. Wise, E.R., Maltsev, S., Davies, E.M., Duer, M.J., Jaeger, C., Loveridge, N., Murray, R.C., Reid,

D.G. (2007) "The organic-mineral interface in bone is predominantly polysaccharide," *Chem. Mater.* 19:5955–5057.

142. Woods, C.A., Kilpatrick, C.W. (2005) *Mammal Species of the World, a Taxonomic and Geographic Reference.* Smithsonian Institution Press, Washington, D.C.

143. Wright, M. (2011) Personal communication, Ivory density: Assuming that in 1 kg of ivory (i.e, approximately 450 cm³) the inorganic and the organic parts represent 80 and 20 %W/W, respectively, the volume occupied by the inorganic and the organic parts would correspond approximately to 56 and 44 %, respectively.

144. Yates, B.C., Espinoza, E.O., Baker, B.W. (2010) "Forensic species identification of elephant (Elephantidae) and giraffe (Giraffidae) tail hair using light microscopy," *Forensic Science, Medicine, and Pathology*, 6:165–171.

145. Yates, B.C., Sims, M.E. (2006) "Tupilak transformations: Traditional Ivory objects as modern souvenirs," *International Council for Archeology*, pp. 230–234.

146. Zioupos, P., Wang, X.T., Currey, J.D. (1996) "Experimental and theoretical quantification of the development of damage in fatigue tests of bone and antler," *Journal of Biomechanics* 29:969 –1002.

147. Αγωγσδ. (1834) "Hints on etiquette and the usages of society with a glance at good habits," Longman, Rees, Orme, Brown, Green, and Longman, London.

Chapter 13
Acknowledgments

I am particularly indebted to Jim Richards at the "Stones 'N Bones Museum" in Sarnia, Ontario, the best small museum in its field in North America, for allowing me to photograph specimens in their care. Ms. C. Sims, Fish and Wildlife Services, Oregon, has been generous with helpful comments on whale ivory. Dr. A. Virag's about to be published research on proboscidian ivory structure will be as helpful to all investigators as it has been to me. Dr. Judith Eger, at the Royal Ontario Museum, has been most helpful in tracking down ivory teeth in their collections. Dr. L.J. Szewciw has been a mine of information about all aspects of whale baleen, for which I am most grateful. Emil Racovita's granddaughter, Ouana Marcu, told me stories about his life and was most generous in giving me his bone scarf fastener. Dr. Rob Dean introduced me to errors in the lore of "apple corers." Dr. Richard Sabin, Senior Curator, at the Natural History Museum, London, was most helpful in distinguishing cementum in *Orca* and *Physeter*. My granddaughter, Robin Locke, generously donated a picture of her tattoos for the enjoyment of all. My friends Ken and Celia McDonald gave me constant encouragement, photographs, and interesting bone specimens.

I am grateful to the following for permission to use their material. Figs. 2.6.2, 2.7. Dr. James T. McMahon, Cleveland Clinic.

Fig. 6.26 B. Professor John Locke, University of Alberta, Edmonton.

Fig. 7.8.2 J. L.J. Szewciw, University of Guelph.

Fig. 7.10.1 C. Fig. 9.3 A. Ken McDonald and to the following for permission to photograph their material.

Fig. 5.10 A, Fig. 5.11 A, Fig. 5.12 A, Fig. 5.13 A. Fig. 6.9 F, H. Fig. 6.15 A, B. Fig. 7.4.1 A. Fig. 7.6.3 A. Fig. 7.6.6 A, B. "Stones 'N Bones Museum," Sarnia.

Fig. 6.6 A. Photograph of part of the *Physeter* Skull from the Tring Museum by kind permission of the Natural History Museum, South Kensington, London.

Fig. 6.7 F. Krocher EK (2007) Skull of *Orcinus orca,* Schaedel Senckenberg museum Frankfurt am Main. Modified from Photograph. Wikimedia Commons. Licensed under the Creative Commons Attribution—Share Alike 2.5 Generic.

Figs. 6.26 D, F, E. The Royal Tyrrell museum, Alberta.

Fig. 7.3.2 A, B, C. Attic Books, London.

Fig. 7.3.2 E, Robin Locke.

Fig. 7.6.7 A, B. Biology Department, Western University.

Fig. 9.6 C, D. Celia MacDonald.

Chapter 14
Conclusion

The change to plastics begun in the 1870s, and completed between the wars, had many consequences. 1. As the mechanized pouring of plastics into moulds required a smaller work force, it put many craftsmen out of work. 2. It created disposable goods, causing a decline in the appreciation of possessions, devaluing everything to the level of disposable plastic, for example the ivory handled carving set in Figure 9.5 E selling for as little as $13 in the interwar years (values are only now rising as everyday objects have become collectors items). 3. Plastics altered the nature of the remaining work force, changing skilled turners and carvers into rare specialist careers.

An aim of this book has been to encourage the reader to value the work of craftsmen in the pre-plastic era. It hopes that every flea market will become his or her own "antiques road show," inexpensive but intellectually as rewarding as a trip to an art history museum. The interest of articles made in the last few centuries is not just that they are made of natural materials rather than plastics, but that many of them are no longer made at all or even that their function is no longer known. The visitor to a flea market is a detective reconstructing a way of life from a glimpse into a largely unknown past.

Chapter 15
Index

Antler, 5, 8, 10, 18-22, 30, 38-54, 70, 142, 144, 182, 184, 194, 195, 200, 204, 212, 214, 215, 227, 229, 255, 256, 258-261, 264-267, 269

Alicorn, 68, 69, 255, 261

Anatomy, 4, 6, 255, 267, 268

Bakelite, 181, 198, 204, 260, 261

Bands, 59, 60, 65, 66, 72-76, 79, 84, 86, 88, 90, 93, 95, 96, 104, 109, 135, 137, 169, 245, 251, 255, 257, 259, 260, 261

Bark, birch, 239, as Ivory 255

Basic multicellular unit (BMU), 255, 259

Beaks, 3, 14, 138, 156

Beam, 38, 40-43, 45-49, 222, 255, 260, 261

Bison, 144, 147, 148, 151, 266

Black corals, 137, 178, 255, 265

Bodkins, 215, 216

Bog Oak, 178, 180, 203, 255

Bolster, 255, 256, 257

Bone:

    Bleaching, 254

    Cancellous bone, 255, 261

    Collagen arrangement, 13

    Curating, 250

    Density, 17, 203

    External, 38

    Fashion, 218

    Form, 18

    Formation, 30

    Growth rings, 21, 23, 59, 75, 84, 90, 104, 148, 151, 169, 210, 257

    Growth, 30

    Jigged, 258

    Laminar Bone, 27, 258

    Long Bones, 26

    Medullary, 164, 259

    Observational Techniques, 51

    Osteonic, 32

    Physical properties, 15

    Profile, 7

    Repair, 249

    Restoring, 251

    Skeleton, 24

    Spongy, 36, 261

    Stress, 19

    Structure, 25, 37

    Toiletry, 218

    Toys, 210

    Trabecular, 261

    Utility of, 208

    Whale, 231

Bovine, 24, 145, 147, 149, 153, 246, 257

Boxwood, 181, 220, 256

Burr, 255, 256, 266

Cachalot, 60, 255

Canines, 13, 55, 57, 61, 65, 75, 77, 82-84, 86, 88, 90, 201, 257, 259

Cap, 255

Capillary network sheets, 24, 25, 27, 28, 35, 37, 255-259, 261

Caprine, 149, 153, 155, 157, 257

Caribou, 38, 40, 42, 44, 48, 228, 229

Cartilage, 26, 36, 137, 214, 255, 256

Celluloid, 181, 204, 255, 260, 261

Cement sheath, 79, 255, 259,

Cement, 35, 55, 58, 62, 65, 75, 81, 102-104, 120, 252, 255, 256, 258, 259

Cementum, 17, 21, 22, 55, 57, 59, 61-66, 70, 73-75, 77-80, 83, 84, 86, 88, 90, 93, 99, 102, 103, 106, 108-111, 113-116, 119-122, 255, 256, 259, 260, 270

Cementum-Dentine Junction, 86, 255, 256

Chattesina, 256

Choil, 256

Ciborium, 256

Circumferential lamellae, 25, 29, 256

Circumferential system, 25, 29, 122, 256

Claws, 3, 14, 126, 134, 136, 138, 140, 156, 160, 208, 216

Collagen, 9, 10-13, 15, 16, 18, 24-27, 29, 34, 37, 43, 51, 57, 58, 69, 104, 123, 124, 128, 129, 133, 134, 222, 251, 255, 256, 258, 261, 262, 268

Complete helicoids, 256

Containers, 128, 131, 133, 178, 193, 205, 210, 228, 229, 234, 238

Coronet, 41, 255, 256

Curls, 81, 86, 243, 256, 262

Cutlery, 100, 102, 144, 181, 183, 193-195, 202, 220, 224, 227, 233, 250, 251, 253, 255, 257, 258, 260, 263, 268

Darwin's cosh, 191, 193, 241

Deer, 20, 30, 32, 35, 38, 39, 40- 42, 44-46, 49, 51, 138, 142, 155, 157, 196, 207, 208, 255, 260, 264, 266, 267

Dentinal tubules, 7, 17-19, 23, 57, 58- 60, 65, 66, 73, 74, 75, 76, 77, 79, 80, 84, 86, 88, 90, 92, 93, 95, 96, 103, 104, 106, 107, 108, 110, 112, 113, 121, 122, 123, 204, 256, 258, 259, 260, 261, 262

Dentine, 7, 9, 10, 11, 12, 13, 18, 19, 22, 55, 57, 58, 59, 61, 62, 65, 66, 70, 74, 75, 77-79, 80, 81, 83, 84, 86, 88, 90, 99, 102-104, 108, 110, 115, 116, 119, 120, 122, 123, 255-258, 260

Dermis, 10, 11, 16, 22, 26, 126, 128, 129, 131, 133, 137, 139, 140, 252, 256, 257, 259, 263

Dudgeon, 256

Ebony, 178, 180, 210

Elephants, 3, 17, 23, 55, 57, 59, 62, 65, 69, 74, 75, 81, 84, 86, 88, 92, 95, 96, 99, 100-103, 108, 115, 116, 119, 120-123, 133, 162, 173, 207, 222, 256, 259, 260, 262, 266, 267

Elk, 40-42, 44, 48, 49, 51, 54, 70, 140, 254, 264

Enamel, 10, 11, 17, 22, 55, 57, 61, 62, 65, 74, 77, 80, 81, 83, 84, 86, 88, 90, 93, 99, 102, 103, 133, 220, 234, 255, 260, 261

Endosteal surface, 25, 30, 32-34, 256, 258

Endosteum, 25, 256

Epidermis, 10, 16, 22, 126, 128, 129, 131, 137, 139, 140, 252, 256, 257, 259, 263

Epiphyseal plate, 36, 256

Epithelium, 10, 55, 57, 58, 65, 70, 86, 122, 123, 126, 256, 257, 261

Feathers, 3, 10, 11, 13, 18, 124, 126, 158, 175-177, 204, 204, 224, 227, 228, 246, 248, 258, 265

Ferrule, 196, 198, 257

Finial, 257

Forks, 5, 40, 42, 193, 194, 195, 220, 233, 245, 257

Goats, 21, 142, 144, 147, 149, 153, 158, 196, 257

Ground substance, 256, 257, 259, 260

Growth bands, 60, 109

Growth layers, 57, 59, 61, 66, 72, 77, 84, 86, 88, 93, 96, 107, 108, 110, 151, 257

Growth rings, 23, 59, 148, 151, 257

Haft, 256, 257, 261

Hair, 3, 9, 10, 11, 13, 16, 18, 41, 124, 126, 128, 131, 142, 155, 156, 157, 158, 158, 160, 161, 162, 164, 165, 166, 169, 175, 183, 184, 191, 193, 198, 200, 203, 224, 227, 229, 233, 238, 239, 242, 243, 245, 258, 263, 267, 269

Haversian Systems, 25

Helices, 122

Helicoidal architecture, 95, 107, 257

Helix, 11, 12, 14, 23, 70, 74, 81, 83, 142, 149, 257

Hippopotamus, 3, 17, 55, 83, 88, 122, 123, 128, 250, 256, 257, 258, 260, 265, 267

Hooves, 3, 13, 14, 95, 124, 126, 138, 140, 142, 144, 150, 156, 160, 193, 214, 217, 231, 237

Horn

    Artifacts, 195, 196, 243

    Beaks, 156

    Bison, 151

    Classification, 144

    Cleaning, 252

    Curves, 23, 142

    Decorative, 212, 213

    Fashion, 218

    Form, 18

    Goats, 153

    Growth, 21, 104

Helices, 23, 142
Identifying, 203
Physical properties, 15
Polishing, 252
Powder horn, 202, 231
    Augustus Smith, 188
Profile, 7
Pronghorn, 155, 157
Restoring, 251
Rhinoceros, 170-175, 246
Sheep, 153
Shoe, 218, 219
Smell, 204
Structure, 11
Toiletry, 218
Unicorn, 69
Use in commerce, 149
Utility of, 229, 230
Horn eyes, 142, 147, 150, 153, 155, 246, 257
Hornbill "ivory," 156, 255, 257
Hydroxyapatite, 11, 15, 57, 258

Inro, 257
Interstitial lamellae, 257, 258
Ivory
    Architectural pattern, 104, 122
    Artifacts, 196, 197, 199, 206, 222, 223
    Bands, 86
    Beads, 253, 254
    Black, 258
    Calcification, 96
    Components, 258
    Composition, 58, 103
    Cracking, 20
    Curating, 251
    Cutlery, 194, 195, 199
    Density, 17, 203
    Dental formulae, 56, 57
    Dentinal tubules, 59, 74, 84, 103, 106, 107, 113, 119, 123
    Elephant, 99, 102, 102
    Form, 18, 55
    Growth (layers), 22, 59, 84, 86, 90, 104
    Helices, 23
    Hippopotamus, 88-97
    Identifying, 204
    Mammoth, 101
    Marine, 258

Mastodon, 101
Matrix, 104
Morse, 259
Narwhal, 70, 72,
Natural Colors, 78
Observational Techniques, 51, 60
Orca, 61, 65
Pearls, 3, 69, 75, 76, 86, 258
Physeter, 60
Physical properties, 15
Repairing, 251
Restoring, 251
Schreger pattern, 108, 109, 115, 119, 120
Sources of, 56, 62
Spherites, 103
Spikes, 186
Stress, 19, 20
Structure, 58, 65, 90, 103, 110, 112, 114
Tagua nut, 180
Teething sticks, 196
Tooth test, 203
Tusks, 86, 100
Unicorn, 69
Utility of, 222
Vegetable, 178, 180, 217, 261
Walrus, 76-78
Warthog, 82
Waves, 95, 122, 262

Jagger, 258
Jambiya, 172, 173, 258
Japanned, 258
Jet, 178, 180, 181, 203, 204, 258, 266

Keratin, 7, 9, 10, 11, 13, 14, 15, 16, 18, 21, 22, 23, 57, 95, 124-128, 131, 134, 137, 138, 140, 142, 145, 147, 149, 151, 153, 155, 157, 160, 162, 164, 166, 168, 169, 170, 173, 174, 175, 188, 203, 238, 242, 248, 252, 255, 257, 258, 260, 261, 262, 263, 264, 267, 268
Kern, 186, 258,

Lamellae, 13, 24, 25, 26, 27, 29, 34, 35, 37, 38, 43, 51, 52, 140, 255, 256, 257, 258, 259, 265
Laminae, 7, 13, 20, 22, 24, 25, 27, 29, 30, 32, 33, 34, 35, 43, 45, 46, 51, 57, 59, 60, 65, 66, 73, 74, 79, 80, 86, 88, 92, 95, 96,

107, 108, 110, 113, 122, 123, 140, 255, 256, 258, 259, 260, 261

Laminar Bone, 7, 13, 20, 24, 25, 26, 27-29, 30, 32, 33, 34, 35, 36, 37, 43, 44, 45, 46, 47, 49, 51, 52, 53, 155, 204, 255, 26, 257, 258, 259

Latten, 258

Leather, 9, 128, 129, 131, 133, 134, 138, 186, 191, 198, 207, 208, 218, 219, 258, 260

Left handed spiral, 83, 258, 260

Mammoths, 3, 23, 77, 99, 101, 102, 103, 115, 116, 118, 119, 120, 121, 260, 264

Marine ivory, 57, 259

Mastodons, 3, 99, 101, 102, 103, 115

Matrix bands, 75, 104

Matrix, 13, 22, 30, 57, 58, 60, 72, 74, 75, 77, 79, 84, 90, 92, 104, 108, 110, 122, 126, 140, 155, 157, 162, 164-166, 168, 174, 175, 241, 256- 259, 266, 261

Medullary bone, 164, 259

Melanocyte, 16, 259

Melanosome, 16, 259

Mesoderm, 10, 11, 26, 256, 259

Moose, 20, 40, 42, 44, 45, 47, 48, 61, 260

Morphology, 4, 6, 8, 259, 263, 264, 265, 266, 268

Morse ivory, 75, 259

Mother of pearl (MoP), 194, 218, 233, 249, 251, 259

Mousing, 259

Muskox, 149, 154

Napkin rings, 181, 206, 207

Narwhal, 3, 23, 57, 59, 65, 68, 69-75, 103, 122, 222, 229, 258, 259, 260, 261, 263, 264, 266,

Needlework tools, 214, 216, 217, 242, 265, 268

Nerve channels, 25, 65, 73, 75, 86, 259

Netsukes, 257, 259

Odontolite, 259

Okimono, 101, 259

Orca, 3, 57, 60, 61, 62, 63, 64, 65, 66, 67, 75, 88, 122, 258, 270

Osteoblast, 25, 259

Osteoclast, 41, 259

Osteocyte, 24, 25, 259

Osteoid, 259

Osteon, 7, 8, 13, 18, 19, 20, 21, 24, 25, 26, 27,

30, 32, 33, 34, 35, 37, 43, 44, 45, 46, 47, 48, 49, 51, 53, 54, 181, 204, 205, 207, 241, 255, 256, 257, 258, 259, 261, 262, 266

Osteonic Bone, 13, 20, 24, 25, 27, 30, 32, 34, 37, 43, 44, 46, 51, 204, 205, 207, 241, 255, 258, 261

Palm tree, 181

Palmate antlers, 40, 42, 47, 259

Papyrus, 129, 131

Parchment, 129, 131, 234, 260

Pearl-like concretions, 59, 75, 76, 260

Peculiars, 260

Pedicles, 40, 41, 260

Periosteum, 25, 27, 35, 260

Peripheral ivory, 260

Phleam, 200, 260

Physeter, 3, 60, 61, 62, 63, 64, 65, 66, 67, 255, 270

Pigs, 3, 17, 22, 23, 40, 57, 59, 75, 79, 80, 81, 82, 83, 84, 86, 88, 92, 122, 129, 133, 138, 162, 243, 256, 258, 259, 261, 262

Plastics, 5, 9, 17, 19, 149, 164, 168, 169, 170, 181, 182, 203, 204, 228, 229, 246, 249, 255, 260, 271

Porcupine, 158, 162, 164, 238, 239

Pricker, 260

Proboscidean tusks, 81, 95, 104, 115, 123, 260

Pronghorn, 150, 155, 157, 257

Pyx, 260

Quills, 3, 158, 162, 162, 164, 228, 239, 248

Rack of antlers, 19, 20, 21, 40, 42, 51, 142, 260

Rhinoceros, 68, 69, 70, 104, 126, 138, 170, 172, 173, 246, 265, 266, 267

Ricasso, 260

Right handed spiral, 83, 258, 260

Rondel or Roundel, 260

Scale tang, 260

Scaliola, 260

Schreger columns, 59, 96, 108, 110, 111, 114, 115, 116, 123, 257, 260, 261

Schreger lines, 121, 260

Schreger Pattern, 59, 60, 81, 86, 96, 102, 106, 109, 110, 114, 115, 116, 119, 120, 121, 260, 267, 268

Scrapers, 201, 207, 208
Scute, 134, 137, 139, 242, 243, 245, 260
Seahorse teeth, 260
Segments, 14, 106, 107, 108, 110, 115, 134, 160, 260
Shagreen, 133, 134, 260
Sheep, 21, 129, 133, 142, 147, 149, 153, 160, 161, 162, 196, 234, 261
Shell, 5, 6, 9, 10, 11, 18, 20-22, 25, 44-49, 51-53, 74, 77, 83, 90, 124, 134-140, 149, 178, 181, 184, 198, 200, 201, 203, 242, 243, 245, 249, 251-253, 255, 259, 260, 261
Shepherd's Purse, 191, 193
Skein, 59, 79, 80, 81, 86, 90, 92, 96, 122, 216, 217, 261
Skin, 9, 10- 12, 15, 16, 21, 41, 51, 52, 62, 77, 126, 128, 129, 131, 133, 134, 137, 138, 140, 142, 144, 156, 158, 160, 162, 169, 175, 178, 207, 208, 216, 227, 229, 250, 256, 258, 261
Smith, Augustus, 186, 188, 202
Spikes, 40, 41, 83, 131, 168, 186, 208
Spongy bone, 18, 20, 25, 27, 30, 32, 33, 36, 37, 43, 44, 45, 46, 47, 48, 49, 51, 54, 155, 205, 213, 214, 255, 261
Stainless steel, 198, 220, 261
Steenbok, 148
Stress, 18, 19, 20, 21, 36, 46, 51, 60, 62, 69, 75, 104, 121, 123, 140, 160, 172, 175, 253, 255, 261,
Swage, 261

Tagua nut, 178, 180, 181, 261
Tang, 250, 251, 253, 255, 260, 261
Teething Sticks, 196, 198, 202
Thermoplastic, 255, 261
Thermoset, 181, 261
Thirled, 261
Tines, 38, 40, 42, 43, 46, 47, 193, 255, 20, 261
Tortoiseshell, 3, 5, 6, 9, 10, 11, 21, 22, 124, 134, 135, 136, 138, 181, 184, 198, 200, 201, 203, 242, 243, 245, 245, 249, 251, 252, 253, 260, 261
Totipotent, 10, 261
Toys, 198, 202, 210, 268
Trabecular bone, 261
Tropocollagen, 11, 12, 261
Tusks

As Ivory, 55
Cementum distribution, 74
Dental formulae, 57
Elephant, 99
Form, 17
Growth, 83
Hippopotamus, 88-92
Lamina orientation, 74
Lifespan, 100
Mammoth, 101
Mastodon, 101
Narwhal, 70
Pigs, 79-82
Schreger pattern, 115
Size, 100
Structure, 77
Tools, 206
Unicorn, 69
Walrus, 75-80

Undercutting, 60, 95, 261
Unicornum falsum, 68, 261
Unicornum verum, 68, 69, 261

Vascular compartment, 261
Vegetable Ivory, 178, 180, 181, 203, 216, 217, 261
Vellum, 3, 128, 129, 131, 248, 261
Volkmann's canals, 29, 262
Vulcanite, 178, 260, 262

Walrus, 3, 17, 57, 59, 65, 75, 76, 77, 78, 79, 80, 90, 207, 208, 210, 212, 222, 224, 227, 228, 229, 256, 258, 259, 260, 265
Waves, 59, 74, 86, 88, 90, 92, 95, 96, 107, 110, 112, 115, 116, 119, 122, 123, 138, 147, 161, 162, 189, 256, 260, 262

Whale Baleen, 126, 164, 165, 166, 168, 169, 203, 241, 264, 267, 268, 270,
Wildebeest, 148
Woggles, 206, 207
Wool, 13, 124, 158, 159, 160, 161, 162, 184, 214, 215, 216, 218, 227, 228, 233, 238, 253, 264